WITHDRAWN

Pathogenesis and Immunology of Treponemal Infection

IMMUNOLOGY SERIES

NOEL R. ROSE
*Professor and Chairman
Department of Immunology and
  Infectious Diseases
The Johns Hopkins University
School of Hygiene and Public Health
Baltimore, Maryland*

1. Mechanisms in Allergy: Reagin-Mediated Hypersensitivity
    Edited by Lawrence Goodfriend, Alec Sehon, and Robert P. Orange
2. Immunopathology: Methods and Techniques
    Edited by Theodore P. Zacharia and Sidney S. Breese, Jr.
3. Immunity and Cancer in Man: An Introduction
    Edited by Arnold E. Reif
4. *Bordetella pertussis:* Immunological and Other Biological Activities
    J. J. Munoz and R. K. Bergman
5. The Lymphocyte: Structure and Function (in two parts)
    Edited by John J. Marchalonis
6. Immunology of Receptors
    Edited by B. Cinader
7. Immediate Hypersensitivity: Modern Concepts and Development
    Edited by Michael K. Bach
8. Theoretical Immunology
    Edited by George I. Bell, Alan S. Perelson. and George H. Pimbley, Jr.
9. Immunodiagnosis of Cancer (in two parts)
    Edited by Ronald B. Herberman and K. Robert McIntire
10. Immunologically Mediated Renal Diseases:
    Criteria for Diagnosis and Treatment
    Edited by Robert T. McCluskey and Giuseppe A. Andres
11. Clinical Immunotherapy
    Edited by Albert F. LoBuglio
12. Mechanisms of Immunity to Virus-Induced Tumors
    Edited by John W. Blasecki

13. Manual of Macrophage Methodology: Collection, Characterization, and Function
    Edited by Herbert B. Herscowitz, Howard T. Holden, Joseph A. Bellanti, and Abdul Ghaffar
14. Suppressor Cells in Human Disease
    Edited by James S. Goodwin
15. Immunological Aspects of Aging
    Edited by Diego Segre and Lester Smith
16. Cellular and Molecular Mechanisms of Immunologic Tolerance
    Edited by Tomáš Hraba and Milan Hašek
17. Immune Regulation: Evolution and Biological Significance
    Edited by Laurens N. Ruben and M. Eric Gershwin
18. Tumor Immunity in Prognosis: The Role of Mononuclear Cell Infiltration
    Edited by Stephen Haskill
19. Immunopharmacology and the Regulation of Leukocyte Function
    Edited by David R. Webb
20. Pathogenesis and Immunology of Treponemal Infection
    Edited by Ronald F. Schell and Daniel M. Musher

Other Volumes in Preparation

Pathogenesis and Immunology of Treponemal Infection

edited by
RONALD F. SCHELL
Department of Medicine
Division of Infectious Diseases and Clinical Microbiology
Hahnemann University School of Medicine
Philadelphia, Pennsylvania

DANIEL M. MUSHER
Departments of Medicine, and Microbiology and Immunology
Baylor College of Medicine, and
Infectious Disease Section
Veterans Administration Medical Center
Houston, Texas

MARCEL DEKKER, INC.   New York and Basel

Library of Congress Cataloging in Publication Data

Main entry under title:

Pathogenesis and immunology of treponemal infection.

    (Immunology series ; v. 20)
    Includes indexes.
    1. Syphilis. 2. Syphilis--Immunological aspects.
3. Treponematosis. I. Schell, Ronald F., [date]
II. Musher, Daniel. III. Series. [DNLM: 1. Treponemal
infections--Immunology. 2. Treponemal infections--
Etiology. W1 IM53K v.20 / WC 422 P297]
RC201.15.P37 1983   616.95'13   82-23547
ISBN 0-8247 1384-2

COPYRIGHT © 1983 by MARCEL DEKKER, INC. ALL RIGHTS RESERVED.

Neither this book nor any part may be reproduced or transmitted in
any form or by any means, electronic or mechanical, including photo-
copying, microfilming, and recording, or by any information storage
and retrieval system, without permission in writing from the publisher.

MARCEL DEKKER, INC.
270 Madison Avenue, New York, New York 10016

Current printing (last digit):
10 9 8 7 6 5 4 3 2 1

PRINTED IN THE UNITED STATES OF AMERICA

Series Editor's Foreword

Despite the fact that it is now some eighty years since Schaudinn identified *Treponema pallidum* as the causative agent of syphilis, a satisfactory understanding of immunity in this disease has not been reached. As early as 1848 Ricord stated that "an individual who had once acquired syphilis was thereafter protected against reinfection." This view was shared by most clinicians of that day. As time went on, however, disquieting reports of reinfection appeared. The second course of syphilis was often as severe as the first. From these observations came the concept that immunity in syphilis lasts only as long as there is active infection.

During the 1920s and 1930s, the question of whether active disease is a precondition for protective immunity was hotly debated. With the introduction of successful therapy in the 1940s, interest in the problem flagged. It seemed quite probable then that the disease could be eradicated by contact tracing and vigorous drug treatment. The recent increased incidence of syphilis in the United States and throughout the world has emphasized the need for more effective control measures. A better understanding of the pathogenesis and immunology of the disease is the first step toward the development of effective immunological prevention.

The present volume reviews our present state of knowledge in this field. The availability of newer experimental forms of syphilis, especially in inbred animals such as hamsters and rabbits, permits a more searching analysis of the problem. Moreover, it is now possible to dissect the immune response into humoral and cellular pathways and to deal with each separately. These approaches should not only increase our understanding of immunity in syphilis but in other chronic infections as well.

Interest in syphilis has waxed and waned, depending on public health policy. It is a matter of some personal gratification to the series editor to see these topics dealt with again, since the biology of

T. pallidum occupied the center of his research effort between the years 1949 and 1951. Perhaps it is time to realize that a sustained effort is needed to tackle the still-pertinent goal of eliminating the "great pox."

Noel R. Rose
Professor and Chairman
Department of Immunology and
Infectious Diseases
The Johns Hopkins University
School of Hygiene and Public Health
Baltimore, Maryland

Foreword

Interest in specific diseases tends to follow long cycles over time; syphilis and other treponemal infections are no exceptions. Coming in the wake of great advances in knowledge of the treponematoses during the first three decades of this century, the discovery and widespread use of penicillin brought the hope that these diseases would finally be reduced to negligible proportions in the panoply of mankind's afflictions. This hope has been only partially realized.

The treponeme is a wily and elusive foe, with great powers of survival. Moreover, man's lifestyle and habits have changed little at the elemental level of intimate human relationships. Added now is a generation of physicians who have had little experience in recognizing and treating syphilis and kindred diseases; the diseases smolder on, surfacing unexpectedly, to confound the diagnostician and the public health practitioner.

All the while, however, a persistent handful of scientists and clinicians throughout the world has continued to study these diseases and expand our knowledge about them. It is timely, therefore, that these new advances be brought together, subjected to critical appraisal, and made a part of modern scientific inquiry, medical practice, and public health. Ronald F. Schell and Daniel M. Musher have done this in *Pathogenesis and Immunology of Treponemal Infection*, with the assistance of a number of other outstanding contributors to the field. Indeed, it is evident that much has happened in the past several decades. Research techniques scarcely dreamed of a generation ago have been brought to bear on old questions, which have, in many instances, been resolved. For research on the treponematoses is not a thing apart from the mainstream of biological inquiry, but borrows from it, and in turn makes its own contribution. This volume will be an indispensable asset to students of syphilis and the treponematoses.

Thomas B. Turner
Dean Emeritus
The Johns Hopkins University School of Medicine
Baltimore, Maryland

Preface

The clinical manifestations of treponemal disease have fascinated physicians for centuries. A long and venerable line of distinguished investigators, including Hunter, Charcot, Hutchinson, and Ehrlich, to name just a few, added to their reputations through studies of this remarkable infection. In recent years, however, the mainstream of immunological, physiological and biochemical research has bypassed treponemal disease; as a result, the nature of the organism and immune response of the host to treponemal infection is still poorly understood.

The exclusion of treponemal disease from modern science was due, to a great extent, to technical problems associated with unique characteristics of the treponemes. The inability to cultivate virulent treponemes discouraged and hindered early investigators. It was extremely difficult to study the onset and evolution of infection-induced immunity, for which accurate counts of organisms in tissue are required. In addition, since virulent treponemes must be maintained in the laboratory by animal transfer and isolated from infected mammalian tissue, any attempt to characterize them immunologically raises the problem of distinguishing treponemal antigens from those of the mammalian host.

To these difficulties one must add the paucity of animal models. Except in hamster, the inbred strains so important for immunological research are not readily available. Finally, as if these formidable technical problems were not enough, the discovery of penicillin further discouraged researchers. The prediction—not borne out by subsequent events—that the treponematoses would be eliminated rapidly by the "wonder drug" reduced enthusiasm for studying them. Following World War II, except for a few devotees whose laboratories continued to work on some problems related to the microbiology and immunology of treponemal infection, treponemes were largely ignored.

During the last decade and a half, investigations carried out in the face of these difficulties accumulated a tremendous amount of new knowledge about *Treponema pallidum*. Fortunately, many investigators have shown the patience, cleverness, and fortitude to circumvent the stumbling blocks.

It has been our intention to emphasize this information. *Pathogenesis and Immunology of Treponemal Infection* will serve as a major reference work, not only for students, but for our colleagues interested in treponemal disease. This volume is divided into three parts. The first section is devoted to the structure, physiology, and metabolism of the treponemes. The clinical description of syphilis and models of treponemal disease are presented in the second section. Finally, the pathogenesis of treponemal disease and mechanisms of protection and immunoregulation are discussed.

Our knowledge about treponemal diseases has advanced greatly, yet there is still much to learn. We have not yet succeeded in cultivating virulent treponemes free of mammalian tissue. We have not defined the mechanisms of virulence, the factors responsible for sustaining the life of treponemes in vivo, nor the mechanisms by which the infected host eventually controls the infection. It is our hope that this book will stimulate further questioning and arouse the curiosity of a new generation of clinicians and investigators.

Ronald F. Schell
Daniel M. Musher

Contents

Series Editor's Foreword-Noel R. Rose		*iii*
Foreword-Thomas B. Turner		*v*
Preface		*vii*
Contributors		*xi*

Part I	Virulent Treponemes	
Chapter 1	Morphology *Kari Hovind-Hougen*	3
Chapter 2	Composition *Russell C. Johnson*	29
Chapter 3	Genetics of *Treponema* *A. Howard Fieldsteel*	39
Chapter 4	Metabolic Activities *C. D. Cox*	57
Chapter 5	In Vitro Cultivation of *Treponema pallidum* *Howard M. Jenkin and Paul L. Sandok*	71
Part II	Treponemal Infections	
Chapter 6	Syphilis and Yaws *Daniel M. Musher and John M. Knox*	101
Chapter 7	Rabbit and Hamster Models of Treponemal Infection *Ronald F. Schell*	121
Part III	The Immune Response	
Chapter 8	Immunopathology of Syphilis *Konrad Wicher and Victoria Wicher*	139
Chapter 9	The Jarisch-Herxheimer Reaction *Edward J. Young*	161
Chapter 10	Toxic Activities of *Treponema pallidum* *T. J. Fitzgerald and L. A. Repesh*	173

Chapter 11	Attachment of Treponemes to Cell Surfaces T. J. Fitzgerald	195
Chapter 12	The Parasitic Strategies of *Treponema pallidum* Joel B. Baseman and John F. Alderete	229
Chapter 13	Humoral Immune Mechanisms in Acquired Syphilis Nancy H. Bishop and James N. Miller	241
Chapter 14	Immunoregulatory Effects in Experimental Syphilis Robert E. Baughn	271
Chapter 15	Histopathology and Immunopathology of Experimental Syphilis Stewart Sell	297
Chapter 16	Cell-Mediated Immunity James D. Folds	315
Chapter 17	T-Cell-Mediated Resistance Ronald F. Schell, John K. Chan, and Jack L. LeFrock	331
Chapter 18	Macrophages and Host Resistance Sheila A. Lukehart	349

Author Index 365
Subject Index 389

Contributors

John F. Alderete, Ph.D. Department of Microbiology, University of Texas Health Science Center, San Antonio, Texas

Joel B. Baseman, Ph.D. Department of Microbiology, University of Texas Health Science Center, San Antonio, Texas

Robert E. Baughn, Ph.D. Departments of Microbiology and Immunology, and Dermatology, Baylor College of Medicine and Syphilis Research Laboratory, Houston Veterans Administration Medical Center, Houston, Texas

Nancy H. Bishop, Ph.D. Department of Biology, California State University, Northridge, Northridge, California

John K. Chan, Ph.D.[*] Department of Medicine, Division of Infectious Diseases and Clinical Microbiology, Hahnemann University School of Medicine, Philadelphia, Pennsylvania

C. D. Cox, Ph.D. Department of Microbiology, University of Massachusetts, Amherst, Massachusetts

A. Howard Fieldsteel Ph.D[†] Life Sciences Division, SRI International, Menlo Park, California

T. J. Fitzgerald, Ph.D. Departments of Medical Microbiology and Immunology, University of Minnesota School of Medicine, Duluth, Minnesota

---

[*]*Present affiliation*: Memorial Hospital Medical Center of Long Beach, Long Beach, California

[†]Deceased

James D. Folds, Ph.D. Department of Bacteriology and Immunology, School of Medicine, University of North Carolina, Chapel Hill, North Carolina

Kari Hovind-Hougen, Ph.D., D.Sc. Department of Biophysics, Statens Seruminstitut, Copenhagen, Denmark

Howard M. Jenkin, Ph.D. The Hormel Institute, University of Minnesota, Austin, Minnesota

Russell C. Johnson, Ph.D. Department of Microbiology, University of Minnesota, Minneapolis, Minnesota

John M. Knox, M.D. Department of Dermatology, Baylor College of Medicine, Houston, Texas

Jack L. LeFrock, M.D. Department of Medicine, Division of Infectious Diseases and Clinical Microbiology, Hahnemann University School of Medicine, Philadelphia, Pennsylvania

Sheila A. Lukehart, Ph.D. Department of Medicine, Division of Infectious Diseases, University of Washington School of Medicine, Seattle, Washington

James N. Miller, Ph.D. Treponemal Research Laboratory, Department of Microbiology and Immunology, UCLA School of Medicine, Los Angeles, California

Daniel M. Musher, M.D. Departments of Medicine, and Microbiology and Immunology, Baylor College of Medicine, and Infectious Disease Section, Veterans Administration Medical Center, Houston, Texas

L. A. Repesh, Ph.D. Departments of Medical Microbiology and Immunology and Biomedical Anatomy, University of Minnesota School of Medicine, Duluth, Minnesota

Paul L. Sandok, Ph.D. Department of Biology, University of North Carolina at Charlotte, Charlotte, North Carolina

Ronald F. Schell, Ph.D. Department of Medicine, Division of Infectious Diseases and Clinical Microbiology, Hahnemann University School of Medicine, Philadelphia, Pennsylvania

Stewart Sell, M.D. Department of Pathology, University of Texas Health Science Center at Houston, Houston, Houston, Texas

Konrad Wicher, Ph.D., D.M.Sc. Division of Laboratories and Research, New York State Department of Health, Albany, and The State University of New York at Buffalo, Buffalo, New York

Contributors

Victoria Wicher, Ph.D. Division of Laboratories and Research, New York State Department of Health, Albany, New York

Edward J. Young, M.D. Departments of Medicine, and Microbiology and Immunology, Baylor College of Medicine, and Infectious Disease Section, Veterans Administration Medical Center, Houston, Texas

Pathogenesis and Immunology of Treponemal Infection

Part I
Virulent Treponemes

1
Morphology

KARI HOVIND-HOUGEN
Statens Seruminstitut
Copenhagen, Denmark

Historical Review 4
Size and Shape 5
Cell Envelope 9
Flagella 13
Cytoplasm 17
Division 19
Other Pathogenic Treponemes 19
Concluding Remarks 20
References 23

Most of the morphological studies on human pathogenic treponemes have been performed on cells of *Treponema pallidum*. The gross morphology of these cells was described by Schaudinn and Hoffmann over 75 years ago (1,2). The existence of flagella and their unusual location inside the outer cell membrane was predicted by Noguchi as early as 1928 (3). This knowledge of the anatomy of the treponemes was achieved by the interpretation of results skillfully obtained by use of the dark-field technique in light microscopy and will be surveyed in a brief historical part of this chapter.

Since the 1940s the pathogenic treponemes have been extensively studied by electron microscopy. An excellent and comprehensive review of these studies with references up to 1965 was given by Wilcox and Guthe (4). Electron microscope studies on cells of *T. pallidum* have generally used the Nichols strain. Some studies

have been extended to other strains, with the result that cells of
T. pallidum were found to be morphologically identical, irrespective
of the strain examined (5, 6 and Hovind-Hougen, unpublished data).

Only a few electron microscope studies have been published on the
morphology of *Treponema pertenue*. Generally they have confirmed
results obtained by dark-field microscopy, showing *T. pertenue* to be
morphologically indistinguishable from *T. pallidum* (6-9). Although
Treponema carateum has only been studied in the electron microscope
with the shadow-casting technique (7,10), which has a rather limited
resolving power and does not show details of the cell interior, it
seems most likely, at present, that these cells are morphologically
similar to those of *T. pallidum* and *T. pertenue*.

Historical Review

The first description of regularly waved spirochetes in the exudates
of primary syphilitic lesions of the genitalia was published by Donné
in 1837 (see Ref. 11), whose observations were confirmed by Vanoye
in 1841 (see Ref. 11). In 1904-1905 Schaudinn and Hoffmann (1), in
a paper on the presence of spirochetes in syphilitic lesions, described
the morphology of the spirochete, which is now known as *Treponema
pallidum*. It was characterized as a thin, spirally wound cell, 4-14 μm
long, and less than 0.25 μm wide; the number of waves per cell varied
between 6 and 14; and the ends of the cells were pointed. When
Castellani (12), in 1904, received the preliminary report from
Schaudinn, he was reminded of the strong resemblance in the clinical
manifestations of parangi (yaws) and syphilis. He also recalled that
earlier the same year he had seen some almost invisible spirochete-like
organisms during the examination of secretions from ulcers in a case
of yaws. Castellani described these spirochetes as extremely thin
cells with tapering ends, 7-20 μm long, and with a variable number of
waves (12).

Noguchi (3) in his famous description of the spirochetes, stated
that cells of *T. pallidum* and *T. pertenue* were morphologically indistinguishable. He thought they were 8-11 μm long and 0.25-0.30 μm
wide with pointed ends; they had regular and rigid waves with a wavelength of 1 μm; and they divided transversely by binary fission.
Noguchi described a spring-like axial filament and a layer of contrac-
tile protoplasm enclosed in a delicate periplast as the essential structures of the treponemal cell. The protoplasmic substance appeared to
be homogeneous. Noguchi also claimed that the axial filament had several characteristics in common with bacterial flagella, i.e., morphology,
staining properties, and function, that of locomation. Thus, according to Noguchi, the only difference between bacterial flagella and the
axial filaments of the spirochetes was that the former are extracellular,
or exogenous, while the latter are intracellular, or endogenous
(p. 465 in Ref. 3).

1. Morphology

Treponema carateum, the cause of pinta was first demonstrated in 1938 by Saenz, Grau Triana, and Armenteros (see Ref. 4). Léon-Blanco (see Ref. 4) described a spirochete which he called *Treponema herrejoni* in lesions from a patient with pinta and found it identical in morphology to *T. pallidum*.

Many of the earlier electron microscope studies concentrated on whether treponemes and other spirochetes were flagellated or not. The reason for this was that the resolution possible with the electron microscope allowed the detection of a number of thin fibrils attached to the spirochetes. Swain (13) made a careful electron microscope study of some spirochetes, including *T. pallidum*. He concluded that there were no true exogenous flagella, but observed a band of fibrils which wound in a spiral fashion around the spirochete and ran along its full length. The number of individual fibrils varied for different species of spirochetes. Cells of *T. pallidum* usually possessed three fibrils, but four were observed on one organism. The diameter of each fibril was 0.02 μm, and the cells were 6-15 μm long, had a mean width of 0.13 μm, and were regularly waved with a wavelength of 0.15 μm. The ends of the cells were tapered. The essential structures of each cell comprised the cell wall, the cytoplasmic body, and the fibrils. In the treponemes these fibrils were situated within the cell membrane.

No differences were revealed in the morphologies of cells of *T. pertenue* and *T. carateum* when compared with cells of *T. pallidum* (7,10). These results were obtained from electron microscope studies of shadow-casted material. Cells of *T. pertenue* were 8-15 μm long, with an average width of 0.13 μm, while those of *T. carateum* were 9-18 μm long and about 0.15 μm wide. Flagellar bundles, consisting of two to four individual flagella, were observed to wind around the cells. Most of the cells had pointed ends.

Pillot and Ryter (14) made an extensive electron microscope study of spirochetes in which ultrathin sectioning and negative-staining techniques were used. Their work represented a breakthrough in modern morphological studies and considerably extended our knowledge about the ultrastructure of these organisms. Subsequent results published by others have confirmed their observations and contributed further information on treponemal ultrastructure.

Size and Shape

Treponemes are unicellular helical rods (15). The cells of *T. pallidum* are 5-15 μm long, the length depending on the stage of growth of the individual cell; i.e., the shortest are the newly divided cells, while the longest comprise two or more fully developed cells held together by a mutual outer envelope. The helical shape is evident in sectioned material, where only sinusoidal pieces of the cells are included in each section (Figs. 1-6) (14,16). Scanning electron microscope studies of critical-point dried cells have also shown the helical shape

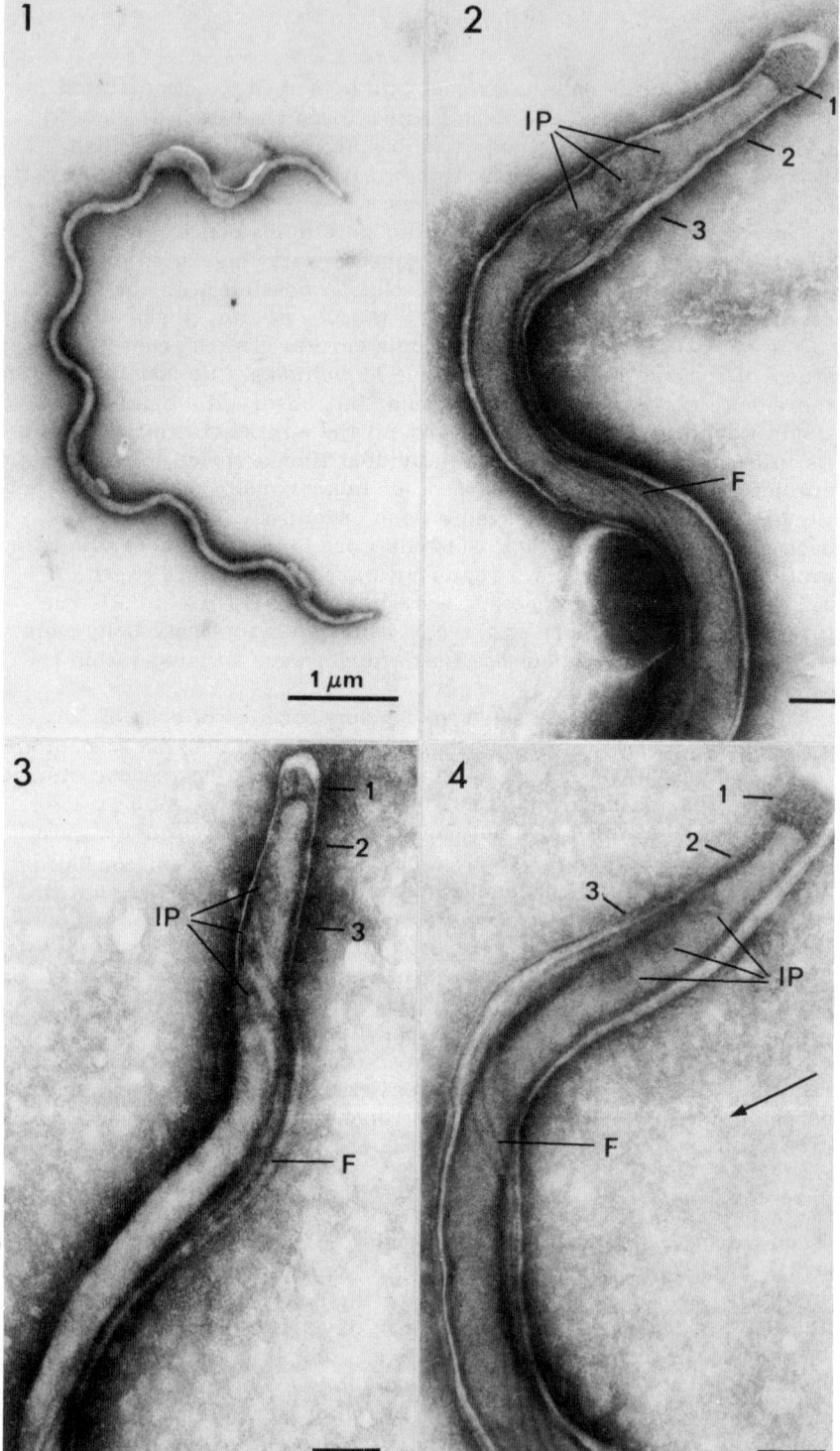

1. Morphology

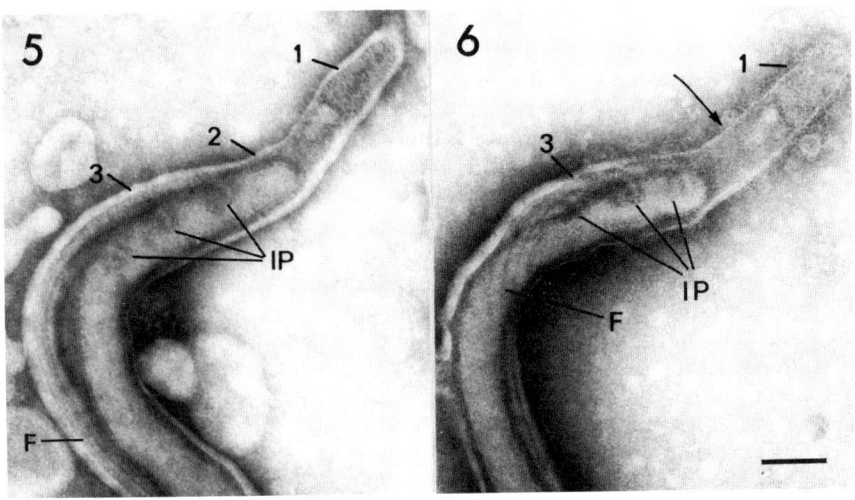

Figures 5 and 6 show cells of *T. pertenue* Gauthier and *T. pallidum* Nichols, respectively. In Fig. 5, Zone 2 of the cell is slightly damaged, and completely lacking in the cell of Fig. 6 (arrow). Zone 1 is preserved as a structural entity in both cells, and the fine striations are well seen. IP denotes the insertion points of the flagella (F). Material negatively stained with 1% ammonium molybdate, pH 7 (× 90,000). Bar in Fig. 6 = 100 nm.

Figure 1 Cell of *T. pallidum* Nichols with regular waves and pointed ends. Material negatively stained with 1% ammonium molybdate, pH 7 (× 15,000).

Figures 2-4 Ends of human pathogenic treponemes showing the three characteristic zones (see text). The insertion points (IP) of the three flagella (F) are situated in a row. Figure 2 clearly shows the fine striations in Zone 1, and fimbriae (arrow) can be discerned on the cell in Fig. 4. Figure 2 shows a cell of *T. pallidum* Nichols, Fig. 3 a cell of *T. pallidum* obtained directly from a human chancre, and Fig. 4 a cell of *T. pertenue* Gauthier. Material negatively stained with 1% ammonium molybdate, pH 7 (× 90,000). Bar = 100 nm.

of each organism (17,18). The cells have a rather constant wavelength of 1.1 µm, measured as the distance from the top of one wave to the top of the next on flat cells lying on a substrate such as the supporting film of a specimen grid (Fig. 1) (19). The wave amplitude is 0.2-0.3 µm and the diameter of the helix is thus about 0.5 µm (19). The cells have pointed ends and the width increases for about one wavelength, from the tip of the cell to where it reaches its maximum width of about 0.15 µm (Figs. 1-4) (9,14,16,19).

The two ends of a cell are morphologically identical. At higher magnifications the ends are seen to consist of three zones, each with a characteristic structure and electron density (Figs. 2 and 3) (9,14, 16,19). The outermost tip constitutes Zone 1, and Zone 2 consists of the outermost part of the cytoplasmic body, i.e., the cell proper, and extends from the end of Zone 1 to the region where the flagella are inserted. Zone 3 is the region of the cell where the flagella are attached to the cell, with their insertion points arranged in a row along the length of the cell.

Zone Differentiation

Zone 1 extends beyond the cytoplasmic membrane and is covered by the outer envelope only. A substructure of fine parallel lines is often observed in this part (Figs. 2,4-6), and this region, the tip, is often preserved as a structural entity in slightly damaged cells (Figs. 5 and 6).

As will be discussed at length in Chap. 10, cells of T. pallidum show a polar attachment to eukaryotic cells in tissue culture (17,18,20) and to the surface membranes of human mononuclear phagocytes (21). No physical derangement of either the surface of the cultured cells or the treponemes can be observed by scanning electron microscopy (17,18). Studies of sections may eventually give insight into whether the terminal portion of human pathogenic treponemes has any role in the attachment of the organisms to host cells; at present, the mechanism for this attachment remains unknown. Spirochetes with polar regions which appear to be specialized for cellular attachment have been demonstrated in association with the surface of the Pyrsonympha cell membrane (22,23). Similarly, all rod- or helix-shaped organisms observed in other studies were found to be attached end on to the epithelium of the stomach or small intestine of man and other mammals (24-27, and H. A. Nielsen et al. and K. Hovind-Hougen et al. unpublished data).

Zone 2 consists of the front-end part of the cytoplasm and is separated from Zone 1 by the cytoplasmic membrane (Figs. 2-4). It is about 0.17 µm long. In this region the cell gradually widens until the full width is obtained around the region of the flagellar insertion. In negatively stained preparations Zone 2 appears to be more electron lucent than the rest of the cell (14,16,19) and is also more easily

1. Morphology

damaged. The first sign of serious damage to a cell is the disappearance of Zone 2, which results in a seemingly empty space between the tip of the cell and the region where the flagella are inserted (Figs. 5 and 6).

Zone 3 consists of the insertion region for the flagella. Undamaged cells of *T. pallidum* and *T. pertenue* always show three flagella inserted subterminally at each end (Figs. 2-6). The flagella are inserted in a row parallel to the long axis of the cell, and the distance between their insertion points is about 0.1 µm. The bundles of flagella, one bundle originating from each end, wind around the cytoplasmic body of the cell. Generally, the flagella are so long that they overlap and interdigitate in the middle region of the cell. The length of each individual flagellum can vary, and consequently, six flagella are present in the middle part of a cell, whereas any number of them, from three to six, can be found more toward the ends (Fig. 2).

Fimbriae

Slender appendages, fimbriae, have been seen to protrude from the cell periphery of cells of *T. pertenue* Gauthier (Fig. 4). Generally they are 1-5 µm long and 2-3 nm wide (9). The presence of fimbriae has not been demonstrated on cells of either *T. pallidum* Nichols or wild strains of *T. pallidum* (Fig. 3); however, fimbriae can only be resolved in optimally stained preparations. Consequently further studies are needed to obtain evidence of the presence or absence of fimbriae, with the possibility of using this as a criterion for differentiation between cells of the two species.

Cell Envelope

The outer envelope of negatively stained human pathogenic treponemes does not possess any surface layer. After treating cells of *T. pallidum* and *T. pertenue* with Teepol (a detergent), sodium deoxycholate, or *Myxobacter* AL-1 protease I, no surface layers were revealed, while similar treatments have shown the presence of such layers on cells of most of the strains of cultivable treponemes examined (19).

Swain (13) discussed the possible presence of a slime layer exterior to the fibrils on cells of *T. pallidum* and concluded that the cells were covered by a delicate outer membrane. He stated, however, that cells of *Borrelia duttoni* and *B. recurrentis* possess a slime layer or a capsule (13). This result was later confirmed by the demonstration of a surface layer covering the outer membrane of cells of various *Borrelia* species (28,29).

The presence of a slime layer or surface coat has been said to be responsible for the time lapse observed before immobilizing antibodies show any effect on the treponemes in the *Treponema pallidum* immobilization (TPI) test (30). Similarly, surface material has been presumed to be responsible for the fact that freshly extracted treponemes are unsuitable for use in agglutination tests (31) and fluorescence treponemal tests (32).

To further study whether cells of *T. pallidum* possess an extracellular layer, Zeigler et al. (33) prepared sections of testis obtained from experimentally infected rabbits after the tissue had been fixed by a method in which ruthenium red is added to the fixative (34), which enhances the electron density of acid mucopolysaccharides. The method has on several occasions made extracellular coats and thin fibrils visible in cell-to-cell or bacteria-to-cell attachments, structures which could not be resolved in material prepared with routine fixation methods (35-38). The micrographs of Zeigler et al. are not easy to interpret, however, because ultrastructural details of the treponemal cells are difficult to observe. Ruthenium red-positive material is seen to be abundant in the tissue intercellular spaces and is also seen to adhere to the surfaces of both the treponeme and tissue cells, but it does not seem to be predominantly associated with the treponemes.

Recently, Fitzgerald et al. (39) published an electron microscope study of treponemes in experimentally infected testicular tissue fixed by a similar procedure. Their micrographs showed treponemes in apposition to the ruthenium red-positive glycocalyx of the tissue cells. The outer membrane of the treponemal cells is only well preserved on some cells, but on these it appears to be symmetric both with respect to electron density and to the width of the two dark lines. Large amounts of ruthenium red-positive material were observed in the intercellular space. The authors concluded that the organisms are predominantly situated in areas that contain relatively large amounts of acid mucopolysaccharides (39), although it should be noted that this is not necessarily the same as showing that the material is actually providing an outer layer for the treponemes. Controls of noninfected rabbit testis processed by the same methods were not included in any of these studies, and micrographs of regions of the infected tissue where no treponemes were present were not given. Such controls would be of interest in establishing the extent of ruthenium red-positive material in the extracellular space of normal rabbit testis tissue and the possible effect of treponemal infection on the synthesis of this material in testis tissue.

My opinion is that until the present time electron microscopy has been unable to provide convincing evidence for the presence of a capsule or slime layer on cells of *T. pallidum*.

Outer Membrane

Sections of cells of *T. pallidum* and *T. pertenue* show that the organisms are surrounded by a triple-layered outer membrane consisting

1. Morphology

of two dark layers with a narrow light gap in between (Figs. 11-16). The two dark layers are of equal electron density, and each is approximately 3 nm wide. This membrane has the same appearance and dimension, irrespective of whether the treponemes are examined (1) after extraction from infected rabbit testis, prior to or after fixation (14,16,40); (2) after perfusion of experimentally infected animals (16,41); or (3) in biopsies of primary and secondary human syphilitic lesions (42,43, and Hovind-Hougen, unpublished data). The outer membrane of *T. pallidum* is also symmetric in sections of material when ruthenium red is added to the fixative (33,39).

Peptidoglycan Layer

The peptidoglycan layer is seen in thin sections of treponemes as a thin, dark line in close apposition to the outer leaflet of the cytoplasmic membrane (Figs. 11 and 13-16).

Indirect evidence for the presence of a peptidoglycan layer in cells of *T. pallidum* and *T. pertenue* has been obtained by treating cells with sodium deoxycholate (DOC) or enzymes. The helical shape of the cells is only slightly influenced by treatment with DOC, while treatment for a few minutes with *Myxobacter* AL-1 protease I makes the shape almost unrecognizable (9,14,44). It is known that protease I isolated from *Myxobacter* AL-1 splits the muramyl-alanine bonds of the peptidoglycan (45), whereas sodium deoxycholate has no effect on these bonds (46).

Further evidence for the presence and position of a peptidoglycan layer in the human pathogenic treponemes has only been obtained by deduction from studies on *Treponema* strain Reiter (47-50) and other spirochetes (46,51-53). Joseph and co-workers isolated the peptidoglycan layer from *Spirochaeta stenostrepta* (46). They found that, when isolated, the layer maintained a helical shape, thus proving its shape-conferring role in the spirochete.

Cytoplasmic Membrane

In sectioned cells of *T. pallidum* and *T. pertenue* the cytoplasmic membrane is seen as a triple-layered membrane about 8 nm wide (Figs. 11-16). Due to the close apposition of the electron-dense peptidoglycan layer to the outer leaflet of the membrane, the cytoplasmic membrane sometimes appears asymmetric, with the outer dark line wider than the inner line. This effect is especially pronounced in sections where the treponemes are sectioned at an oblique angle. The membrane is regarded as equivalent to the cytoplasmic membrane of other bacteria, although it has never been isolated from treponemes or from other spirochetes (51).

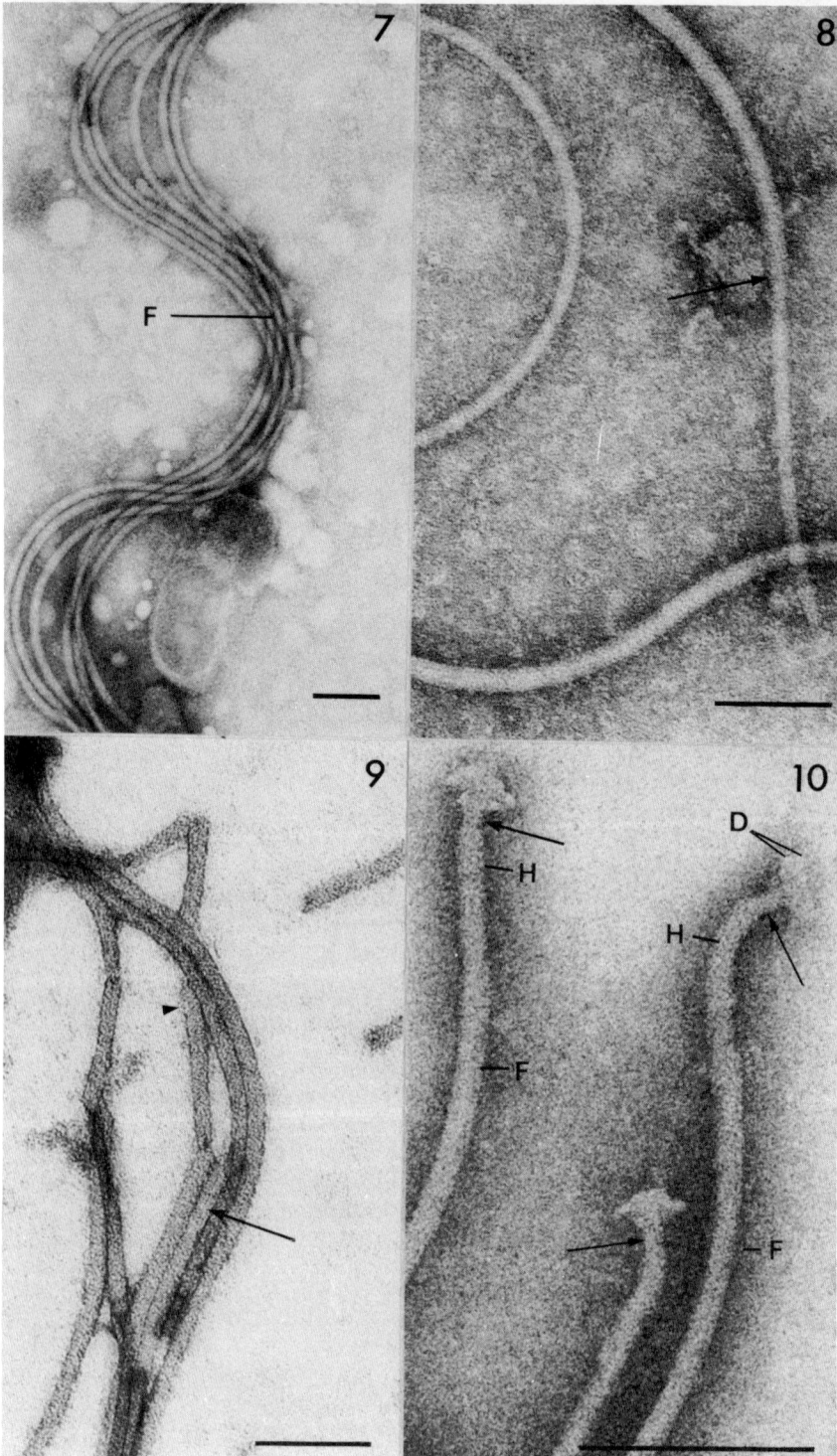

1. Morphology

Flagella

Instead of the term *axial filament* the term *flagellum* should be used, because this filament is structurally and chemically similar to flagella of other bacteria [Subcommittee on the Taxonomy of the Spirochetes, unpublished data (54)].

The flagella lie between the outer membrane and the peptidoglycan layer (Figs. 2-6, 11, 13, 14, and 16); consequently the ultrastructure of negatively stained flagella can only be studied on flagella liberated from the organisms. Flagella are isolated by gentle treatment of the treponemes with agents which affect the outer envelope (9,19,44). A flagellum consists of three structural components: the filament, the hook, and the basal body (Fig. 10).

The Filament

The filament of a free flagellum possesses a sinusoidal outline with a wavelength and an amplitude similar to those of the undamaged treponeme (Fig. 7). It is composed of a core, about 10 nm wide, covered by a sheath, so that the total width amounts to about 17 nm (Fig. 8). The sheath does not extend along the full length of the

---

Figures 7-10 show preparations of flagella obtained from cells of *T. pallidum* Nichols. All bars = 100 nm.

Figure 7 The filaments of free flagella (F) are sinusoidal in shape and show approximately the same wavelength and amplitude as a treponemal cell. Material negatively stained with 1% ammonium molybdate, pH 7 ($\times$ 90,000).

Figure 8 Flagellar filaments with and without sheath. A flagellum shows the distal end unsheathed; the arrow marks the end of the sheath. Material negatively stained with 1% ammonium molybdate, pH 7 ($\times$ 160,000).

Figure 9 The sheathed flagella show a hexagonal (arrowhead) or a linear (arrow) arrangement of their substructures. Double stained with 1% uranyl acetate, pH 3, followed by 1% ammonium molybdate, pH 7 ($\times$ 160,000). (*Source*: Reference 16.)

Figure 10 The basal knob of a flagellum consists of two thin discs (D) in close apposition to each other. The pair of discs is connected by a rod (arrows) to the hook (H). Note that the rod shows a substructure different from that of the hook. Note also that each has a substructure different from that of the sheathed flagellum (F). Material negatively stained with 1% ammonium molybdate, pH 7 ($\times$ 320,000). (*Source*: Reference 44.)

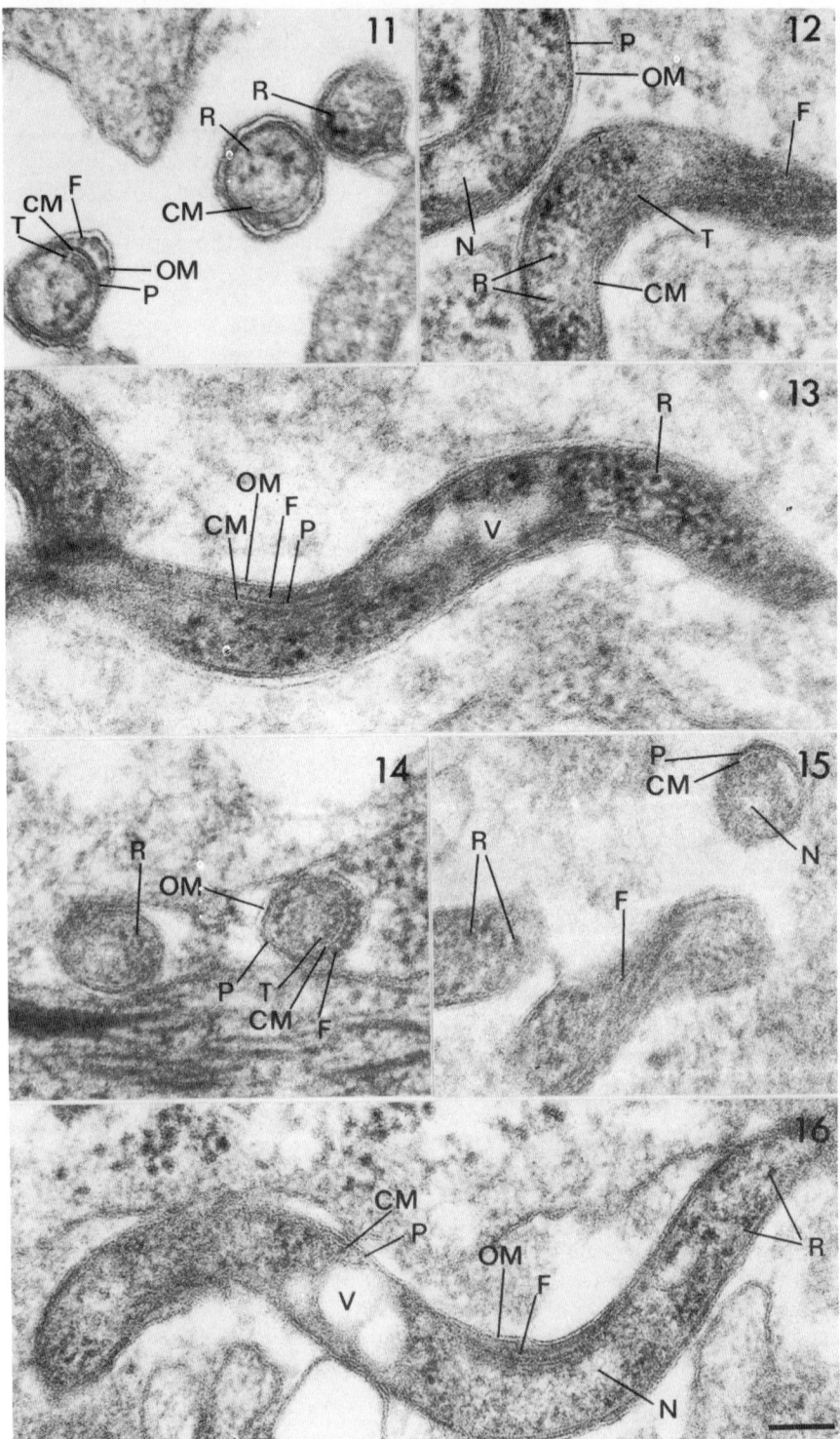

1. Morphology

filament but leaves the distal 0.3-0.5 µm unsheathed (Fig. 8). Examination of sheathed filaments at high magnification shows a substructure which seems to consist of longitudinally arranged subfibrils with a diameter of about 3 nm (Fig. 9). The sheath is vulnerable to various chemicals such as trypsin, 6 M urea, and 0.05 M glycine (19) and can also be removed by extensively washing the flagella with distilled water. There are no reports on the substructure of the core of a flagellum.

The flagella are readily recognizable in sectioned cells. In transverse sections they are observed in the periplasmic space between the outer membrane and the outer part of the peptidoglycan-cytoplasmic membrane complex of the cell (Figs. 11 and 14). In some of these transversely sectioned cells the circumference of the flagella seems to be slightly more electron dense than the core (Fig. 7 in Ref. 9). Whether this part represents the sheath of the filament is not known. In more longitudinally sectioned cells the filaments appear to be of a homogeneous electron density (Figs. 12, 13, 15, and 16). In sectioned cells the width of the flagellum is approximately 18 nm.

The Hook

An abrupt change in the fine structure of the filament is seen to occur at the point of its connection to the hook-shaped structure (Fig. 10). The hook has a honeycombed substructure and is about 50 nm long and approximately 15 nm wide (9,44).

The Basal Body

The basal body consists of a pair of discs which are connected to the hook by a structure called the rod (Fig. 10). The rod is about 13 nm long and 9 nm wide and shows a substructure of fine longitudinal striations (Fig. 10). Its substructural appearance is thus clearly

---

Figures 11-16 Thin-sectioned cells of human pathogenic treponemes are surrounded by a triple-layered outer membrane (OM). The peptidoglycan layer (P) is seen in close apposition to the outer leaflet of the cytoplasmic membrane (CM). Flagella (F) are situated between the outer membrane and the cytoplasmic membrane (Figs. 11-16). Cytoplasmic tubules (T) are discerned in the cytoplasm just underneath the flagella and close to the inner leaflet of the cytoplasmic membrane (Figs. 11, 14). Ribosomes (R) and nuclear regions (N) are seen in the cytoplasm, and vacuoles (V) may also be found (Figs. 13, 16). Figures 11-13 show cells of *T. pertenue* Gauthier in situ in lymph nodes of experimentally infected hamsters and Figs. 14-16 show cells of *T. pallidum* in skin lesions from patients with secondary syphilis (× 90,000). Bar in Fig. 16 = 100 nm.

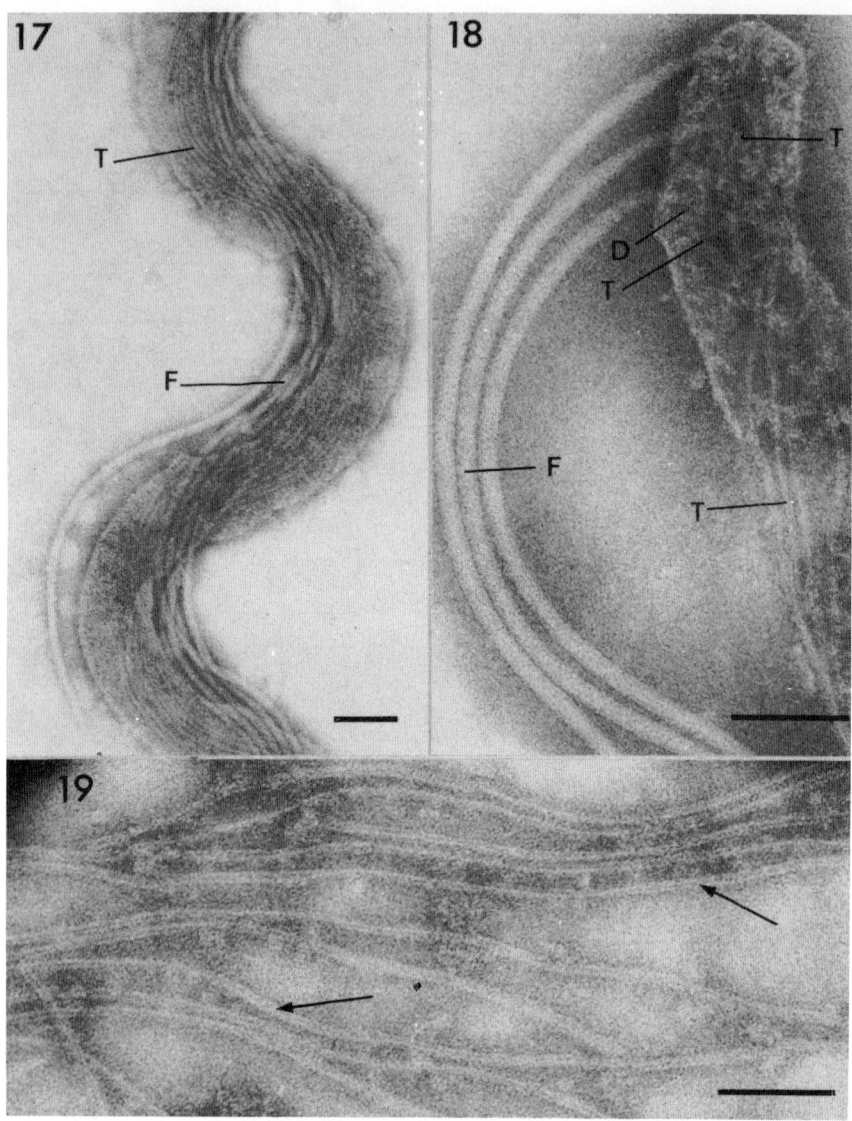

Figures 17-19 were obtained from cells of *T. pallidum* Nichols treated in various ways. Material negatively stained with 1% ammonium molybdate, pH 7. Bars = 100 nm. The cell in Figure 17 was accidently damaged during preparation for electron microscopy. Note the bundle of cytoplasmic tubules (T) winding around the cell in much the same way as the flagella (F) (× 90,000).

Figures 18 and 19 show cells treated with *Myxobacter* AL-1 protease I. In Figure 18, the front part of the cytoplasmic tubules (T) seems to be in close connection to the basal discs (D) of the flagella (F) (× 160,000). In Figure 19, cytoplasmic tubules show uniform width. Electron-dense stain has penetrated the lumen of the tubules (arrows) (× 160,000). (*Source:* Reference 44.)

1. Morphology

different from those of the hook and the flagellar filament. The pair of discs are in close apposition to each other, and both discs have a diameter of 30-35 nm (Fig. 10) (19,44).

Insertion regions of the flagella have not been observed with certainty in sectioned material. It is to be hoped that some fortunate researcher will locate a section that will show the substructure of the terminal part of the flagellum so that a better understanding of the position of the discs in relation to the peptidoglycan layer and the cytoplasmic membrane of the treponemal cell can be obtained.

The structures and dimensions of the flagella of the treponemes are similar to corresponding structures and dimensions of flagella isolated from gram-positive bacteria (19,55,56). DePamphilis and Adler (56) suggested that the flagella from gram-positive bacteria were anchored to the cytoplasmic membrane by the proximal disc. In the case of treponemes one disc might be anchored in the peptidoglycan layer, and the other in the cytoplasmic membrane; or the upper disc might be anchored in the cytoplasmic membrane, and the lower situated just beneath this.

Cytoplasm

Ribosomes and Nuclear Regions

Ribosomes, mesosomes, nuclear regions, and cytoplasmic tubules are recognized in the cytoplasmic matrix of *T. pallidum* and *T. pertenue* Figs. 11-13 and 14-16) (8,9,16,40,57,58). The ribosomes are rather evenly distributed in the cytoplasm as slightly irregular dense dots with a diameter of 0.01 µm (Fig. 11-16). The whorled type of mesosome has been observed and the occasional continuity of this structure with the cytoplasmic membrane has also been seen (Fig. 10 in Ref. 19). Nuclear regions are distinguishable in the cytoplasmic matrix as electron-lucent parts in which delicate strands, probably strands of DNA, are present (Figs. 12 and 16). A few vacuoles are sometimes observed in the cytoplasm of the organisms (Figs. 13 and 16). In general; it can be concluded that except for the presence of cytoplasmic tubules, the cytoplasm of the cells of *T. pallidum* and *T. pertenue* appears to be similar to that of most gram-negative bacteria.

Cytoplasmic Tubules

Bundles of thin fibrils were revealed in negatively stained cells of *T. pallidum* and *T. pertenue* which were accidently damaged during preparation for electron microscopy (Fig. 17) (8,9,44,59). Similar bundles were also observed in cells treated with sodium deoxycholate or *Myxobacter* AL-1 protease I (Figs. 18 and 19) (9,44). A treponeme contains two bundles of these fibrils, one originating from each end of the cell, and each bundle consists of six to eight individual fibrils. The diameter of each fibril is 7-8 nm. The bundles wind around the cell in much the same way as do the flagella, and the fibrils are so long that they overlap in the middle region of the cell. The tubular character of the fibrils is revealed in micrographs of high magnification by the penetration of negative-staining material into the central regions of the fibrils (Fig. 19). The front end of the tubules is frequently seen in close apposition to the basal knob of the flagella (Fig. 18). It is thus tempting to speculate whether these tubules are in some way anchored to or connected with one or both discs of the basal knob.

In sectioned cells the cytoplasmic tubules are observed in the cytoplasm just underneath the flagella and close to the inner leaflet of the cytoplasmic membrane (19,40,41,57-60). In transverse sections they are found to be arranged in a single row, thus demonstrating that individual tubules interdigitate when they overlap in the middle region of the cell (Figs. 11 and 14). Some reports describe the tubules as comma or wedge shaped (57), elongated (8), or ovoid (59) when observed in sectioned cells. The exact shape of these very thin tubules, however, is difficult to determine from sections. The tubules will appear circular only when sectioned perfectly transversely. Any deviation from this orientation will depict the tubules as wedge- or ovoid-shaped structures. Below is a schematic representation of the appearance of circular cytoplasmic tubules in cells transversely sectioned at planes A and B.

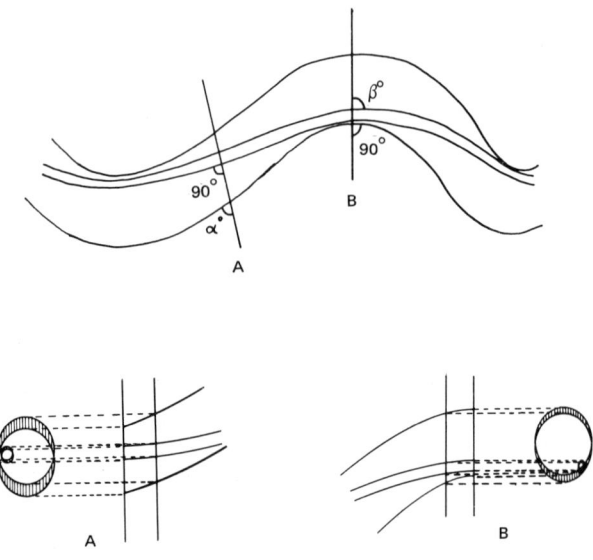

1. Morphology

A represents a section at right angles to the tubule but not to the cell. On a micrograph the cell will appear oblong, but the tubule approximately circular.

B represents a section at right angles to the cell but not to the tubule. On a micrograph the cell will appear approximately circular, but the tubule oblong. However, the tubule appears wedge-shaped because it is partly masked by the cytoplasmic membrane. The finding that tubules in negatively stained material are of uniform width suggests that they are cylindrical.

Division

Cells of *T. pallidum* and *T. pertenue* divide transversely by binary fission. In the light microscope, dividing cells are recognized as long U- or V-shaped cells wriggling around a point in the middle region of the cell. In the electron microscope the first sign of a forthcoming division is the presence of short flagella inserted in the middle region of the cell (Fig. 20). The free ends of the new flagella are directed away from each other, toward the ends of the old cell. At this stage no evidence for the formation of a septum or any other partition is found. At a later stage the two daughter cells are separated by an invagination of the cytoplasmic membrane, but both new cells are still enclosed in a mutual outer envelope (Fig. 21). The diameter of the cell appears to be somewhat smaller at the ·division site. From this point on, the ends of the newly formed cells seem to elongate and become more pointed before the cells finally separate. No evidence has ever been found for the origin of the outermost striated tip of cells of *T. pallidum* and *T. pertenue,* nor has further elucidation of the division process been obtained from studies of sectioned material.

Other Pathogenic Treponemes

Treponema para-luis cuniculi

The morphology of *Treponema para-luis cuniculi* has been found to be identical to that of *T. pallidum* (Fig. 22) (61,62).

Treponema hyodysenteriae

The morphology of *Treponema hyodysenteriae* differs very much from that of other pathogenic treponemes and all other treponemes examined as well. The main differences are in the size and shape of the cells (Fig. 23) (63 and Hovind-Hougen, unpublished data) and also in their mode of division (Fig. 24). Cells of *T. hyodysenteriae* divide in a manner similar to that of cells of the genus *Borrelia*, which they also resemble by not possessing cytoplasmic tubules (Fig. 25). This similarity to *Borrelia* is probably of some importance for the classifi-

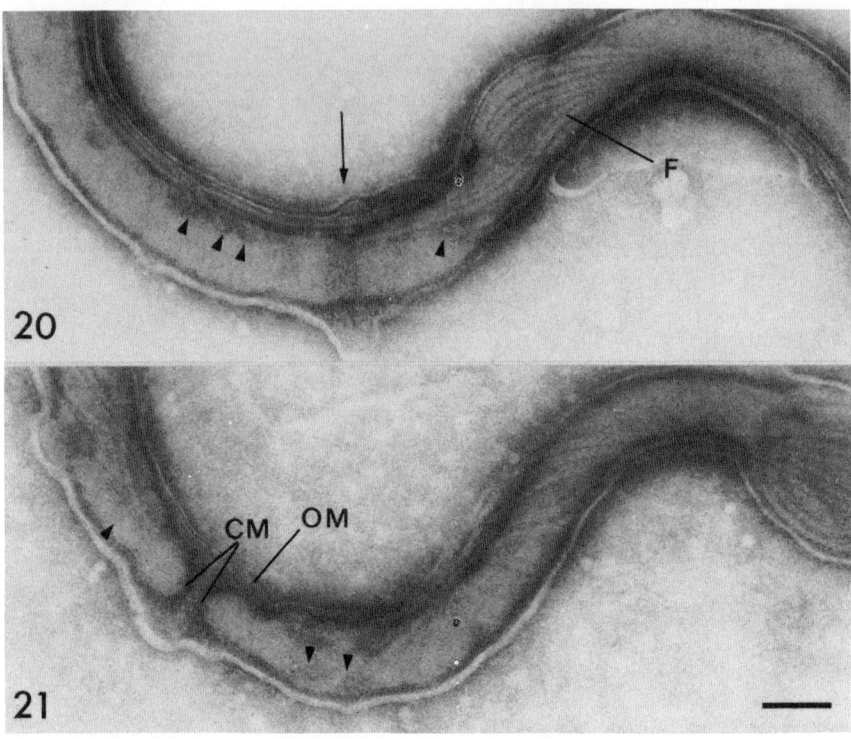

Figures 20 and 21 show dividing cells of *T. pallidum* Nichols. Material negatively stained with 1% ammonium molybdate, pH 7.

Figure 20 A cell at an early stage of the division process. The insertion points of the new flagella are seen (arrowheads). The flagella (F) of the mother cell cross the division site (arrow) so that eight flagella are present there (× 90,000).

Figure 21 A cell at a later stage of the division process. The daughter cells are completely separated by their cytoplasmic membranes (CM) inside a mutual outer membrane (OM). Note the insertion points of the new flagella (arrowheads) (× 90,000). Bar = 100 nm.

cation of these organisms, since the presence of cytoplasmic tubules is regarded as a morphological criterion for the genus *Treponema* (19,51,54).

Concluding Remarks

Very little information is available on the role of the different anatomical structures of human pathogenic treponemes in the pathogenesis of disease. Our knowledge about which treponemal structures are

1. Morphology

efficient antigens for obtaining an immune response is equally limited (Chap. 12). As will be discussed in Chap. 11, the attachment of treponemes to cell surfaces may be an important factor in the establishment of disease and the initiation of an immune response in the host. It is probable that the specialized end structure of the treponeme is of importance for the attachment. Scanning electron microscopy has not, however, provided more detailed information than the demonstration of a universal end-on attachment (17). Ordinary scanning electron microscopy has a rather limited resolution and can only yield structural details of surfaces. Further information about the mechanism of attachment of treponemal cells must most likely await traditional transmission electron microscope studies of negatively stained and of sectioned material.

For many infectious diseases the degree of pathogenicity of a microorganism depends on surface components which are able to react, or prevent reactions, with specialized sites on cell surfaces of the host (Chaps. 11 and 12). Naturally, the envelope of *T. pallidum* cells has received considerable attention in studies on the pathogenicity and immunity of syphilis. Immunoimmobilized cells in the *Treponema pallidum* immobilization (TPI) test (Chap. 13) present a swollen periplasmic space and an outer membrane covered with a layer of fuzzy material (64). In addition, human IgG globulins are attached to the surface of immobilized treponemes after incubation with human syphilitic serum and unheated guinea pig serum (65). In contrast, no IgG can be demonstrated on the motile cells obtained after incubation with the same human serum and heat-treated guinea pig serum (65). These results clearly show that antigenic sites are present on the outer membrane of *T. pallidum* cells. However, heat-labile substance(s), presumably complement, appear to be required for the antigen-antibody reaction to take place.

The host organism is able to produce antibodies against a great variety of morphologically identifiable parasite structures. Antibodies against specific organelles of cells of *Treponema* strain Reiter have been demonstrated in human syphilitic sera (66,67). The Reiter strain has been extensively used for pilot studies, mainly because it is easy to cultivate and cells can thus be obtained in large quantities. However, the results of these studies must be evaluated with great caution because the Reiter cells differ from those of *T. pallidum* not only by being cultivable, but they are also morphologically different from *T. pallidum* cells and, last but not least, nonpathogenic.

Antibodies against different characteristic cell structures can be visualized in the electron microscope by the negative-staining technique (67-69). Elucidation of the structure and function as well as the pathogenicity of human pathogenic treponemes is important to our understanding of the immunity of treponemal infections. I am convinced that the electron microscope will be an important research tool in future work along these lines.

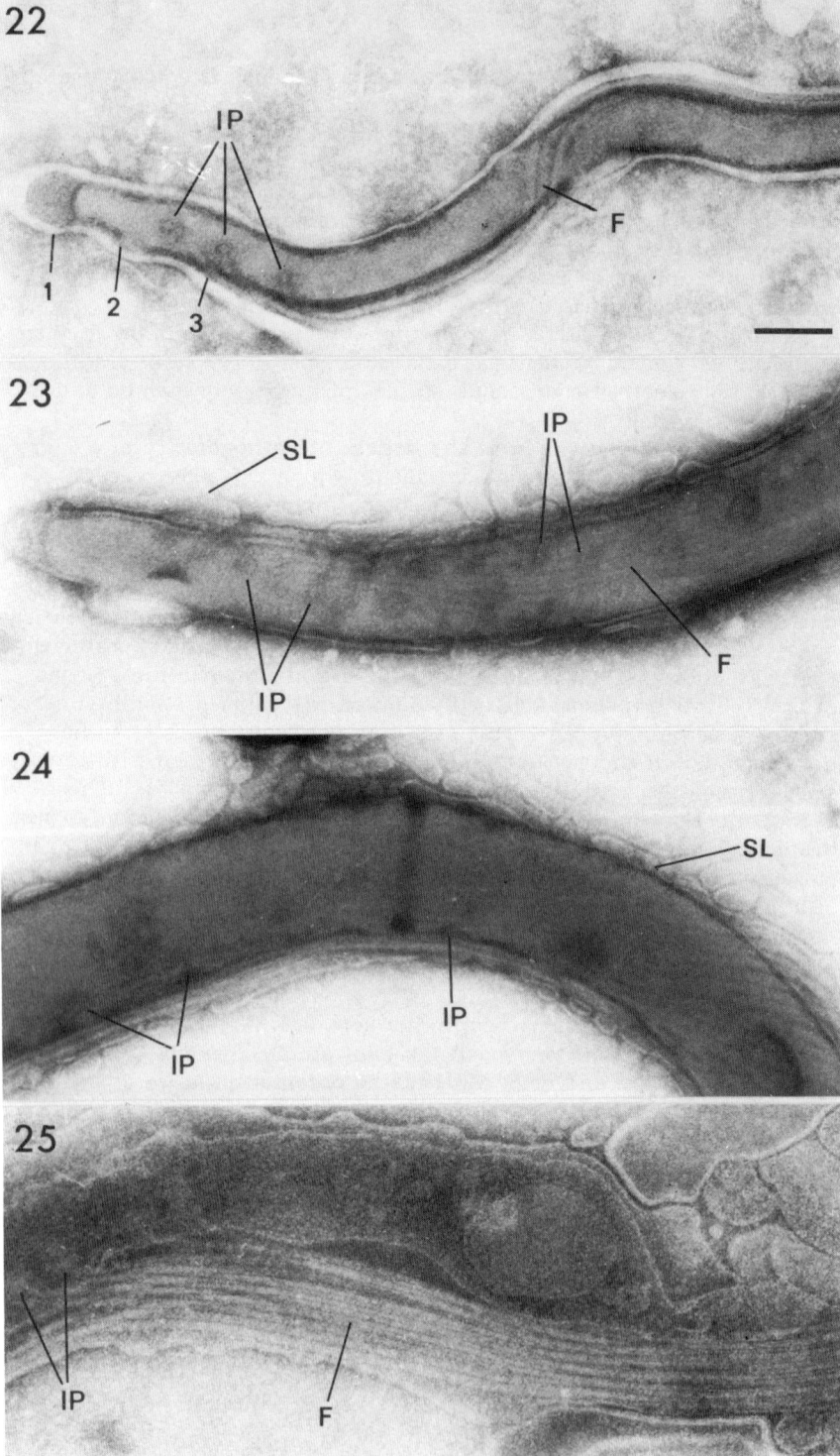

1. Morphology

Acknowledgments

I want to express my sincere gratitude to Dr. A. Birch-Andersen for his valuable cooperation during my work and for his constructive criticism in the preparation of this manuscript. I also thank Dr. H. A. Nielsen for helpful advice; H. Ravn, J. Berg, and F. Laursen for their excellent assistance in electron microscopy; A. G. Overgaard for expert photographic work ; and G. Seidenfaden and A. Thorborg for their great help with the typing and retyping of the manuscript.

References

1. F. Schaudinn and E. Hoffmann. Vorläufiger Bericht über das Vorkommen von Spirochaeten in syphilitischen Krankheitsprodukten und bei Papillomen. *Arb. Gesund. Amte (Berlin)* 22:527-534 (1904-1905).
2. F. Schaudinn and E. Hoffmann. Über Spirochaetenbefunde im Lymphdrüsensaft Syphilitischer. *Dtsch. Med. Wochenschr.* 31:711-714 (1905).

Figure 22 A cell of *T. cuniculi* which demonstrates that the end of the cell is morphologically identical to that of a human pathogenic treponeme (see Figs. 2-4). Zones 1, 2, and 3 (see text) are clearly seen. IP denotes the insertion points of the flagella (F). Material negatively stained with 1% ammonium molybdate, pH 7 (× 90,000). Bar = 100 nm. (*Source*: Reference 61.)

Figures 23-25 Cells of *T. hyodysenteriae* strain B 78.

Figure 23 An end of a cell is shown where IP denotes insertion points of some of the flagella (F). Note the presence of a surface layer (SL) on the cell. Material negatively stained with 1% ammonium molybdate, pH 7 (× 90,000).

Figure 24 The division site of a dividing cell. The ends of the daughter cells appear truncated. IP denotes insertion points of the new flagella and SL the regularly structured surface layer. Note the difference in mode of division compared to *T. pallidum* (Figs. 20-21) (× 90,000).

Figure 25 A cell accidently damaged during preparation for electron microscopy. IP denotes insertion points of the flagella (F) (× 90,000).

3. H. Noguchi. The spirochetes. In *The New Knowledge of Bacteriology and Immunology* (E. O. Jordan and I. S. Falk, Eds.). The University of Chicago Press, Chicago, 1928, pp. 452-497.
4. R. R. Willcox and T. Guthe. *Treponema pallidum*. A bibliographic review of the morphology, culture and survival of *T. pallidum* and associated organisms. *Bull WHO Suppl*. 35:9-35 (1966).
5. J. A. Sykes, J. N. Miller, and A. J. Kalan. *Treponema pallidum* within cells of a primary chancre from a human female. *Br. J. Vener. Dis.* 50:40-44 (1974).
6. E. Mölbert. Vergleichende elektronenmikroskopische Untersuchungen zur Morphologie von *Treponema pallidum, Treponema pertenue* and Reiter Spirochäten. *Zschr. Hyg.* 142:510-515 (1956).
7. J. J. Angulo, J. H. L. Watson, C. C. Wedderburn, F. Léon-Blanco, and G. Varela. Electron micrography of treponemes from cases of yaws, pinta and the so-called Cuban form of pinta. *Am. J. Trop. Med.* 31:458-478 (1951).
8. N. M. Ovčinnikov and V. V. Delektorskij. *Treponema pertenue* under the electron microscope. *Br. J. Vener. Dis.* 46:349-379 (1970).
9 K. Hovind-Hougen, A. Birch-Andersen, and H. J. Skovgaard Jensen. Ultrastructure of cells of *Treponema pertenue* obtained from experimentally infected hamsters. *Acta Pathol. Microbiol. Scand. B* 84:101-108 (1976).
10. J. H. L. Watson, J. J. Angulo, F. Léon-Blanco, G. Varela, and C. C. Wedderburn. Electron microscopic observations of flagellation in some species of the genus *Treponema* Schaudinn. *J. Bacteriol.* 61:455-461 (1951).
11. R. E. Campbell and P. D. Rosahn. The morphology and staining characteristics of *Treponema pallidum*. Review of the literature and description of a new technique for staining the organism in tissues. *Yale J. Biol. Med.* 22:527-543 (1950).
12. A. Castellani. On the presence of spirochetes in two cases of ulcerated parangi (yaws). *Br. Med. J.* 2:1280 (1905).
13. R. H. A. Swain. Electron microscopic studies of the morphology of pathogenic spirochetes. *J. Pathol. Bacteriol.* 69:117-128 (1955).
14. J. Pillot and A. Ryter. Structure des spirochètes. I. Etude des genres *Treponema, Borrelia* et *Leptospira* au microscope électronique. *Ann. Inst. Pasteur* 108:791-804 (1965).
15. R. M. Smibert. *Treponema* Schaudinn 1905. In *Bergey's Manual of Determiniative Bacteriology* (R. E. Buchanan and N. E. Gibbons, Eds.), 8th ed., The Williams & Wilkins Co., Baltimore, 1974, p. 175.
16. O. B. Jepsen, K. Hovind-Hougen, and A. Birch-Andersen. Electron microscopy of *Treponema pallidum* Nichols. *Acta Pathol. Microbiol. Scand.* 74:241-258 (1968).

1. Morphology

17. T. J. Fitzgerald, P. Cleveland, R. C. Johnson, J. N. Miller, and J. A. Sykes. Scanning electron microscopy of *Treponmea pallidum* (Nichols strain) attached to cultured mammalian cells. *J. Bacteriol.* 130:1333-1344 (1977).
18. N. S. Hayes, K. E. Muse, A. M. Collier, and J. B. Baseman. Parasitism by virulent *Treponema pallidum* of host cell surfaces. *Infect. Immun.* 17:174-186 (1977).
19. K. Hovind-Hougen. Determination by means of electron microscopy of morphological criteria of value for classification of some spirochetes, in particular treponemes. *Acta Pathol. Microbiol. Scand., B Suppl.* 255:3-27 (1976).
20. T. J. Fitzgerald, R. C. Johnson, J. N. Miller, and J. A. Sykes. Characterization of the attachment of *Treponema pallidum* (Nichols strain) to cultured mammalian cells and the potential relationship of attachment to pathogenicity. *Infect. Immun.* 18:467-478 (1977).
21. B. D. Brause and R. B. Roberts. Attachment of virulent *Treponema pallidum* to human mononuclear phagocytes. *Br. J. Vener. Dis.* 54:218-224 (1978).
22. H. E. Smith and H. J. Arnott. Epi- and endobiotic bacteria associated with *Pyrsonympha vertens*, a symbiotic protozoon of the termite *Reticulitermes flavipes*. *Trans. Am. Microsc. Soc.* 93:180-194 (1974).
23. R. A. Bloodgood, K. R. Miller, T. P. Fitzharris, and J. R. McIntosh. The ultrastructure of *Pyrsonympha* and its associated microorganisms. *J. Morphol.* 143:77-105 (1974).
24. D. L. Harris, R. D. Glock, and J. M. Kinyon. Intestinal treponematoses. In *The Biology of Parasitic Spirochetes* (R. C. Johnson, Ed.), Academic, New York 1976, pp. 277-293.
25. F. D. Lee, A. Kraszewski, J. Gordan, J. G. R. Howie, D. McSeveney, and W. A. Hanlard. Intestinal spirochaetosis. *Gut* 12:126-133 (1971).
26. D. C. Savage and R. V. Blumershine. Surface-surface associations in microbial communities populating epithelial habitats in the murine gastrointestinal ecosystem: Scanning electron microscopy. *Infect. Immun.* 10:240-250 (1974).
27. A. Takeuchi and J. A. Zeller. Ultrastructural identification of spirochetes and flagellated microbes at the brush border of the large intestinal epithelium of the Rhesus monkey. *Infect. Immun.* 6:1008-1018 (1972).
28. K. Hovind-Hougen. Electron microscopy of *Borrelia merionesi* and *Borrelia recurrentis*. *Acta Pathol. Microbiol. Scand., B* 82:799-809 (1974).
29. Y. Karimi, K. Hovind-Hougen, A. Birch-Andersen, and M. Asmar. *Borrelia persica* and *B. baltazardi* sp. nov.: Experimental pathogenicity for some animals and comparison of the ultrastructure. *Ann. Microbiol. Inst. Pasteur, 130B*:157-168 (1979).

30. M. J. Seldeen. The immobilization of *Treponema pallidum* by antibody and complement. A study of certain factors influencing the measurement of immobilizing antibody, Ph. D. thesis, The Johns Hopkins University, Baltimore, Maryland (1953).
31. P. H. Hardy and E. E. Nell. Study of the antigenic structure of *Treponema pallidum* by specific agglutination. *Am. J. Hyg.* 66:160-172 (1957).
32. M. Metzger and J. Ruczkowska. Influence of lysozyme upon the reactivity on *Treponema pallidum* in the FTA-reaction. *Arch. Immunol. Ther. Exp.* 12:702-708 (1964).
33. J. A. Zeigler, A. M. Jones, R. H. Jones, and K. M. Kubica. Demonstration of extracellular material at the surface of pathogenic *T. pallidum* cells. *Br. J. Vener. Dis.* 52:1-8 (1976).
34. J. H. Luft. Ruthenium red and violet. I. Chemistry, purification, methods of use for electron microscopy and mechanism of action. *Anat. Rec.* 171:347-368 (1971).
35. D. E. Akin. Ultrastructure of rumen bacterial attachment to forage cell walls. *Appl. Environ. Microbiol.* 31:562-568 (1976).
36. M. Fletcher and G. D. Floodgate. An electron-microscopic demonstration of an acidic polysaccharide involved in the adhesion of a marine bacterium to solid surfaces. *J. Gen. Microbiol.* 74:325-334 (1973).
37. J. A. Breznak and H. S. Pankratz. In situ morphology of the gut microbiota of wood-eating termites *(Reticulitermes flavipes* (Kollar) and *Coptotermes formosanus* Shiraki). *Appl. Environ. Microbiol.* 33:406-426 (1977).
38. B. E. Brooker and R. Fuller. Adhesion of lactobacilli to the chicken crop epithelium. *J. Ultrastruct. Res.* 52:21-31 (1975).
39. T. J. Fitzgerald, R. C. Johnson, and D. M. Ritzi. Relationship of *Treponema pallidum* to acidic mucopolysaccharides. *Infect. Immun.* 24:252-260 (1979).
40. N. M. Ovčinnikov and V. V. Delektorskij. Current concepts of the morphology and biology of *Treponema pallidum* based on electron microscopy. *Br. J. Vener. Dis.* 47:315-328 (1971).
41. R. C. Johnson, D. M. Ritzi, and B. P. Livermore. Outer envelope of virulent *Treponema pallidum*. *Infect. Immun.* 8:291-295 (1973).
42. H. A. Azar, T. D. Pham and A. K. Kurban. An electron microscopic study of a syphilitic chancre. *Arch. Pathol.* 90:143-150 (1970).
43. J. Metz and G. Metz. Die Lokalisation von *Treponema pallidum* in Hautefflorezenzen der Lues I und II. *Dtsch. Med. Wochenschr.* 97:626-627 (1972).
44. K. Hovind-Hougen. Further observations on the ultrastructure of *Treponema pallidum* Nichols. *Acta.Pathol. Microbiol. Scand. B* 80:297-304 (1972).

1. Morphology

45. P. E. Kolenbrander and J. C. Ensign. Isolation and chemical structure of the peptidoglycan of *Spirillum serpens* cell walls. *J. Bacteriol.* 95:201-210 (1968).
46. R. Joseph, S. C. Holt, and E. Canale-Parola. Peptidoglycan of free-living anaerobic spirochetes. *J. Bacteriol.* 115:426-435 (1973).
47. J. Pillot. Contribution à l'étude du genre Treponema: Structures anatomique et antigénique. D.Sc. thesis. Université de Paris, France, 1965.
48. R. Tinelli and J. Pillot. Etude de la composition du glycopeptide de *Treponema reiteri*. *C. R. Acad. Sci.* 263:739-741 (1966).
49. M. S. Wachter and R. C. Johnson. Treponeme outer envelope: chemical analysis (39151). *Proc. Soc. Exp. Biol. Med.* 151:97-100 (1976).
50. I. Azuma, T. Taniyama, Y. Yamamura, Y. Yanagihara, Y. Hattori, S. Yasuda, and I. Mifuchi. Chemical studies on the cell walls of *Leptospira biflexa* strain Urawa and *Treponema pallidum* strain Reiter. *Jpn. J. Microbiol.* 19:45-51 (1975).
51. S. C. Holt. Anatomy and chemistry of spirochetes. *Microbiol. Rev.* 42:114-160 (1978).
52. C. D. Ginger. Isolation and characterization of muramic acid from two spirochaetes: *Borrelia duttoni* and *Leptospira biflexa*. *Nature* 199:159 (1963).
53. R. Yanagawa and S. Faine. Morphological and serological analysis of leptospiral structure. *Nature* 211:823-826 (1966).
54. R. C. Johnson. The spirochetes. *Annu. Rev. Microbiol.* 31:89-106 (1977).
55. D. Abram, H. Koffler, and A. E. Vatter. Basal structure and attachment of flagella in cells of *Proteus vulgaris*. *J. Bacteriol.* 90:1337-1354 (1965).
56. M. L. DePamphilis and J. Adler. Fine structure and isolation of the hook-basal body complex of flagella from *Escherichia coli* and *Bacillus subtilis*. *J. Bacteriol.* 105:384-395 (1971).
57. R. H. A. Swain and N. Anderson. The ultra-structure of species of *Treponemas* and *Borreliae*, in *The Fine Morphology of Spirochaetas* (B. Babudieri, ed.), Leonardo Edizioni Scientifiche, Roma, 1972, pp. 113-139.
58. N. M. Ovčinnikov and V. V. Delektorskij. Further studies of the morphology of *Treponema pallidum* under the electron microscope. *Br. J. Vener. Dis.* 45:87-116 (1969).
59. S. E. Wiegand, P. L. Strobel, and L. H. Glassman. Electron microscopic anatomy of pathogenic *Treponema pallidum*. *J. Invest. Dermatol.* 58:186-204 (1972).
60. G. Klingmüller, Y. Ishibashi, and K. Radke. Der elektronenmikroskopische Aufbau des *Treponema pallidum*. *Arch. Klin. Exp. Dermatol.* 233:197-205 (1968).

61. K. Hovind-Hougen, A. Birch-Andersen, and H.-J. Skovgaard Jensen. Electron microscopy of *Treponema cuniculi*. *Acta Pathol. Microbiol. Scand. B.* 81:15-26 (1973).
62. J. L. Smith and B. R. Pesetsky. The current status of *Treponema cuniculi*. Review of the literature. *Br. J. Vener. Dis.* 43:117-127 (1967).
63. J. M. Kinyon and D. L. Harris. *Treponema innocens*, a new species of intestinal bacteria, and emended description of the type strain of *Treponema hyodysenteriae* Harris et al. *Int. J. Syst. Bacteriol.* 29:102-109 (1979).
64. K. Hovind-Hougen, H. A. Nielsen, and A. Birch-Andersen. Electron microscopy of treponemes subjected to the *Treponema pallidum* immobilization (TPI) test. 1. Comparison of immunoimmobilized cells and control cells. *Acta Pathol. Microbiol. Scand. C* 87:217-222 (1979).
65. K. Hovind-Hougen, A. Birch-Andersen, and H. A. Nielsen. Electron microscopy of treponemes subjected to the *Treponema pallidum* immobilization (TPI) test. 2. Immunoelectron microscopy. *Acta Pathol. Microbiol. Scand. C* 87:263-268 (1979).
66. P. H. Hardy, W. R. Frederichs, and E. E. Nell. Isolation and antigenic characteristics of axial filaments from the Reiter treponeme. *Infect. Immun.* 11:380-386 (1975).
67. N. S. Pedersen, C. S. Petersen, N. H. Axelsen, A. Birch-Andersen, and K. Hovind-Hougen. Isolation of heat-stabile antigen from *Treponema reiter*, using an immunoadsorbent with antibodies from syphilitic patients. *Scand. J. Immunol.* 14:137-144 (1981).
68. I. Ørskov, F. Ørskov, and A. Birch-Andersen. Comparison of *Escherichia coli* fimbrial antigen F7 with type 1 fimbriae. *Infect. Immun.* 27:657-666 (1980).
69. A. M. Lawn. Simple immunological labelling method for electron microscopy and its application to the study of filamentous appendages of bacteria. *Nature* 214:1151-1152 (1967).

2
Composition

RUSSELL C. JOHNSON
University of Minnesota
Minneapolis, Minnesota

Surface Mucopolysaccharides 30
Protein Content 30
Lipids 31
Deoxyribonucleic Acid Base 32
Individual Structures 32
References 34

There is a paucity of information on the chemical composition of *Treponema pallidum* and other treponemes pathogenic for humans. To a great extent, this is due to the inability to cultivate adequate numbers of these treponemes in vitro and the difficulty in separating host tissue from *T. pallidum* harvested from testicularly infected rabbits.

Meaningful chemical analyses of *T. pallidum* require cell preparations free of contaminating host tissue. Since the only reliable way to obtain large numbers of *T. pallidum* is from infected rabbit testes, there is a problem concerning the purity of the harvested treponemes. Several approaches to overcoming this difficulty have been explored. A reduction in the amount of contaminating host tissue in treponeme cell preparations has been accomplished by the administration of corticosteroids to the infected rabbits (1,2). This steroid treatment decreased cellular infiltration into the testicular syphilomas and increased the yield of *T. pallidum*. It is important that the treponemes are harvested at the time of maximal orchitis and before the testes become hemorrhagic (1,2). Density-gradient centrifugation (3), continuous-flow zonal centrifugation in cesium chloride gradients (4), a discontinuous gradient of sodium and meglumine diatrizoates (5), and continuous-particle electrophoresis (6) have been utilized to remove rabbit tissue from treponemal cells. Unfortunately, these techniques result in nonviable cells whose structures or components may have been lost or modified. Separation of *T. pallidum* from tissue cell and debris has also been accomplished by filtration. Initially membrane filters were used that retained many of the treponemes (7); however, the use of Nucleopore filters (0.8-μm pore size) allowed almost complete recovery of *T. pallidum* while removing all observable tissue cells (8). The combination of differential centrifugation and Nucleopore filtration results in a relatively "clean" preparation of *T. pallidum* that retain their physiological activity. Unwashed treponemes have host proteins adsorbed on their surface (9). Some of the host proteins are loosely associated with the cell surface and can be removed by washing the cells. Other host proteins are tightly bound to the cell surface and require protease digestion for their removal, which also removes some treponemal proteins (9; see Chap. 12).

Surface Mucopolysaccharides

Electron microscope studies of *T. pallidum* stained with ruthenium red suggested the presence of a surface layer of acidic mucopolysaccharide material (10,11). Acid bovine serum albumin (BSA) combined with acidic mucopolysaccharide results in the formation of a precipitate (12). A bead-type precipitate was observed on the surface of *T. pallidum* treated with acid BSA, providing additional evidence for the presence of a surface layer of acidic mucopolysaccharide (13). Partial identification of the surface mucopolysaccharide was accomplished with plant lectins. Wheat germ agglutinin and soybean agglutinin react with N-acetyl-D-glucosamine (a component of hyaluronic acid) and N-acetyl-D-galactosamine (a component of chondroitin sulfate), respectively. Both plant lectins agglutinated freshly harvested *T. pallidum*, suggesting that the surface-associated mucopolysaccharide may be a complex of hyaluronic acid and chondroiton sulfate or similar acidic mucopolysaccharides (13). This surface layer of mucopolysaccharide may be responsible for the relatively poor serological activity of freshly harvested *T. pallidum* in the agglutination test (14; see Chap. 11).

Protein Content

The protein content of *T. pallidum* has been determined by several investigators (2,4). It would appear that the protein content of the treponemes reported may be a reflection of the "purity" of the cell preparation. Thomas et al. (4), utilizing continuous-flow zonal centrifugation, reported a protein content of 5.9×10^{-7} μg per treponeme. Hardy and Nell (2), using differential centrigution, obtained

2. Composition

an average value of 1.9×10^{-7} µg protein per treponeme. The lowest protein value per treponeme was reported by Matthews et al. (15). They combined differential centrifugation, Nucleopore filtration, and Hypaque gradients to purify their cell preparation and obtained a protein concentration of 0.56×10^{-7} µg per cell.

Lipids

Spirochetes have a high lipid content. Approximately 20% of the cell weight is comprised of lipids, the bulk of which are in polar form. Studies on the lipid composition of members of the genera *Spirochaeta*, *Leptospira*, and *Borrelia* and the nonpathogenic treponemes indicate that the lipid composition appears to be quite characteristic for the genera of spirochetes studied (16,17). Glycolipids are present in the *Spirochaeta*, *Borrelia*, and *Treponema*, but absent in the *Leptospira*. These glycolipids consist of only the monoglycosyldiglyceride type; no diglycosyl or triglycosyl forms were observed (16,17). The lipid composition of *Borrelia hermsii* is similar to that of the *Treponema*. The major exception to this is that *B. hermsii* synthesizes the lipid cholesteryl glucoside (17). This lipid has been reported in only one other bacterial genus, the *Mycoplasma* (18).

The lipid composition of *T. pallidum* has been investigated (15,19,20). Organisms cultivated in complex media (e.g., serum containing) or harvested from host tissues will incorporate or adsorb lipids from medium components or host tissue, markedly limiting the value of these analyses. Accordingly, in evaluating lipid composition studies of *T. pallidum* harvested from rabbit testes the presence of absence of lipid components in host tissue becomes extremely important. Vaczi et al. (19) reported that the phospholipid composition of *T. pallidum* (Budapest strain) was quite complex, consisting of 11 to 13 components. No quantitative data on these components was given, and monoglycosyldiglyceride, a glycolipid comprising 22-50% of the nonpathogenic treponemes studied (16,20-23), was identified neither (19) in *T. pallidum* nor in the nonpathogenic treponemes examined. Smibert (20) reported the lipid composition of the Beckman diagnostic fluorescent treponemal antibody test antigen, which consists of electrophoretically purified *T. pallidum*. The total lipid consisted of 41% phospholipid, 37% glycolipid, and 22% neutral lipid. Matthews et al. (15) studied the lipid composition of *T. pallidum* purified by differential centrifugation, filtration through Nucleopore membranes, and sedimentation in Hypaque density gradients. Total lipids consisted of 32.2% neutral lipids, primarily cholesterol, and 67.8% phospholipid. The phospholipids contained phosphatidylcholine (32.1%), sphingomyelin (14.8%), cardiolipin (13.0%), phosphatidylethanolamine (6.2%), phosphatidylinositol serine (1.2%), and lysophosphatidylcholine (0.4%). It may be that the antibodies directed against the cardiolipin component of *T. pallidum* are those reactive in the Venereal Disease Research Laboratories (VDRL) test. It should be noted that cholesterol and these phospholipids are also present in rabbit testicular tissue. However, the lipids of the nonpathogenic treponemes *Treponema phagedenis*, *Treponema denticola*, and *Treponema scolidontum*, cultivated in lipid-defined media, also have phosphatidylcholine as their major phospholipid and contain cardiolipin and phosphatidylethanolamine (16). A significant finding of Matthews et al. (15) is the absence of the glycolipid monoglycosyldiglyceride. Since this glycolipid comprises on the average 48.7% of the polar lipids of the treponemes (16), it suggests that *T. pallidum* is not closely related to the nonpathogenic treponemes studied to date. This observation is in agreement with the genetic studies of Miao and Fieldsteel (24). They reported that there was a total lack of DNA homology between *T. pallidum* and five nonpathogenic treponemes (biotypes of *Treponema phagedenis* and *Treponema refringens*) (Chap. 3).

The nonpathogenic treponemes lack the ability to synthesize, chain-elongate, β-oxidize, or desaturate fatty acids (22,23,25). Accordingly, they must be provided saturated and unsaturated long-chain fatty acids that are incorporated unaltered into the treponemal lipids. Thus, the fatty acid composition of the nonpathogenic treponemes is the same as the composition of the culture medium (23). *Treponema pallidum* appears to share this property with the nonpathogenic treponemes, since it contains the same fatty acids as the tissue from which it was harvested (15).

Deoxyribonucleic Acid Base

The DNA of *Treponema pallidum* has a guanine plus cytosine content of 52.4-53.7% (24) (see Chap. 3). This is higher than the guanine plus cytosine content of the nonpathogenic treponemes *T. refringens* (41.5%) and *T. phagedenis* (38-39%), which are genetically distinct from *T. pallidum* (24). *Treponema hyodysenteriae* is a cultivable pathogenic treponeme that, when in combination with other intestinal bacteria, causes swine dysentery (26). This pathogenic treponeme has DNA with a very low guanine plus cytosine content of 25.8% and does not share DNA homology with *T. pallidum* (27).

Individual Structures

The Outer Envelope

Treponema pallidum is similar to other spirochetes in possessing an outer membrane or outer envelope (28). The function of the outer envelope is not known, but an intact outer envelope is necessary for spirochete viability. Damage to the outer envelope of *Leptospira* by antibody and complement results in the leakage of intracellular components and cell death (29). The outer envelope of spirochetes is quite elastic. When the cell is subjected to adverse conditions blebs appear on the surface, due to the separation of the outer envelope from the underlying protoplasmic cylinder. When the nonpathogenic treponemes are exposed to hypotonic solutions, the outer envelope separates from the protoplasmic cylinder and the cell assumes a spherical shape (30). The sperical forms of spirochetes are nonviable. The outer envelope can be readily removed from these spherical forms of treponemes by the solubilizing activity of low concentrations (0.7 mM) of the detergent sodium dodecyl sulfate (31). However, the protoplasmic cylinder maintains its spiral shape and appears intact upon examination with the electron microscope. Removal of the sodium dodecyl sulfate by dialysis, followed by the addition of divalent or trivalent cations, results in the reaggregation of the treponemal outer envelope (31). The outer envelope aggregate recovered averaged 14.6% of the whole-cell dry weight. The reaggregated outer envelope of *T. phagedenis* biotype Kazan 5 had the following composition: lipid, 4-5%; protein, 60-73%; and carbohydrate, 1-2% (32). Muramic acid was not detected in the outer envelope but was present in the protoplasmic cylinder (32). Although the treponemal outer envelope may resemble the outer envelope of gram-negative bacteria such as *Escherichia coli*, classical endotoxin was not detected in biotype Kazan 5 (33). Jackson and Zey (34) extracted material from *T. phagedenis* Nichols, which, as judged by electron microscopy, has morphological features similar to those found in lipopolysaccharide. However, *T. pallidum* is not known to contain endotoxin.

Preliminary studies with *T. pallidum* strain Nichols harvested from rabbit testes have shown that its outer envelope is solubilized by low concentrations of sodium dodecyl sulfate and reaggregated by removal of the detergent followed by the addition of divalent cations. The outer envelope of parasitic leptospires can be removed in a manner similar to that described for the treponemes, with the exception that cations are not required for reaggregation (35). Animals vaccinated with the leptospiral outer envelope are immune to challenge (36) and possess antibodies that are protective. If the outer envelope of *T. pallidum* contains the protective antigens, then the potential exists for the development of an outer-envelope vaccine for syphilis, once successful in vitro cultivation of this spirochete has been accomplished.

Flagella (Axial Filaments)

The flagella of spirochetes are similar morphologically and chemically to those of other bacteria, but differ from them in that they are not extracellular. Although the spirochete flagella are located between the cell wall and the outer envelope, they are responsible for the motility of *Leptospira* (37) and *Spirocheata* (38) and presumably other spirochetes. The flagella of *Treponema zeulzerae* consist largely of protein (mol wt 37,000) and, like other bacterial flagella, are completely devoid of half-cystine (39). Hardy et al. (40) studied the flagella protein of *T. phagedenis* biotype Reiter and concluded that it was probably the so-called "Reiter protein" of syphilic serology. Since large amounts of *T. pallidum* cells are not presently available, the chemical nature of the flagella of this organism has not been determined.

The Cell Wall

Although the cell-wall composition of *T. pallidum* has not been determined as yet, it is probable that its peptidoglycan will contain the diamino acid ornithine. The basis for this assumption are the reports on the cell-wall composition of the nonpathogenic treponemes (41) *Spirochaeta* (42) and *Borrelia* (43). All these spirochetes have ornithine as a component of their peptidoglycan. Only the obligately aerobic spirochetes, the *Leptospira*, have α, ε-diaminopimelic acid rather than ornithine in their peptidoglycan (41).

References

1. T. B. Turner and D. H. Hollander, Studies on the mechanism of action of cortisone in experimental syphilis. *Am. J. Syp.* 38:371-378 (1954).
2. P. H. Hardy and E. E. Nell. Isolation and purification of *T. pallidum* from syphilitic lesions in the rabbit. *Infect. Immun.* 11:1296-1299 (1975).
3. T. Ratheu and C. J. Pfau. Purification of the pathogenic *Treponema pallidum* by density gradient centrifugation. *Scand. J. Clin. Lab. Invest.* 17:130-134 (1965).
4. M. L. Thomas, J. W. Clark, G. B. Cline, N. G. Anderson, and H. Russell. Separation of *Treponema pallidum* from tissue substances by continuous-flow zonal centrifugation. *Appl. Microbiol.* 23:714-720 (1972).
5. J. B. Baseman, J. C. Nichols, J. W. Rumpp, and N. S. Hayes. Purification of *Treponema pallidum* from infected rabbit tissue: resolution into two treponemal populations. *Infect. Immun.* 10:1062-1067 (1974).
6. J. D. Schmale, D. S. Kellogg, Jr., C. E. Miller, P. Schammel, and J. O. Thayer. Separation of *Treponema pallidum* from tissue debris through continuous particle electrophoresis. *Appl. Microbiol.* 19:287-289 (1970).
7. F. W. Chandler, Jr., and J. W. Clark, Jr.. Passage of *Treponema pallidum* through membrane filters of various pore sizes. *Appl. Microbiol.* 19:326-328 (1970).

2. Composition

8. N. L. Schiller and C. D. Cox. Catabolism of glucose and fatty acids by virulent Treponema pallidum. Infect. Immun. 16:60-68 (1977).
9. J. F. Alderete and J. B. Baseman. Surface-associated host proteins on virulent Treponema pallidum. Infect. Immun. 26:1048-1056 (1979).
10. J. A. Zeigler, A. M. Jones, R. H. Jones, and K. M. Kubica. Demonstration of extracellular material at the surface of pathogenic T. pallidum cells. Br. J. Vener. Dis. 52:1-8 (1976).
11. T. J. Fitzgerald, P. Cleveland, R. C. Johnson, J. N. Miller, and J. A. Sykes. Scanning electron microscopy of Treponema pallidum (Nichols strain) attached to cultured mammalian cells. J. Bacteriol. 130:1333-1344 (1977).
12. A. N. Ibrahim and M. M. Streitfeld. The microassay of hyaluronic acid concentration and hyaluronidase activity by capillary turbidity (CT) and capillary turbidity reduction (CTR) tests. Anal. Biochem. 56:428-434 (1973).
13. T. J. Fritzgerald and R. C. Johnson. Surface mucopolysaccharides of Treponema pallidum. Infect. Immun. 24:244-251 (1979).
14. P. H. Hardy, Jr., and E. E. Nell. Specific agglutination of Treponema pallidum by sera from rabbits and human beings with treponemal infections. J. Exp. Med. 101:367-382 (1955).
15. H. M. Matthews, T. K. Yang, and H. M. Jenkin. Unique lipid composition of Treponema pallidum (Nichols virulent strain). Infect. Immun. 24:713-719 (1979).
16. B. P. Livermore and R. C. Johnson. Lipids of the Spirochaetales: comparison of the lipids of several members of the genera Spirochaeta, Treponema and Leptospira. J. Bacteriol. 120:1268-1273 (1974).
17. B. P. Livermore, R. F. Bey, and R. E. Johnson. Lipid metabolism of Borrelia hermsi. Infect. Immun. 20:215-220 (1978).
18. G. H. Rothblat and P. F. Smith. Nonsaponfiable lipids of representative pleuropneumonia-like organisms. J. Bacteriol. 82:479-491 (1961).
19. L. Vaczi, K. Kiraly, and A. Rethy. Lipid composition of treponemal strains. Acta Microbiol. Acad. Sci. Hung. 13:79-84 (1966).
20. R. M. Smibert. Cultivation, composition and physiology of avirulent treponemes. In The Biology of Parasitic Spirochetes (R. C. Johnson, Ed.), Academic, New York, 1976, pp. 49-56.
21. B. P. Livermore and R. C. Johnson. The lipids of four unusual non-pathogenic host-associated spirochetes. Can. J. Microbiol. 21:1877-1880 (1975).
22. H. Meyer and F. Meyer. Lipid metabolism in the parasitic and free-living spirochetes Treponema pallidum (Reiter) and Treponema zuelzerae. Biochem. Biophys. Acta. 231:93-106 (1971).
23. R. C. Johnson, B. P. Livermore, H. M. Jenkin, and L. Eggebraten. Lipids of Treponema pallidum Kazan 5. Infect. Immun. 2:606-609 (1970).

24. R. Miao and A. H. Fieldsteel. Genetics of *Treponema*: Relationship between *Treponema pallidum* and five cultivable treponemes. *J. Bacteriol. 133*:101-107 (1978).
25. S. L. Allen, R. C. Johnson, and D. Peterson. Metabolism of common substrates by the Reiter strain of *Treponema pallidum*. *Infect. Immun. 3*:727-734 (1971).
26. R. D. Glock and D. L. Harris. Swine dysentery II. Characterization of lesions in pigs inoculated with *Treponema hyodysenteriae* in pure and mixed culture. *Vet. Med. Small Anim. Clin.* 67:65-68 (1972).
27. R. M. Miao, A. H. Fieldsteel, and D. L. Harris. Genetics of *Treponema hyodysenteriae* and its relationship to *Treponema pallidum*. *Infect. Immun. 22*:736-739 (1978).
28. R. C. Johnson, D. M. Ritzi, and B. P. Livermore. Outer envelope of virulent *Treponema pallidum*. *Infect. Immun. 8*:291-295 (1973).
29. R. C. Johnson and L. H. Muschel. Antileptospiral activity of serum. I. Normal and immune serum. *J. Bacteriol. 91*:1403-1409 (1966).
30. P. H. Hardy, Jr., and E. E. Nell. Influence of osmotic pressure on the morphology of the Reiter treponeme. *J. Bacteriol. 82*:967-978 (1961).
31. R. C. Johnson, M. S. Wachter, and D. M. Ritzi. Treponeme outer envelope: Solubilization and reaggregation. *Infect. Immun.* 7:249-258 (1973).
32. M. S. Wachter and R. C. Johnson. Treponeme outer envelope: chemical analysis. *Proc. Soc. Exp. Biol. Med. 151*:97-100 (1976).
33. R. C. Johnson. Comparative spirochete physiology and cellular composition. In *The Biology of Parasitic Spirochetes* (R. C. Johnson, Ed.), Academic, New York, pp. 39-48.
34. S. W. Jackson and P, N. Zey. Ultrastructure of lipopolysaccaride isolated from *Treponema pallidum*. *J. Bacteriol. 114*:838-844 (1973).
35. N. E. Auran, R. C. Johnson, and D. M. Ritzi. Isolation of the outer sheath of parasitic *Leptospira* and its immunogenic properties in hamsters. *Infect. Immun. 5*:968-975 (1972).
36. R. F. Bey, N. E. Auran, and R. C. Johnson. Immunogenicity of whole cell and outer envelope leptospiral vaccines in hamsters. *Infect. Immun. 10*:1051-1056 (1974).
37. D. B. Bromley and N. W. Charon. Axial filament involvement in the motility of *Leptospira interrogans*. *J. Bacteriol. 137*:1406-1412 (1979).
38. B. J. Paster and E. Canale-Parola. Involvement of periplasmic fibrils in motility of spirochetes. *J. Bacteriol. 141*:359-364 (1980).
39. M. A. Bharier and S. C. Rittenberg. Chemistry of axial filaments of *Treponema zuelzerae*. *J. Bacteriol. 105*:422-429 (1971).

40. P. H. Hardy, Jr., W. R. Fredericks, and E. E. Nell. Isolation and antigenic characteristics of axial filaments from the Reiter treponeme. *Infect. Immun.* *11*:380-386 (1975).
41. I. Azuma, T. Taniyama, Y. Yamamura, Y. Yanagihara, S. Hattori, S. Yasuda, and I. Mifuchi. Chemical studies on the cell walls of *Leptospira biflexa* strain Urawa and *Treponema pallidum* strain Reiter. *Jap. J. Microbiol.* *19*:45-51 (1975).
42. R. Joseph, S. C. Holt, and E. Canale-Parola. Peptidoglycan of free-living anaerobic spirochetes. *J. Bacteriol.* *115*:426-435 (1973).
43. E. Klaviter and R. C. Johnson. Isolation of the outer envelope, chemical components and ultrastructure of *Borrelia hermsi* grown in vitro. *Acta Trop.* *36*:123-131 (1979).

3
Genetics of *Treponema*

A. HOWARD FIELDSTEEL[†]
SRI International
Menlo Park, California

Deoxyribonucleic Acid Base Composition of Treponemes 40
Genetic Relationship between *Treponema pallidum* and the
 Cultivable Treponemes 42
Relationship between *Treponema pallidum* and *Treponema
 hyodysenteriae* 47
Genetic Relationship between *Treponema pallidum* and
 Treponema pertenue 49
References 52

It is generally recognized that three species of treponemes are pathogenic for humans. These species cause four clinically distinct diseases (1-4). The first of these organisms to be described was *Treponema pallidum*, the etiologic agent of venereal syphilis (5-7). The unnamed species of treponeme that causes nonvenereal endemic syphilis, or bejel, is considered to be a subspecies or variant of *T. pallidum* (8). *Treponema pertenue*, the causative agent of yaws, was discovered by Castellani (9) in 1905, the same year that *T. pallidum* was discovered. *Treponema carateum*, the etiologic agent of pinta, was not described until 1938 (10). The origin and relationship of these treponemes are obscure but have been a matter of speculation for many years. Hudson (2) believed that one organism (*T. pallidum*) was the causative agent of all four diseases and that clinical distinctions were due to both environmental and host influences. Hackett (1) also believed that the

---
[†]The field of treponemal research lost one of its great leaders with the death of Dr. A. Howard Fieldsteel on May 21, 1982.

four human treponematoses were closely related, but he theorized that they originated from an animal that harbored an infectious agent from which mutants arose, the first being *T. carateum*, followed by the organisms causing yaws, endemic syphilis, and finally venereal syphilis. He also considered that the changes were a result of environmental pressures. Willcox (3) proposed a third theory which combined the other two concepts. He postulated that the *Treponemata* originally arose from free-living treponemes in water and were acquired by man as commensal saprophytes, and that environmental circumstances led to the selection of mutants best suited for transmission under the prevailing circumstances.

To more closely define the pathogenic treponemes, attempts were initiated to cultivate them in vivo and in vitro. A number of well-documented virulent strains of *T. pallidum* and *T. pertenue* have been isolated and studied in a variety of animal hosts, most often in rabbits (11,12). However, it was apparent that to carry out definitive studies involving parameters other than pathogenesis, the treponemes that were pathogenic for man would have to be cultivated in vitro; and as a natural sequel to the discovery of the causative agents of syphilis and yaws, attempts were made to cultivate these bacteria on artificial media. Almost immediately, claims were made for the cultivation of *T. pallidum* (13-15), but none of the cultivable organisms were virulent. Noguchi (16) claimed to have cultivated *T. pallidum* that was pathogenic for rabbits, but the isolate supposedly lost its virulence during in vitro cultivation. Many other claims have been made for in vitro cultivation, as Willcox and Guthe indicated in their thorough review (12). However, none of the strains isolated in vitro were pathogenic for any animal hosts, nor have any of them ever been shown to have a causal relationship to treponemal disease in humans. Furthermore, in serologic studies of the Nichols, Noguchi, Reiter, Kazan, and Kroo strains, Eagle and Germuth (17) found that these fell into three distinct serological groups, but they were all morphologically and antigenically different from *T. pallidum*.

Deoxyribonucleic Acid Base Composition of Treponemes

Until recently, the inability to cultivate the pathogenic treponemes infecting humans has precluded the use of biochemical and genetic analyses for determining genetic relationships. However, it has been known for many years that determination of the composition of deoxyribonucleic acid (DNA), expressed as the mole percentage of guanine plus cytosine (G+C), can reveal important predictive information about taxonomic and genetic relationships among microorganisms (18-22). Although the G+C content of DNA may differ considerably at the genus or family level, ranging between 24 and 75 mol %, it usually varies by no more than 6% within one bacterial species. A difference of 10% or more between the G+C contents of two species in the same genus indi-

3. Genetics of Treponema

cates that they probably have different genetic compositions and will show little, if any, sequence homology.

Several investigators have determined the DNA base composition of cultivable treponemes that at one time or another were purported to be *T. pallidum*. For example, Marmur et al. first reported the G+C content of *T. pallidum* to be 34-36 mol % (23). Although no reference to the strain of the organism was made, undoubtedly they were referring to one of the cultivable treponemes, and not *T. pallidum*. Rathlev and Pfau reported the G+C content of *Treponema phagedenis* biotype Reiter to be 38 mol % (24). Canale-Parola et al. (25) obtained identical results with the Reiter treponeme (37.8 mol %) and further demonstrated that *Treponema refringens* biotype Nichols had a G+C content of 41.3 mol %. Smibert (26,27) has reported G+C values for *T. phagedenis* as being 38-40 mol %, *T. refringens* biotype Noguchi as 39-43 mol %, and *T. refringens* biotype Nichols as 37-40 mol %.

In 1978, Miao and Fieldsteel (28) carried out the first study to determine whether the pathogenic Nichols strain of *T. pallidum* is genetically related to cultivable treponemes. The results of their study comparing the G+C contents of these treponemes are presented in Table 1. For comparative purposes, the results of other investigators' studies on the cultivable treponemes are also tabulated. The cultivable treponemes appear to fall into two groups: *T. phagedenis* and its bio-

Table 1 Guanine Plus Cytosine (G+C) Content of DNA Obtained from Various Treponemes

Source of DNA	G+C content of DNA (mol %)	
	Refs. 23-27	Ref. 28
T. pallidum (Nichols), virulent	–	52.4–53.7
T. phagedenis	38–40	39.0
T. phagedenis biotype Reiter	37.8–38.0	39.0
T. phagedenis biotype Kazan 5	–	38.0
T. refringens biotype Noguchi	39–43	41.5
T. refringens biotype Nichols	37–41.3	–
Rabbit testis, normal	–	42.2
E. coli (standard)		50.0[a]

[a]The T_m (that temperature corresponding to the midpoint of the thermal denaturation curve of the DNA) of each DNA species was measured against that of *Escherichia coli*. The G+C content was then calculated from the relationship 0.41°C/1% G+C, with the DNA of *E. coli* being defined as 50.0% G+C.

types in one group and *T. refringens* and its biotypes in another. The most striking point is that the noncultivable virulent Nichols strain of *T. pallidum* contained 52.4-53.7 mol % G+C and thus appeared to be unrelated to the cultivable nonpathogenic treponemes. Furthermore, it should be noted that the base composition of DNA extracted from a normal rabbit testis was 42.2 mol %. All of the DNA species gave smooth thermal denaturation curves, with no evidence for the presence of satellite DNAs.

Miao et al. (29) also sought to determine whether a genetic relationship existed between *T. pallidum* and strains of *Treponema hyodysenteriae*, the causative agent of swine dysentery. Because *T. hyodysenteriae* was the only pathogenic treponeme that had been cultivated in vitro, it was of interest to determine whether pathogenic and nonpathogenic strains of *T. hyodysenteriae* appeared related to either the cultivable nonpathogenic human-derived treponemes or the noncultivable pathogenic *T. pallidum* (Nichols). Because initial assays indicated that strains of *T. hyodysenteriae* had unusually low G+C contents, measurements had to be made with *Clostridium perfringens* DNA (26.5 mol % G+C) as a standard (21), rather than *Escherichia coli* as previously used (Table 1). All of the *T. hyodysenteriae* strains tested contained 25.7-25.9 mol % G+C, and all of the DNA species gave similar denaturation curves, with no indication of the presence of satellite DNAs. It seems likely that these possible genetic code-limit organisms (30) are unrelated to either the cultivable nonpathogenic or noncultivable pathogenic human-derived treponemes. It is interesting to note that in an investigation of *Treponema succinifaciens*, an anaerobic spirochete occurring in the intestines of healthy pigs (31), Cwyk and Canale-Parola (32) found that the G+C content was 36 mol %. This is significantly different from the G+C content of the DNA from *T. hyodysenteriae*, but it not unlike that of other cultivable *Treponema* species.

Genetic Relationship between *Treponema pallidum* and the Cultivable Treponemes

Although G+C values (in mol %) are most important for the classification and identification of bacteria, similarity of DNA base composition does not necessarily imply identity of genetic composition. Even within given taxonomic groups of bacteria, DNA analysis can yield important information. This is especially true for organisms that are phenotypically similar. To supplement studies on G+C base composition, hybridization of single-strand DNA from different sources often provides specific physicochemical means for determining genetic relatedness among bacterial and other species (23,33,34). Nucleic acid hybridization techniques have been used extensively to determine relatedness among many bacterial and viral species; however, they have only been used to a limited extent with respect to *Treponema*. Smibert has stated that based on DNA homology, *T. phagedenis* var.

3. Genetics of Treponema

reiteri is identical to the Reiter treponeme (35). He has also stated that the Reiter strains of *T. phagedenis* show a very high homology with DNA from the English Reiter and Kazan strains and a very low homology with DNA from strains of *T. refringens* and *Treponema denticola* (27).

As noted earlier, Miao and Fieldsteel (28) showed that, on the basis of the G+C content of the DNA they were able to determine that *T. pallidum* (Nichols), *T. refringens*, and *T. phagedenis* fell into three general categories. These investigators then carried out definitive studies to determine the extent of DNA sequence homology among *Treponema*, as determined by DNA-DNA saturation reassociation assays. Initially, the reassociation kinetics of DNA from pathogenic *T. pallidum* and three cultivable nonpathogenic treponemes were determined by measuring the reassociation of trace amounts of ^{125}I-labeled DNA with known concentrations of unlabeled, totally homologous DNA. The reactions were analyzed by chromatography on hydroxyapatite columns. The reassociation kinetics of *T. pallidum*, *T. phagedenis* biotype Reiter, and *T. refringens* biotype Noguchi are shown in Fig. 1. The data are expressed in C_0t values (34), i.e., the concentration of DNA in moles of nucleotides per liter multiplied by the time in seconds required for reassociation. The C_0t values are those for the unlabeled

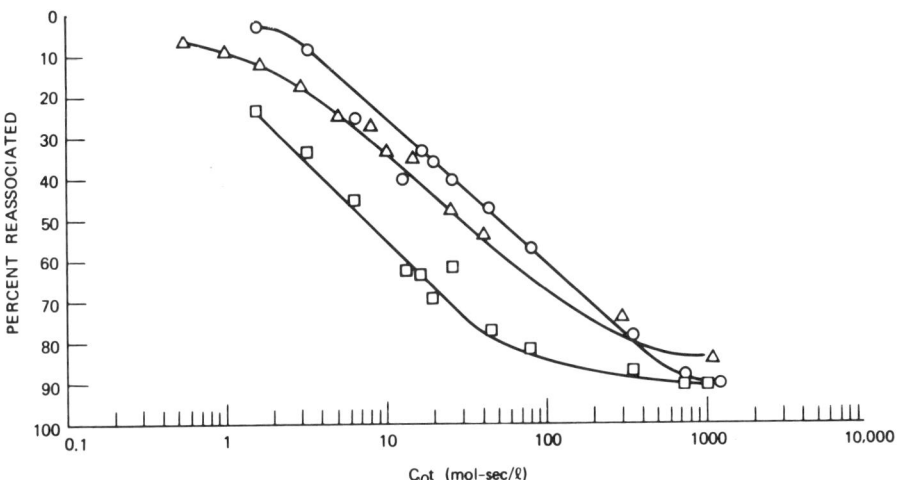

Figure 1 Reassociation kinetics of treponemal DNAs. Trace amounts of ^{125}I-labeled DNA were reassociated in the presence of an excess amount of unlabeled, totally homologous DNA at 60°C. At intervals, samples were analyzed on hydroxyapatite columns. C_0t values are for the unlabeled DNA. Values for $C_0t_{\frac{1}{2}}$ were *T. pallidum* (△), 29 mol-sec/liter; *T. phagedenis* biotype Reiter (o), 50 mol-sec/liter; and *T. refringens* biotype Noguchi (□), 7.5 mol-sec/liter. (From Ref. 28.)

homologous DNA. The maximum C_0t value for [^{125}I] DNA alone was 0.02 mol-sec/liter when the C_0t value for unlabeled DNA was 1000 mol-sec/liter. The reassociation of [^{125}I] DNA was therefore completely dependent on the reassociation of the unlabeled homologous DNA species. The maximum level of reassociation was 85-90% and the baseline level was 2-5% for *T. pallidum* and *T. phagedenis* biotype Reiter. The data in Fig. 1 show that the $C_0t_{\frac{1}{2}}$ (50% reassociation) values were different for each of the DNA species tested. The smallest value, 7.5 mol-sec/liter, was for *T. refringens* biotype Noguchi. The $C_0t_{\frac{1}{2}}$ values for *T. pallidum* and *T. phagedenis* biotype Reiter DNAs were 29 and 50 mol-sec/liter, respectively.

The kinetics of reassociation for DNA from *T. phagedenis* biotype Reiter and *T. phagedenis*, as analyzed by nuclease S1 digestion, are shown in Fig. 2. In these experiments, trace amounts of [^{125}I] DNA were again added to a large excess of unlabeled homologous DNA. The kinetics of reassociation for *T. phagedenis* biotype Reiter DNA were virtually identical, whether the products were analyzed by chromatography on hydroxyapatite columns ($C_0t_{\frac{1}{2}}$, 50 mol-sec/liter; Fig. 1) or by resistance to nuclease S1 digestion ($C_0t_{\frac{1}{2}}$, 52 mol-sec/liter; Fig. 2). The $C_0t_{\frac{1}{2}}$ value for *T. phagedenis* DNA (28 mol-sec/liter; Fig. 1) was about the same as that for *T. pallidum* DNA (29 mol-sec/liter; Fig. 1). Both reactions, whether analyzed by hydroxyapatite or nuclease S1, followed second-order kinetics. The maximum levels of reassociation ranged from 85 to 90% of the total DNA and occurred at C_0t values of 300 (*T. refringens* biotype Noguchi), 600 (*T. pallidum* and *T. phagedenis*), and 1000 mol-sec/liter *T. phagedenis* biotype Reiter).

The virtually complete reassociation of each [^{125}I] DNA with unlabeled homologous DNA in the reassociation kinetics assays showed that the [^{125}I] DNAs were accurate probes. Furthermore, the shape of the reassociation kinetics curve of the *T. pallidum* DNA indicated that there was little or no contamination with other DNA, such as that from rabbit testis. This was further confirmed when no spectrophotometrically detectable amounts of any contaminating DNA were observed in the thermal denaturation assays.

Saturation reassociation assays were then utilized to determine the maximum extent of DNA sequence homology between the five cultivable nonpathogenic treponemes and pathogenic *T. pallidum* (Nichols). In this assay, a constant amount of ^{125}I-labeled probe DNA was reassociated for a fixed length of time to minimize self-association. Simultaneous reactions, run in the presence of increasing amounts of test DNA, were used as a direct measure of the extent of sequence homology between the two DNA species. After 72 hrs of incubation in the standard reaction mixture, there was 2% or less self-reassociation; this value matches the base-line levels determined in the reassociation kinetic studies.

3. Genetics of Treponema

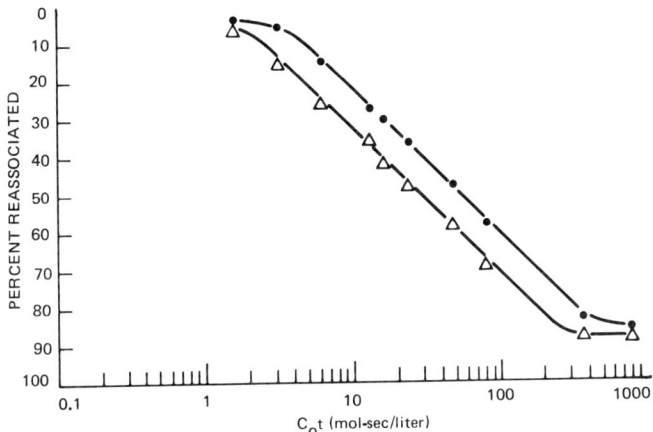

Figure 2 Reassociation kinetics of DNA from *T. phagedenis* biotype Reiter and *T. phagedenis*. Trace amounts of ^{125}I-labeled DNA were added to an excess amount of unlabeled homologous DNA at 60°C. At intervals, samples were analyzed by nuclease S1 digestion. Values for $C_0 t_{\frac{1}{2}}$ were *T. phagedenis* biotype Reiter (●), 52 mol-sec/liter; and *T. phagedenis* (△), 28 mol-sec/liter. (From Ref. 28.)

Saturation reassociation assays were performed with *T. pallidum* [^{125}I] DNA and unlabeled DNA from *T. pallidum*, *T. phagedenis* biotype Reiter, *T. phagedenis* biotype Kazan 5, *T. phagedenis*, *T. refringens* biotype Noguchi, and *T. refringens* biotype Nichols; salmon sperm DNA was used as a control. The reassociation maximum was 85%, which occurred when labeled *T. pallidum* DNA was reacted with the unlabeled *T. pallidum* DNA. The lowest reassociation was 2%, with salmon sperm DNA. The reassociation with the DNA from the five cultivable treponemes was about 5%, which indicated that the cultivable treponemes shared virtually no sequence homology with *T. pallidum* and were therefore genetically unrelated to this species. These results are summarized in Table 2. Miao and Fieldsteel (28) then utilized ^{125}I-labeled DNA from the five cultivable treponemes as probes in saturation reassociation assays against the corresponding unlabeled DNA from these organisms. Analysis was carried out by nuclease S1 digestion. The reassociation of *T. phagedenis* biotype Reiter [^{125}I] DNA in the presence of salmon sperm DNA was 2%, whereas it approached 100% in the presence of homologous Reiter DNA. Next, *T. phagedenis* biotype Kazan 5 DNA was reassociated with *T. phagedenis* biotype Reiter [^{125}I] DNA and about 100% reassociation was detected, indicating that *T. phagedenis* biotype Kazan 5 possessed all of the DNA

Table 2 Maximum Levels of Reassociation of ^{125}I-Labeled DNA from T. pallidum and Various Cultivable Treponemes with Unlabeled DNA

[^{125}I] DNA	Percentage of reassociation with unlabled DNA[a]						
	SS[b]	Tp(N)	Re	K5	Pd	Ng	Ni
Tp(N)	2	100	5	5	5	5	5
Re	2	ND[c]	100	100	54	5	5
K5	2	ND	93	100	57	2	2
Pd	1	ND	100	93	100	1	1
Ng	1	ND	1	1	1	100	90

[a]Saturation reassociation assays were performed with each ^{125}I-labeled DNA and the indicated unlabeled DNA. The maximum level of reassociation in each assay is shown. The level of reassociation with the homologous test DNA, which ranged from 85 to 97%, was taken as 100%. In all instances, reassociation reached a plateau level.
[b]SS, Salmon sperm; Tp(N), T. pallidum (Nichols); Re, T. phagedenis biotype Reiter; K5, T. phagedenis biotype Kazan 5; Pd, T. phagedenis; Ng, T. refringens biotype Noguchi; Ni, T. refringens biotype Nichols.
[c]ND = Not done.
Source: Adapted from Ref. 28.

sequences present in the former and that the two organisms were essentially identical. The reassociation level of T. phagedenis biotype Reiter [^{125}I] DNA was 54% with T. phagedenis DNA, but was 5% with T. refringens biotype Noguchi or Nichols DNA. These results were confirmed by measuring the saturation of T. phagedenis biotype Kazan 5 [^{125}I] DNA with the unlabeled DNA of the other cultivable treponemes. The data indicate 93% homology between Kazan 5 and Reiter DNA, but no homology between Kazan 5 and either Noguchi or Nichols. It is interesting that T. phagedenis DNA possessed only 57% of the sequences in Kazan 5 DNA. The degree of DNA sequence homology among the T. phagedenis biotypes was extended by using T. phagedenis [^{125}I] DNA as the probe. The data indicated that the Reiter biotype contained all the sequences of T. phagedenis and that the Kazan 5 biotype contained at least 93% of the sequences of T. phagedenis. There was no homology between Noguchi [^{125}I] DNA and Reiter, Kazan 5, or T. phagedenis DNA, but Nichols DNA had at least 90% of the sequences present in Noguchi DNA.

The molecular weights of the DNAs of these two treponemes were calculated from the C_0t curves and by saturation reassociation assays, and they were in agreement. The estimated double-strand molecular weight of the DNAs of *T. pallidum* and *T. phagedenis* genomes was 9.05×10^9; the corresponding value for the DNAs of *E. coli* and *T. refringens* biotype Noguchi was approximately 2.5×10^9. The molecular weight of *T. phagedenis* was 56% that of *T. phagedenis* biotype Reiter (1.62×10^{10}). The difference in the molecular weights of the genomes of *T. phagedenis* and its biotype Reiter is extraordinary. Although *T. phagedenis* contained only 54-56% of the sequences present in biotypes Reiter and Kazan 5, both biotypes contained all the sequences present in *T. phagedenis*. None of the treponemal genomes contained repeated sequences. This may be evidence that deletion of the DNA has occurred in *T. phagedenis,* or that the Kazan 5 and Reiter biotypes have gained some unique DNA sequences via unknown recombinational events.

The complete lack of homology between *T. pallidum* and the five nonpathogenic cultivable treponemes appears to support the hypothesis that the latter were probably contaminants in the clinical specimens from which they were originally isolated and bear no relationship to the pathogenesis of syphilis. This lack of homology appears to conflict with the fact that there are known antigenic relationships among the treponemes. However, it should be pointed out that the limit of resolution with the *T. pallidum* [^{125}I] DNA preparation is only 5% of the entire genome, or 4.5×10^8 daltons, which is enough DNA to code for approximately 450 proteins. Therefore, the sequences coding for the shared antigens may not be detected by this procedure. With the *T. phagedenis* biotype Reiter DNA the limit of detection was about 0.5%, or 8×10^7 daltons of DNA, which could code for 80 proteins. Although immunological assays detect a small degree of relatedness among antigens, DNA-DNA hybridization has the advantage of being quantitative, easily interpreted, and giving the total extent of homology.

Relationship between *Treponema pallidum* and *Treponema hyodysenteriae*

As discussed above, strains of *T. hyodysenteriae* have base compositions of 25.7-25.9 mol % G+C, compared to a range of 37-53.7 mol % for the treponemes isolated from humans (29). It seems unlikely, therefore, that a relationship exists between *T. hyodysenteriae* and *T. pallidum* or the cultivable treponemes isolated from humans. However, because *T. hyodysenteriae* is the only known cultivable pathogenic treponeme (36-38), Miao et al. performed a series of experiments to determine whether *T. hyodysenteriae* was a possible genetic link because the noncultivable pathogenic treponemes and the cultivable nonpathogenic treponemes (29). Using DNA-DNA saturation reassociation assays, they studied the relationship between *T. pallidum*

(Nichols) and pathogenic and nonpathogenic isolates of *T. hyodysenteriae*, as well as between *T. hyodsyenteriae*, *T. phagedenis*, and *T. refringens* (Table 3). When *T. pallidum* [^{125}I] DNA was used as a probe with unlabeled DNA from two pathogenic strains (B 204 and A-1) and two nonpathogenic strains (B 256 and 4/71) of *T. hyodysenteriae*, there was no reassociation (<5%) of *T. pallidum* DNA with the DNA from any of the *T. hyodysenteriae* strains, whereas >95% reassociation occurred with unlabeled homologous DNA. When ^{125}I-probes were prepared from the DNA of *T. hyodysenteriae* strain B 204, A-1, or B 256, less than 5% reassociation occurred in the presence of DNA from *T. pallidum*, *T. phagedenis* biotype Reiter, or *T. refringens* biotype Noguchi. Moreover, unlabeled homologous *T. hyodysenteriae* DNA yielded greater than 95% reassociation of [^{125}I] DNA.

The extent of DNA sequence homology among the swine treponemes was also determined. The maximum extent of reassociation of B 204 [^{125}I] DNA in the presence of DNA from B 204, A-1, B 256, 4/71, or salmon sperm are also summarized in Table 3. The level of reassociation in the presence of homologous DNA was >95%, whereas reassociation with salmon sperm DNA was <2%. Reassociation in the presence of A-1 DNA was 80%, indicating that the two pathogenic isolates of *T. hyodysenteriae*, B 204 and A-1, were closely related but not identical. The level of reassociation in the presence of DNA from the nonpathogenic isolates of *T. hyodysenteriae*, B 256 and 4/71, was only

Table 3 Maximum Levels of Reassociation of ^{125}I-Labeled DNA from *T. pallidum* and *T. hyodysenteriae* with Homologous and Heterologous Unlabeled DNA

[^{125}I] DNA	Percentage of reassociation with unlabeled DNA[a]							
	SS[b]	Tp(N)	B 204	A-1	B 256	4/71	Re	Ng
Tp(N)	<2	>95	<5	<5	<5	<5	5	5
B 204	<2	<5	>95	80	28	28	<5	<5
A-1	<2	<5	80	>95	28	28	<5	<5
B 256	<2	<5	28	28	100	90	<5	<5

[a]Saturation reassociation assays were performed with each ^{125}I-labeled DNA and the indicated unlabeled DNA. The maximum level of reassociation in each assay is shown.
[b]SS, Salmon sperm; Tp(N), *T. pallidum* (Nichols); B 204 and A-1, pathogenic strains of *T. hyodysenteriae*; B 256 and 4/71, nonpathogenic strains of *T. hyodysenteriae*; Re, *T. phagedenis* biotype Reiter; Ng, *T. refringens* biotype Noguchi.
Source: Adapted from Ref. 29.

3. Genetics of Treponema

28%. The same results were obtained by measuring the extent of reassociation of A-1 [^{125}I] DNA in the presence of the various DNA species. The homology between the two nonpathogenic isolates of *T. hyodysenteriae*, measured using B 256 [^{125}I] DNA as the probe, was 90% between B 256 and 4/71 and 28% between B 256 and either B 204 or A-1.

From the saturation reassociation data, it is apparent that the four strains of swine treponemes are genetically distinct from the human treponemes, pathogenic *T. pallidum* (Nichols) and nonpathogenic *T. phagedenis* biotype Reiter and *T. refringens* biotype Noguchi. The two pathogenic isolates *T. hyodysenteriae* B 204 and A-1 appeared to be related at the species level (>75% homology) but were not identical. The nonpathogenic strains B 256 and 4/71 appeared to be nearly identical. Moreover, the pathogenic and nonpathogenic isolates were clearly within the same genus (28% homology) but appeared to be distinct species. Although the genome complexities of the swine isolates were not determined, the reassociation assays indicated that all these strains have about the same size genome. Based on these results and biochemical characteristics, Kinyon and Harris (39) have proposed the term *T. hyodysenteriae* for the pathogenic swine isolates (204, A-1, etc.) and *T. innocens* for the nonpathogenic swine isolates (B 256, 4/71, etc.).

The very large differences in DNA base composition between *T. pallidum* and the swine treponemes, together with the results of the reassociation assays, indicate that the swine organisms could be assigned to a different genus. At present, it is uncertain as to which established genus, if any, these organisms belong.

Genetic Relationship between *Treponema pallidum* and *Treponema pertenue*

Because of the inability to cultivate the pathogenic treponemes that infect humans, classification of these treponemes has been based largely on morphological and clinical descriptions. However, DNA-DNA saturation reassociation assays have also been applied by Miao and Fieldsteel (40) to measure the degree of DNA sequence homology among different strains of *T. pallidum* (Nichols and KKJ) and a strain of *T. pertenue* (Gauthier) which was isolated in hamsters in 1960 from a Nigerian child with yaws (41). *Treponema pertenue* [^{125}I] DNA was reassociated with an excess amount of unlabeled homologous *T. pertenue* DNA, and the kinetics of reassociation were determined (Fig. 3). The reaction followed second-order kinetics and had a $C_0t_{\frac{1}{2}}$ value of 26 mol-sec/liter, which was almost identical to that for *T. pallidum* (Nichols) (29 mol-sec/liter) under the same conditions. No repetitive sequences were present in either treponemal genome, and the molecular weight

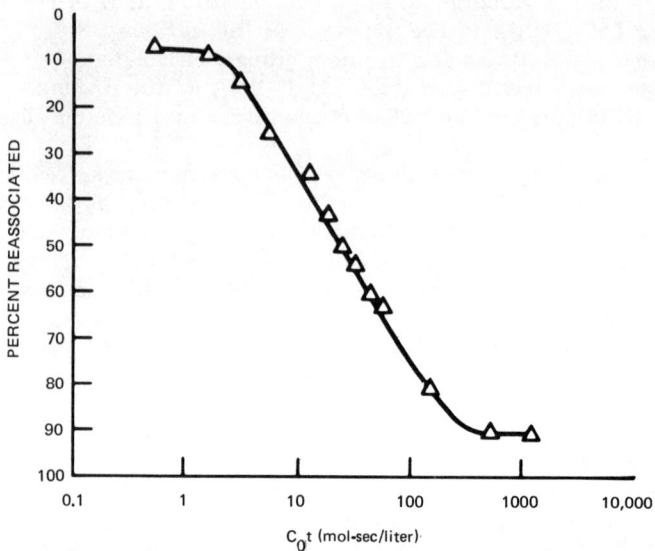

Figure 3 Kinetics of reassociation of [^{125}I]-labeled *T. pertenue* (Gauthier) DNA. Trace amounts of ^{125}I-labeled DNA were reassociated in the presence of excess unlabeled, homologous DNA at 60°C. At intervals, samples were diluted into 2 ml of S1 buffer and 1000 units of endonuclease S1 per milliliter. The mixture was incubated at 37°C for 2 hrs. Acid-precipitable [^{125}I] DNA was collected on Millipore filters, and the percentage of reassociation was calculated as the ratio of S1-resistant radioactivity to the total radioactivity in each sample. Total radioactivity was the acid-precipitable radioactivity in a duplicate sample without endonuclease S1 in the digestion mixture. C_0t values are for the unlabeled DNA. (From Ref. 40.)

of DNA from *T. pertenue* (Gauthier) and *T. pallidum* (Nichols) were calculated to be 9×10^9; this compares with *E. coli*, which has a DNA molecular weight of 2.5×10^9 (23).

Saturation reassociation assays using *T. pallidum* (Nichols), *T. pallidum* (KKJ), and *T. pertenue* (Gauthier) [^{125}I] DNAs were performed in the presence of unlabeled DNA from these organisms as well as DNA from *T. phagedenis* biotype Reiter, *T. refringens* biotype Noguchi, and salmon sperm. The results are summarized in Table 4. It seems likely that the two strains of *T. pallidum* and *T. pertenue* are idnetical within the limits of resolution of this technique and might be regarded as a single species. However, it should be noted that the strains differ from each other biologically (11,41) in that *T. pertenue* (Gauthier) produced treponeme-containing indurated lesions after

3. Genetics of Treponema

intracutaneous inoculation into the shaved groin of Syrian hamsters, whereas the strains of *T. pallidum* produced no such signs of infection after similar inoculation into hamsters (40). Like *T. pallidum*, *T. pertenue* had no DNA sequence homology with salmon sperm, *T. phagedenis* biotype Reiter, or *T. refringens* biotype Noguchi. These data should not necessarily be interpreted as an indication that similar biochemical functions are expressed in the three pathogenic treponemes, but only that they have the same biochemical potentials, as demonstrated by the close homology of their DNAs.

These results suggest that very little genetic drift has occurred among the pathogenic treponemes of human origin. Whether lack of genetic drift is related to the pathogenicity of the human treponemes is unknown; however, this degree of stability is remarkable. Continuous passage of *T. pallidum* in rabbits did not appear to give rise to detectable changes in DNA sequence, since *T. pallidum* (Nichols) has been passaged continuously in rabbit testes for more than 65 years, whereas *T. pallidum* (KKJ) is a relatively recent isolate, having undergone only eight passages in rabbit testes. Even more remarkable is the fact that *T. pallidum* (Nichols) has retained its ability to produce clinical syphilis in humans after 62 years of passage in rabbits (42).

Another indication of the unusual stability of *T. pallidum* is the fact that no evidence has yet been presented that it is any less susceptible to penicillin today than when penicillin therapy was first utilized in

Table 4 Maximum Levels of Reassociation of ^{125}I-Labeled DNAs from Pathogenic and Human-Derived Treponemes and Unlabeled DNA

[^{125}I] DNA	Percentage of reassociation with unlabeled DNA[a]					
	SS[b]	Tp(N)	Tp(K)	Tpt	Re	Ng
Tp(N)	2	100	100	100	5	5
Tp(K)	2	100	100	100	2	2
Tpt	2	100	ND[c]	100	2	2

[a]Saturation reassociation assays were performed with each ^{125}I-labeled DNA and the indicated DNA. The maximum level of reassociation with the homologous DNA, which ranged from 91 to 99%, was taken as 100%. In all cases reassociation reached a plateau level.
[b]SS, Salmon sperm; Tp(N) and Tp(K), *T. pallidum* (Nichols) and *T. pallidum* (KKJ); Tpt, *T. pertenue*; Re, *T. phagedenis* biotype Reiter; Ng, *T. refringens* biotype Noguchi.
[c]ND = Not done.
Source: Adapted from Ref. 40.

syphilis therapy in 1942 (43). On the other hand, the nonpathogenic cultivable treponemes of human origin and the pathogenic cultivable treponemes of swine exhibited about 10% genetic drift. Although it was not possible to obtain unequivocal evidence, the homology studies of Miao and Fieldsteel (40) on *T. pallidum* and *T. pertenue* seem to support Hudson's view (2) that syphilis and yaws are probably caused by the same organisms.

The procedures utilizing the introduction of ^{125}I into purified DNA should be applicable to the analysis of the genetic relationships between any organisms from which microgram quantities of DNA can be obtained. They should be especially useful in the identification of treponemes grown in vitro and putatively identified as *T. pallidum*.

Acknowledgments

The work carried out in the author's laboratory was supported by Public Health Service contract N01 AI 42536 and grant R01 AI 115113 from the National Institute of Allergy and Infectious Diseases.

References

1. C. J. Hackett. On the origin of the human treponematoses. *Bull. WHO* 29:7-41 (1963).
2. E. R. Hudson. Treponematoses and African slavery. *Br. J. Vener. Dis.* 40:43-52 (1963).
3. R. R. Willcox. The treponemal evolution. *St. John's Hosp. Dermatol. Soc. Trans.* 58:21-27 (1972).
4. R. R. Willcox. Changing patterns of treponemal disease. *Br. J. Vener. Dis.* 50:169-178 (1974).
5. F. Schaudinn and E. Hoffmann. Vorläufiger Bericht über des Vorkommen von Spirochäten in Syphilitischen Krankheitsprodukten und bei Papillomen. *Arb. Gesund Amte (Berl.)* 22:527-534 (1904-1905).
6. F. Schaudinn and E. Hoffmann. Über Spirochätenbefunde im Lymphdrusensaft syphilitischer. *Dtsch. Med. Wochenschr.* 31:711-714 (1905).
7. F. Schaudinn and E. Hoffmann. Über Spirochaeta pallida bei Syphilis und die Unterschiede dieser Form gegenüber anderen Arten Dieser Gattung. *Berl. Klin. Wochenschr.* 42:673-675 (1905).
8. World Health Organization. Treponematoses research. Report of a WHO Scientific Group. *WHO Tech. Rep. Ser.* 455:1-91 (1970).
9. A. Castellani. On the presence of spirochaetes in two cases of ulcerated parangi (yaws). *Br. Med. J.* 2:1280 (1905).
10. B. J. G. Saenz, J. G. Triana, and J. A. Armenteros. Demonstración de un treponema en el borde activo de un caso de

pinta de las manos y pies y en la linfa de ganglios superficiales (reporte preliminar). *Arch. Med. Interna* 4:112-117 (1938).
11. T. B. Turner and D. H. Hollander. Biology of the treponematoses. *WHO Monogr. Ser.* 35:1-278 (1957).
12. R. R. Willcox and T. Guthe. *Treponema Pallidum*. A bibliographical review of the morphology, culture and survival of *T. pallidum* and associated organisms. *Bull. WHO Suppl.* 35:1-169 (1966).
13. G. Volpino and A. Fontana. Einige Veruntersuchungen über künstliche Kultivierung der *Spirochaeta pallida* (Schaudinn). *Zentralbl. Bakteriol. I. Abteil. Orig.* 42:666-669 (1906).
14. J. Schereschewsky. Züchtung er *Spirochaeta pallida* (Schaudinn). *Dtsch. Med. Wochenschr.* 35:835 (1909).
15. J. Schereschewsky. Weitere Mittleilung über die Züchtung der *Spirochaeta pallida*. *Dtsch. Med. Wochenschr.* 35:1260-1261 (1909).
16. H. Noguchi. A method for the pure cultivation of pathogenic *Treponema pallidum (Spirochaeta pallida)*. *J. Exp. Med.* 14:99-108 (1911).
17. H. Eagle and F. G. Germuth. Serological relationships between five cultured strains of supposed *T. pallidum* (Noguchi, Kroó, Nichols, Reiter, and Kazan) and two strains of mouth treponemata. *J. Immunol.* 60:223-239 (1948).
18. K. Y. Lee, R. Wahl, and E. Barbu. Contenu en bases puriques et pyramidiques des acides désoxyribonucléiques des bactéries. *Ann. Inst. Pasteur Paris* 91:212-224 (1956).
19. J. Marmur and P. Doty. Heterogeneity in deoxyribonucleic acids. I. Dependence on composition of the configurational stability of deoxyribonucleic acids. *Nature* 183:1427-1429 (1959).
20. N. Sueoka. Variation and heterogeneity of base composition of deoxyribonucleic acids: A compilation of old and new data. *J. Mol. Biol.* 3:31-40 (1961).
21. J. Marmur and P. Doty. Determination of the base composition of deoxyribonucleic acid from its thermal denaturation temperature. *J. Mol. Biol.* 5:109-118 (1962).
22. L. R. Hill. An index to deoxyribonucleic acid base composition of bacterial species. *J. Gen. Microbiol.* 44:419-437 (1966).
23. J. Marmur, S. Falkow, and M. Mandel. New approaches to bacterial taxonomy. *Ann. Rev. Microbiol.* 17:329-372 (1963).
24. T. Rathlev and C. J. Pfau. The nucleic acids from Reiter's treponemes. *Arch. Biochem. Biophys.* 106:343-347 (1964).
25. E. Canale-Parola, Z. Udris, and M. Mandel. The classification of free-living spirochetes. *Arch. Microbiol.* 63:385-397 (1968).
26. R. M. Smibert. *Spirochaetales*, a review. In *Critical Reviews of Microbiology* (A. I. Laskin and H. Lechevalier, Eds.), Vol. 3, CRC Press, Cleveland, Ohio, 1975, pp. 491-552.

27. R. M. Smibert. In *Bergey's Manual of Determinative Bacteriology* (R. E. Buchanan and N. E. Biggons, Eds.), 8th ed., The Williams & Wilkins Co., Baltimore, 1974, pp. 167-195.
28. R. Miao and A. H. Fieldsteel. Genetics of *Treponema*: Relationship between *Treponema pallidum* and five cultivable treponemes. *J. Bacteriol. 133*:101-107 (1978).
29. R. M. Miao, A. H. Fieldsteel, and D. L. Harris. Genetics of *Treponema*: Characterization of *Treponema hyodysenteriae* and its relationship to *Treponema pallidum. Infect. Immun.* 22:736-739 (1978).
30. C. R. Woese and M. A. Bleyman. Genetic code limit organisms— Do they exist? *J. Mol. Evol. 1*:223-229 (1972).
31. D. L. Harris and J. M. Kinyon. Significance of anaerobic spirochetes in the intestines of animals. *Am. J. Clin. Nutr.* 27:1297-1304 (1974).
32. W. M. Cwyk and E. Canale-Parola. *Treponema succinifaciens* sp. nov., an anaerobic spirochete from the swine intestine. *Arch. Microbiol. 122*:231-239 (1979).
33. B. J. McCarthy and E. T. Bolton. An approach to the measurement of genetic relatedness among organisms. *Proc. Nat. Acad. Sci. USA 50*:156-164 (1963).
34. R. J. Britten and D. E. Kohne. Nucleotide sequence repetition in DNA. *Carnegie Inst. Washington Year 65*:78-105 (1966).
35. J. M. Miller, V. H. Falcone, B. Golden, C. W. Israel, U. S. G. Kuhn III, and R. M. Smibert. Spirochetes in body fluids and tissues. In *Manual of Investigative Methods* (J. N. Miller, Ed.), Charles C. Thomas, Springfield, 1971, pp. 3-69.
36. R. D. Glock and D. L. Harris. Swine dysentery. II. Characterization of lesions in pigs inoculated with *Treponema hyodysenteriae* in pure and mixed culture. *Vet. Med. Small. Anim. Clin.* 67: 65-68 (1972).
37. A. H. Hamdy and M. W. Glenn. Transmission of swine dysentery with *Treponema hyodysenteriae* and *Vibrio coli. Am. J. Vet. Res.* 35:791-797 (1974).
38. J. M. Kinyon, D. L. Harris, and R. D. Glock. Enteropathogenicity of various isolates of *Treponema hyodysenteriae. Infect. Immun.* 15:638-646 (1977).
39. J. M. Kinyon and D. L. Harris. *Treponema innocens*, a new species of intestinal bacteria, and emended description of the type strains of *Treponema hyodysenteriae. Int. J. Syst. Bacteriol.* 29:102-109 (1979).
40. R. M. Miao and A. H. Fieldsteel. Genetic relationship between *Treponema pallidum* and *Treponema pertenue*, two noncultivable human pathogens. *J. Bacteriol. 141*:427-429 (1980).
41. K. Hovind-Hougen, A. Birch-Andersen, and H-J. S. Jensen. Ultrastructure of cells of *Treponema pertenue* obtained from

experimentally infected hamsters. *Acta Pathol. Microbiol. Scand. 84B*:101-108 (1976).
42. T. J. Fitzgerald, R. C. Johnson, and M. Smith. Accidental laboratory infection with *Treponema pallidum*, Nichols strain. *J. Am. Vener. Dis. Assoc.* 3:76-78 (1976).
43. O. Idsøe, T. Guthe, and R. R. Willcox. Penicillin in the treatment of syphilis. *Bull WHO Suppl.* 47:1-68 (1972).

4
Metabolic Activities

C. D. COX
University of Massachusetts
Amherst, Massachusetts

Catabolism and Energy Generation 58
Anabolic Activities 63
References 66

When the metabolic activities of virulent treponemes were briefly reviewed in 1970 (1) the available information was both meager and highly speculative. This was because most of the data had been obtained from experiments designed to prolong survival of the noncultivable virulent treponemes or from experiments utilizing cultivable indigenous spirochetes which are now known to be unrelated to syphilis. Survival studies were important because *Treponema pallidum* could not then be cultivated on laboratory media, a situation which has not changed. Evidence indicated that glucose (2) and pyruvate (3) prolonged survival and that a low redox potential was required (3,4). The latter finding has been supported by more recent publications (5,6). The anaerobic stature of *T. pallidum* (7) was apparently based upon earlier experiments which showed that the viability of virulent *T. pallidum* decreased more rapidly in air than in atmospheres of N_2 and H_2 (8,9), and on companion investigations on anaerobic nonpathogenic indigenous spirochetes, especially the Reiter treponeme (10). Unfortunately, such information did not lead to in vitro cultivation.

The continued inability to cultivate the treponemes responsible for syphilis, yaws, and pinta has been chiefly responsible for our serious lack of knowledge concerning their metabolic activities. *Treponema hyodysenteriae* has been associated with swine dysentery and has been cultivated on solid (16) and liquid (17) media; however, it has not yet been subjected to extensive metabolic study.

In recent years highly sensitive radioactive, polarographic, and spectrophotometric assays have permitted more revealing experiments on the metabolic activities of virulent *T. pallidum*. Data from such experiments on these treponemes extracted from infected tissue assumed even greater significance because procedures were used which negated or reduced metabolic contributions of eukaryotic cells. Such procedures involved selective centrifugation and filtration (11-14) and the use of selective metabolic inhibitors (15). Recent information has been based on the use of the Nichols virulent strain of *T. pallidum* and constitutes the basis for the remainder of this review.

The anaerobic nature of *T. pallidum* was questioned in 1974 (11), when the first evidence for O_2 consumption by virulent *T. pallidum* was reported. Treponemes were freshly extracted from testicles of infected rabbits, and O_2 measurements were made with a Clark-type electrode. Oxygen consumption was found to be dependent on the number of treponemes, and the rate was similar to that of the known aerobic *Leptospira*. Optimum O_2 uptake occurred at a temperature near 38°C. O_2 consumption was inhibited by micromolar levels of cyanide and by azide, amytal, and chlorpromazine, suggesting a role for a cytochrome-dependent terminal electron transport system. Evidence for uncoupling of oxidative phosphorylation was suggested by slight and transient stimulation of O_2 uptake in millimolar levels of cyanide and levels of chlorpromazine higher than those which inhibited uptake. Subsequently, evidence was presented which suggested that various concentrations of O_2 enhanced survival and motility (18-21), as well as metabolic activity (15). O_2 consumption has recently been shown to be glucose dependent, and O_2 was determined to be the major electron acceptor during the oxidative metabolism of glucose (57). The initial rate of respiration was independent of the dissolved O_2 concentration, but the respiration rate decreased upon prolonged incubation at the high dissolved O_2 concentration of 0.20 μmol/ml. These treponemes consumed O_2 to a low dissolved O_2 concentration of 0.01 μmol/ml when respiration ceased. Thus the respiration by this treponeme would seem to be influenced by the concentration of dissolved O_2 and the length of incubation.

Catabolism and Energy Generation

Of 22 carbon sources studied, only glucose and pyruvate were clearly degraded to CO_2 (12,13). It is interesting to note that the amount of glucose decarboxylated was directly correlated with the concentration of O_2 up to 20% (15). Fatty acids were not catabolized by β-oxidation (13). Data from the use of differentially labeled glucose in conjunction with enzymatic analyses on cell-free extracts of *T. pallidum* indicated

4. Metabolic Activities

that glucose was degraded by a combination of the Embden-Meyerhoff-Parnas (EMP) and hexose monophosphate shunt (HMP) pathways (13). The HMP pathway provides a source of NADPH, as well as pentose and triose phosphates required for biosynthesis; the EMP pathway probably functions as the major energy-yielding pathway. However, CO_2 was evolved from only the carboxyl position of pyruvate, suggesting the absence of a functioning Krebs cycle (12,13). Enzymatic analyses confirmed this suggestion and revealed only isocitrate dehydrogenase and malate dehydrogenase activities among the possible Krebs cycle enzymes (13). The absense of isocitrate lyase activity would also suggest the absence of a glyoxalate shunt. Certainly the absence of a functioning Krebs cycle would indicate a limited capacity for energy generation in the absence of other energy-generating systems to be discussed later. However, negative findings should be interpreted with caution, and a Krebs cycle may indeed be functioning in T. pallidum in vivo.

Incomplete oxidation of glucose by cell-free extracts of T. pallidum resulted in the end products CO_2, acetate, and lactate, with the acetate:lactate ratio depending on the O_2 tension (15,57). A comparison of acetate and lactate accumulation at intermediate and high dissolved O_2 concentrations indicated that acetate formation paralleled O_2 consumption, although lactate formation was relatively independent of O_2 metabolism (57). Although the NADH-dependent lactate dehydrogenase is known to catalyze the reduction of pyruvate to lactate, the mechanism for pyruvate oxidation to acetate and CO_2 by T. pallidum was not understood until 1979 (22), when evidence was presented that pyruvate decarboxylation was dependent upon O_2 and inorganic phosphate and that CO_2 evolution and O_2 consumption during pyruvate oxidation followed similar kinetics. These and other data indicated that the overall oxidation of pyruvate utilized O_2 and inorganic phosphate and yielded CO_2, acetyl phosphate, and H_2O_2. Phosphotransacetylase and acetate kinase activities were also found which could catalyze the formation of acetyl CoA and ATP, respectively, from acetyl phosphate. Thus pyruvate metabolism could be coupled to substrate level phosphorylation, offsetting perhaps to some degree any deficiencies resulting from the lack of a functioning Krebs cycle. However, production of lactate under experimental conditions (15) suggests that these treponemes may utilize pyruvate as a terminal electron acceptor. Any formation of lactate during aerobic metabolism would be expected to reduce the amount of puruvate and NADH available for energy generation. Regulation of NADH oxidation or pyruvate reduction may present a problem for this treponeme under existing conditions of in vitro maintenance.

A recent report (57) has presented the first evidence for the inactivation of a treponemal enzyme, pyruvate oxidase, under high dissolved O_2 concentrations. Several dehydrogenases were not affected. Inactivation of this key enzyme would deprive this treponeme of both energy and a key metabolic intermediate. In other bacterial systems, including aerobic, microaerophilic, and anaerobic bacteria, O_2 has been reported to inactivate enzymes important for substrate degradation (57). Maintenance of these treponemes at low dissolved O_2 concentrations resulted in a shift from oxidative to fermentative degradation of glucose and a loss of motility, whereas incubation at high dissolved O_2 concentrations inactivated pyruvate oxidase and rapidly removed motility. It would seem that optimal respiration, pyruvate oxidase activity, and motility proceed only under intermediate concentrations of dissolved O_2, which fits previous evidence reported on survival and motility (18-21). These data would seem to provide a helpful base for future attempts to cultivate this treponeme on laboratory media.

Evidence for a physiologically functioning flavoprotein-cytochrome electron transport system (14), coupled to O_2 consumption and oxidative phosphorylation (23), left no doubt of the capability of virulent *T. pallidum* for aerobic respiration. Reduced-minus-oxidized difference spectra of sonically disrupted virulent *T. pallidum* revealed cytochromes of the b and c types and large amounts of flavoprotein. Difference spectra of the carbon monoxide-binding pigment identified cytochrome o as the terminal oxidase. There was a clear distinction between a c-type cytochrome at 553 nm and a b-type cytochrome at 558 nm. A trough in the 455-nm region indicated large amounts of flavoproteins in *T. pallidum*, as have been observed in *Spirochaeta aurantia* (24), *Treponema hyodysenteriae* (25), and *Leptospira* (26). The lack of an a- or c-type cytochrome in carbon monoxide-bound spectra suggests that cytochrome o functions as the only cytochrome oxidase in *T. pallidum*. Cytochrome o is a b-type cytochrome (27) and may be identical to cytochrome b_{558}, as has been proposed for *S. aurantia* (24). However, there is still the possibility that another b-type cytochrome is present in addition to cytochrome o, such as has been discussed for *S. aurantia* (24) and *Leptospira* (26). The presence of c-type cytochromes in *T. pallidum* along with cytochrome b_{558} places this treponeme in an intermediate position between the "unicytochrome" of *S. aurantia* (24) and the leptospires, which have c-, o-, and a-type cytochromes as well (26).

Cytochromes were not reduced when using either succinate or pyruvate with or without cofactors, or when malate, isocitrate, or lactate was used without pyridine nucleotides (14). The inability of pyruvate to reduce cytochromes physiologically fits the lack of a tricarboxylic acid cycle (13). The inability of succinate to physiologically reduce cytochromes fits the lack of oxoglutarate dehydrogenase and succinate dehydrogenase (13) but may present a potential problem, since succinyl-coenzyme A is instrumental in protoporphyrin synthesis (28).
If *T. pallidum* is unable to synthesize heme, tissue porphyrins may serve as the source of ready-made prosthetic groups. Heme may well be needed for in vitro growth.

4. Metabolic Activities

A previously undetected cytochrome c with an α maximum at 550 nm appeared when malate, isocitrate, or lactate plus pyridine nucleotides were used to physiologically reduce the cytochromes (14). Furthermore, there was no appearance of a trough at 455 nm, indicative of flavoprotein reduction. The cytochrome c_{550} was stable in 8.5 mM H_2O_2 and could be repeatedly reduced after being oxidized by H_2O_2. Cytochromes c_{553} and b_{558} could not again be physiologically reduced after oxidation with H_2O_2, and after their inactivation only cytochrome c_{550} was reduced with NADH. However, cytochromes c_{553} and b_{558} were able to be reduced with dithionite after H_2O_2 oxidation. Cytochrome c_{550} did not appear to bind carbon monoxide and therefore would not seem to function as a terminal oxidase. That malate plus NAD and isocitrate plus NADP were able to physiologically reduce cytochrome c_{550} would argue for the importance of malate and isocitrate dehydrogenases despite the absence of a tricarboxylic acid cycle (13). The high levels of malate dehydrogenase previously found could suggest that this enzyme is a major source of reducing power. However, whether or not c_{550} participates in electron transport during normal NADH oxidation is not known, since it could easily be masked by the larger c_{553} peak.

The absence of concomitant flavoprotein reduction when cytochrome c_{550} was reduced by malate, isocitrate, or lactate plus pyridine nucleotides would seem to be important (14). A lactate dehydrogenase that donates electrons directly to cytochrome c has been reported in acetic acid bacteria (29,30), and a malate dehydrogenase in *Micrococcus lysodeikticus* (31) donates electrons directly to vitamin K_2. The malate vitamin K reductase of *Mycobacterium phlei* also donates electrons directly from malate into the respiratory chain and also bypasses the flavoproteins (32). Thus one could speculate that *T. pallidum* cytochrome c_{550} may be the electron acceptor of a membrane-bound dehydrogenase or quinone. However, cytochrome c_{550} does not appear to be a terminal oxidase, and its interaction with other electron carriers remains to be determined. The ability of c_{550} to be repeatedly oxidized by H_2O_2 and then reduced physiologically suggests that it might function with a cytochrome c peroxidase, as has been described for *Pseudomonas fluorescens* (33,34). In the latter system, the reduced cytochrome c donated electrons to H_2O_2 to yield two H_2O, and cytochrome peroxidase was thought to function optimally at low O_2 tensions. Another possibility is that cytochrome c_{550} normally interacts with c_{553} and b_{558}, but that during sonic disruption the dehydrogenases and c_{550} may become separated from the other cytochrome components. Some dehydrogenases are known to form complexes with c-type cytochromes (35,36), and a spatial disorientation caused by ultrasound, lysis, or osmotic shock could prevent the oxidation of substrates and subsequent cytochrome reduction (31,37,38). Further elaboration of the role of cytochrome c_{550} must probably await cultivation of the treponemes in vitro so that enzyme systems can be isolated.

Washing whole treponemes with 200 mM NaCl removed *T. pallidum* cytochromes (14). A single wash removed all detectable c-type cytochromes, and two washes accompanied by vigorous agitation effectively removed the b-type cytochrome as well. In both cases, treponemes remained intact, as observed by dark-field microscopy, and flavoproteins were detected in the usual amounts. These observations are reminiscent of previous reports for *Haemophilus parainfluenzae* cytochrome c_1 (39) and various other gram-negative bacterial as well as mitochondrial c-type cytochromes (40-42).

NADH has been shown to cause cytochrome reduction, O_2 uptake, and ATP formation in *T. pallidum* extracts (23). Some oxidation of NADH appeared to be cyanide insensitive and could stimulate O_2 consumption through the action of a flavoprotein oxidase. However, the evidence indicated that only a small fraction of the NADH oxidase activity was cyanide insensitive, which would seem to indicate that aerobic respiration in *T. pallidum* occurs mainly through the action of NADH dehydrogenase coupled to terminal electron transport and not through the action of a flavoprotein oxidase. Reduction of cytochromes by NADPH indicated that NADPH oxidation also proceeded through a dehydrogenase coupled to the mainstream electron transport chain. This evidence suggests that *T. pallidum* could derive a large amount of energy from terminal electron transport coupled to oxidative phosphorylation. How well this system functions under the pO_2 of tissue in the host is unknown at this time. However, one could conclude that the inability to cultivate this microorganism is probably not due to intrinsic problems with energy metabolism.

In considering the difficulties which this treponeme displays in growing on laboratory media, one would seem to be faced with the significance of its ability to regulate its metabolic activities under both high and low concentrations of dissolved O_2. *Treponema pallidum* has been shown to produce H_2O_2 during the oxidation of pyruvate and NADH (22). In addition, previously observed reduced flavoproteins and cyanide resistant respiration (14,23) are known to be potential sites for superoxide radical generation. *T. pallidum* has recently been shown to possess activities for superoxide dismutase and catalase but not peroxidase (59). The superoxide dismutase was shown to be the copper-zinc type and was identified electrophoretically to be of rabbit origin, which is consistent with a previous finding that a surface coat of host proteins exists on this treponeme (60). The catalase activity may represent either an additional host-derived protein or an intrinsic treponeme enzyme. Although the rabbit superoxide dismutase associated with *T. pallidum* was enzymatically active, one cannot rule out the possibility that its presence in *T. pallidum* may be fortuitous. However, one must also consider the possibility that rabbit superoxide dismutase, as well as catalase, does function for the benefit of *T. pallidum*. Resolution of the cellular location of rabbit superoxide

4. Metabolic Activities

dismutase would be helpful in evaluating the functional role of this enzyme. Rabbit superoxide dismutase associated with the outermost surface of the treponeme could prevent cellular damage by catalyzing the dismutation of superoxide radicals generated extracellularly and/or by shielding key outer membrane components from oxidation. The enzyme might also catalyze the dismutation of any intracellular superoxide radicals which may have diffused to the exterior of the cell. It is difficult to envision such diffusion occurring without concomitant cellular damage; however, one must remember that this treponeme has not yet been cultivated on laboratory media. The numerous host proteins that have been detected previously were either loosely or avidly associated with the treponeme surface, and the presence of noncompetitive binding sites was suggested (60). The mechanism of binding of rabbit superoxide dismutase to *T. pallidum* is as yet unknown. If the enzyme were loosely adsorbed to the treponeme surface, it might readily dissociate upon extraction of cells from tissue or during maintenance in vitro. Also, the level of the enzyme detected may only be a fraction of that required by this treponeme for protection against oxidized intermediates of O_2 when removed from tissue.

Anabolic Activities

Virulent *T. pallidum* has been shown to incorporate radiolabeled amino acids into protein in a linear fashion for at least 24 hr after extraction from infected rabbit testicles (43,44). Incorporation proceeded optimally at 34°C and pH 7.6 and was inhibited by erythromycin but not cyclohexamide. Several amino acids were incorporated at various efficiencies, which correlated with the size of unlabeled extracellular amino acid pools in the testicular extracts (43). This would suggest that most exogenous amino acids were utilized for protein synthesis by this treponeme. Optimal incorporation of amino acids occurred under 10-20% O_2 concentrations, and marked reduction of protein synthesis occurred with higher and lower O_2 concentrations and under anaerobic conditions (15). The capacity of these treponemes for synthesizing a wide range of high-molecular-weight proteins under atmospheric conditions was confirmed by the use of acrylamide gel autoradiography (45).

Ribosomal RNA synthesis has been observed by measuring the incorporation of [^{3}H]uridine and uracil into trichloroacetic acid-precipitable material from freshly harvested *T. pallidum* (46). In another report (44) [2-^{14}C]uracil, but not [2-^{14}C]uridine was incorporated into whole cells of *T. pallidum*. The reason for the discrepancy with uridine is not clear. In the earlier report (46), the significance of the finding of incorporation was magnified by evidence that radiolabeled treponemal 23S, 16S, and 4-5S RNA classes coelectrophoresed with similar molecules of *Escherichia coli* RNA. Incorporation of [^{3}H]uridine was sensitive to actinomycin D, a specific inhibitor of RNA synthesis. Maximal incorporation of [^{3}H]uridine occurred in an atmosphere of 20% O_2, and incorporation was greatly reduced at lower O_2 concentrations.

Temperature effects on RNA synthesis by *T. pallidum* (43,46) were different from those exerted on protein synthesis (43,44). The optimal temperature for protein synthesis in vitro was 34°C, whereas the maximal level of continual RNA synthesis during a 24-hr incubation occurred at 37°C. The highest levels of uridine incorporation were obtained at 39°C, but a reduction in total counts per minute between 8 and 24 hr suggests that this is not a physiologically favorable incubation temperature. Utilization of [^{3}H]uridine at 25 and 33°C was not markedly different from that observed at 37°C, but small temperature variations exerted a profound influence on protein synthesis (43).

Of considerable interest is the difference between protein (43) and RNA (46) synthesis in the persistence of linearity in both processes. Whereas protein synthesis remained linear over at least 24 hr, RNA synthesis was linear for only 2 to 4 hr. Further net accumulation occurred between 4 and 24 hr of incubation, but a slight decrease in total counts per minute occurred in the interval between 24 and 48 hr. This decrease does not appear to be the result of cell death, since the majority of treponemes remained actively motile. One is confronted with the obvious question of whether these treponemes actually began to shut down RNA synthesis after 2 to 4 hr, or whether the decrease was caused by ribonuclease activity. The 1:1 ratio of 23S to 16S rRNA extracted from *T. pallidum* compared to the usual 2:1 ratio obtained with *E. coli* on polyacrylamide gels also could be consistent with greater lability of 23s rRNA molecules to ribonuclease (47).

Comparison of findings among different experiments is difficult, and holding or maintenance conditions could be expected to be very important. Nevertheless, the possibility of a shutdown in RNA synthesis within a few hours after extraction from tissue does not seem to be consistent with a recent report (18) that *T. pallidum* can maintain virulence for 2 to 3 weeks in vitro without an increase in cell numbers. Final resolution of this important problem will probably depend upon future pulse-chase experiments.

Treponema pallidum is apparently capable of synthesizing DNA from exogenously supplied adenine (48) and uridine but not thymidine (49). Thymidine kinase activity was not found. DNA polymerase activities and generation times of several bacteria were generally found to correlate, and low levels of DNA polymerase activity were found which fit the in vivo generation time for *T. pallidum*. DNA synthesis continued for 24 hr after removal from host tissue, after which an increase in DNA synthesis ceased even though the treponemes remained motile. Interpretation of the significance of these findings is similar to that for RNA synthesis. Certainly DNA synthesis could not be expected to continue if cells were not committed to division, and DNA synthesis for 24 hr could have proceeded under prior in vivo commitment. More

4. Metabolic Activities

work is clearly needed; nevertheless, virulent *T. pallidum* clearly seems to be capable of DNA, as well as RNA, synthesis for at least a few hours after removal from infected tissue. In view of our inability to cultivate *T. pallidum* in vitro, correlative investigations between nucleic acid synthesis and degradation with time after removal of the treponemes from their in vivo environment would seem to be most appropriate, and suitable assay procedures are now available.

Virulent *T. pallidum* has recently been shown to incorporate glucose into material which precipitates with trichloracetic acid (50). These studies were performed under atmospheric conditions on treponemes suspended in phosphate-buffered saline containing glutathione. The amount of incorporation was proportional to the number of treponemes and was estimated to equal 33% of the glucose oxidized over a 90-min period. Using the in vivo generation time for *T. pallidum* of 33 hr (51,52) the corresponding instantaneous growth constant ($a = \ln 2/t_D$) would be 0.021 per hour (53). Assuming that half the dry cell weight of *T. pallidum* represents protein, the dry cell weight could be estimated to be 3.8×10^{-13} (54) or 0.56×10^{-13} g (55). One could calculate that over a 90-min period 3.8×10^8 treponemes (1.44×10^{-4} or 2.13×10^{-5} g of cells) incorporated 0.2 µg of glucose, which would represent from 4 to 30% of the cell material needed to be synthesized during cell growth over this time. This compares with glucose incorporated into 35.7% of cellular material of the Reiter treponeme (56). This calculated range of values represents a significant amount of incorporation, especially with the presumption that the treponemes were also capable of utilizing other carbon sources for biosynthesis (43,45,46), and with the knowledge that these experiments were performed under nonpermissive growth conditions. These results and calculations indicate that *T. pallidum* possesses considerable biosynthetic capability in a simple maintenance medium over a period of at least 90 min after harvest from tissue.

Of particular significance has been the recent report that glucose carbons are incorporated by *T. pallidum* into lipids, nucleic acids, and proteins (58). Glucose carbons were found mainly in phospholipids and glycolipids but not in cholesterol or free fatty acids. However, it should be noted that this spirochete has the enzymes necessary to synthesize acetyl coenzyme A from glucose (22). Free fatty acids had previously been shown to be incorporated but not oxidized (13). Chromatographic separation of the phospholipids showed that 70% of the glucose carbons migrated with phosphatidylcholine, and 10% with phosphatidylglycerol, but none with cardiolipin or phosphatidylethanolamine. Glucose carbons were incorporated into only the ribose and deoxyribose moieties of nucleic acids, which is consistent with the ability of this spirochete to incorporate nitrogenous bases into nucleic acids (48,44). Distribution of glucose carbons among the common amino acids in proteins was confined to aspartate. Baseman and Hayes (43) found that all amino acids tested were incorporated to varying degrees, but the amount of [^{14}C]aspartate incorporated was low. The ability of *T. pallidum* to synthesize aspartate from glucose suggests that a limited uptake of free aspartate could be responsible for the low amount of [^{14}C]aspartate observed to be incorporated. It is also possible that *T. pallidum* may utilize both mechanisms for the assimilation of aspartate.

A glimpse into the metabolism of virulent *T. pallidum* became possible in the last few years. One must keep in mind that all of these interesting findings have been obtained using whole treponemes, or their cell-free extracts, studied within a few hours after extraction from infected tissue. The possibility certainly exists that the treponemes at this time were metabolically changing to the influence of the in vitro environmental conditions imposed upon them after removal from tissue. Nevertheless, the significance of the recent observations on metabolic activity seems to be enhanced because the influence of eukaryotic metabolism has apparently been negated or minimized. Within this context, acquisition of existing information on the metabolism of a microorganism that cannot be cultivated in vitro is particularly noteworthy, and such information should be valuable as a basis for its eventual in vitro cultivation.

The emerging picture of *T. pallidum* is one of a spirochete capable of aerobic respiration and glycolysis and possessing a physiologically functioning flavoprotein-cytochrome terminal transport of electrons to O_2, coupled to oxidative phosphorylation. Inability to obtain evidence for a functioning Krebs cycle may be real or artifactual; nevertheless, *T. pallidum* still seems to have adequate energy-generating potential for growth in vitro. Amino acids, adenine, uracil, and glucose are incorporated into macromolecular components, and we must conclude that this treponeme has considerable biosynthetic capability for at least the first few hours after removal from infected tissue. This picture certainly does not fit that of its present classification as the type species of a strictly anaerobic genus (7) and in time should warrant some taxonomic attention. Existing information does not rule out a facultative status, or the possibility that this treponeme may have more than one physiological mode depending upon its environment. Indeed, the ability, or inability, to control or adjust its physiology with environmental change or stress may prove to be as crucial to *T. pallidum* as such problems are to man.

References

1. World Health Organization. Treponematoses Research. *WHO Tech. Rep. Ser.* 455:1-91 (1970).
2. G. E. Kimm, R. H. Allen, H. J. Worton, and J. F. Morgan. Enhancement of survival in vitro of *Treponema pallidum* by addition of glucose and magnesium. *J. Bacteriol.* 80:726-727 (1960).

4. Metabolic Activities

3. R. A. Nelson, Jr. Factors affecting the survival of Treponema pallidum in vitro. Am. J. Hyg. 48:120-132 (1948).
4. M. Metzger and W. Smogor. Study of the effect of pH and Eh values of the Nelson-Diesendruck medium on the survival of virulent Treponema pallidum. Arch. Immunol. Ther. Exp. 14:445-453 (1966).
5. S. R. Graves, P. L. Sandok, H. M. Jenkin, and R. C. Johnson. Retention of motility and virulence of Treponema pallidum (Nichols Strain) in vitro. Infect. Immun. 12:1116-1120 (1975).
6. P. L. Sandok, H. M. Jenkin, S. R. Graves, and S. T. Knight. Retention of motility of Treponema pallidum (Nichols Virulent Strain) in an anaerobic cell culture system and in a cell-free system. J. Clin. Microbiol. 3:72-74 (1976).
7. Bergey's Manual of Determinative Bacteriology. (J. G. Holt, Ed.). 8th Ed. Williams & Wilkins Co., Baltimore, 1977.
8. R. A. Nelson and H. G. Steinman. Factors affecting the survival of Treponema pallidum in vitro. Proc. Soc. Exp. Biol. Med. 68:588 (1948).
9. R. R. Willcox and T. Guthe. Treponema pallidum. Suppl. WHO 35:87 (1966).
10. H. Eagle and H. G. Steinman. The nutritional requirements of Treponemata. J. Bacteriol. 56:163-176 (1948).
11. C. D. Cox and M. K. Barber. Oxygen uptake by Treponema pallidum. Infect. Immun. 10:123-127 (1974).
12. J. C. Nichols and J. B. Baseman. Carbon sources utilized by virulent Treponema pallidum. Infect. Immun. 12:1044-1050 (1975).
13. N. L. Schiller and C. D. Cox. Catabolism of glucose and fatty acids by virulent Treponema pallidum. Infect. Immun. 16:60-68 (1977).
14. P. G. Lysko and C. D. Cox. Terminal electron transport in Treponema pallidum. Infect. Immun. 16:885-890 (1977).
15. J. B. Baseman, J. C. Nichols, and N. S. Hayes. Virulent Treponema pallidum: Aerobe or anaerobe. Infect. Immun. 13:704-711 (1976).
16. D. L. Harris, J. Kinyon, M. T. Mullin, and R. D. Glock. Isolation and propagation of spirochetes from the colon of swine dysentery affected pigs. Can. J. Comp. Med. 36:74-76 (1972).
17. J. M. Kinyon and D. L. Harris. Growth of Treponema hyodysenteriae in liquid medium. Vet. Rec. 95:219-220 (1974).
18. A. H. Fieldsteel, F. A. Becker, and J. G. Stout. Prolonged Survival of virulent Treponema pallidum (Nichols strain) in cell-free and tissue culture systems. Infect. Immun. 18:173-182 (1977).
19. P. L. Sandok, H. M. Jenkin, H. M. Matthews, and M. S. Roberts. Unsustained multiplication of Treponema pallidum (Nichols virulent strain) in vitro in the presence of oxygen. Infect. Immun. 19:421-429 (1978).

20. S. J. Norris, J. N. Miller, J. A. Sykes, and T. J. Fitzgerald. Influence of oxygen tension, sulfhydryl compounds, and serum on the motility and virulence of *Treponema pallidum* (Nichols strain) in a cell-free system. *Infect. Immun.* 22:689-697 (1978).
21. W. S. K. Chalmers and D. Taylor-Robinson. The effect of reducing and other agents on the motility of *Treponema pallidum* in an acellular medium. *J. Gen. Microbiol.* 114:443-447 (1979).
22. J. T. Barbieri and C. D. Cox. Pyruvate oxidation by *Treponema pallidum*. *Infect. Immun.* 25:157-163 (1979).
23. P. G. Lysko and C. D. Cox. Respiration and oxidative phosphorylation in *Treponema pallidum*. *Infect. Immun.* 21:462-473 (1978).
24. J. A. Breznak and E. Canale-Parola. Metabolism of *Spirochaeta aurantia*. II. Aerobic oxidation of carbohydrates. *Arch. Mikrobiol.* 83:278-292 (1972).
25. R. A. Harris, D. L. Harris, and J. M. Kinyon. *Abstr. Annu. Meet. Am. Soc. Microbiol.* 58 (1976).
26. J. B. Baseman and C. D. Cox. Terminal electron transport in *Leptospira*. *J. Bacteriol.* 97:1001-1004 (1969).
27. S. S. Deeb and L. P. Hager. Crystalline cytochrome b_1 from *Escherichia coli*. *J. Biol. Chem.* 239:1024-1031 (1964).
28. J. Lascelles. Tetrapyrrole synthesis in microorganisms. In *The Bacteria, Vol. 3 (I. C. Gunsalus and R. Y. Stanier, Eds.)*, Academic, New York, 1962, pp. 335-372.
29. J. Deley. Comparative carbohydrate metabolism and localization of enzymes in *Pseudomonas* and related microorganisms. *J. Appl. Bacteriol.* 23:400-441 (1960).
30. J. Deley and J. Schel. Studies on the metabolism of *Acetobacter peroxydans*. II. The enzymatic mechanism of lactate metabolism. *Biochim. Biophys. Acta.* 35:154-165 (1959).
31. N. S. Gel'man, M. A. Lukoyanova, I. G. Zhukova, and A. I. Oparin. The electron (hydrogen) transport chain in the cytoplasmic membranes of *Micrococcus lysodeikticus*. *Biolhimiya.* 28:801-807 (1963).
32. N. S. Cohen and A. F. Brodie. Multiple forms of cytochrome b in *Mycobacterium phlei*: Kinetics of reduction. *J. Bacteriol.* 123:162-173 (1975).
33. H. M. Lenhoff and N. O. Kaplan. A cytochrome peroxidase from *Pseudomonas fluorescens*. *J. Biol. Chem.* 220:967-982 (1956).
34. H. M. Lenhoff, D. J. D. Nicholas, and N. O. Kaplan. Effects of oxygen, iron, and molybdenum on routes of electron transfer in *Pseudomonas fluorescens*. *J. Biol. Chem.* 220:983-995 (1956).
35. Y. Iwasaki. Components of the electron-transferring system in *Acetobacter suboxydans* and reconstruction of the lactate oxidation system. *Plant Cell Physiol.* 1:207-220 (1960).

36. T. Nakayama. Studies on acetic acid bacteria. IV. Purification and properties of a new type of alcohol dehydrogenase, alcohol-cytochrome-553 reductase. *J. Biochem.* 49:240-251 (1961).
37. L. Smith. Structure of the bacterial respiratory chain system. Respiration of *Bacillus subtilis* spheroplasts as a function of the osmotic pressure of the medium. *Biochim. Biophys. Acta.* 62: 145-152 (1962).
38. D. C. White. Differential synthesis of five primary electron transport dehydrogenases in *Hemophilus parainfluenzae*. *J. Biol. Chem.* 239:2055-2060 (1964).
39. L. Smith and D. C. White. Structure of the respiratory chain system as indicated by studies with *Hemophilus parainfluenzae*. *J. Biol. Chem.* 237:1337-1341 (1962).
40. C. W. Forsberg, J. W. Costerton, and R. A. MacLeod. Quantitation, chemical characteristics, and ultrastructure of the three outer cell wall layers of a gram-negative bacterium. *J. Bacteriol.* 104:1354-1368 (1970).
41. T. Fujita and R. Sato. Studies on soluble cytochromes in *Enterobacteriaceae*. III. Localization of cytochrome c-552 in the surface layer of cells. *J. Biochem.* 60:568-577 (1966).
42. W. T. Garrard. Selective release of proteins from *Spirillum intersonii* by tris (hydroxymethyl) aminomethane and ethylenediaminetetraacetate. *J. Bacteriol.* 105:93-100 (1971).
43. J. B. Baseman and N. S. Hayes. Protein synthesis by *Treponema pallidum* extracted from infected rabbit tissue. *Infect. Immun.* 10:1350-1355 (1974).
44. P. L. Sandok and H. M. Jenkin. Radiolabeling of *Treponema pallidum* (Nichols virulent strain) in vitro with precursors for protein and RNA biosynthesis. *Infect. Immun.* 22:22-28 (1978).
45. J. B. Baseman and N. S. Hayes. Anabolic potential of virulent *Treponema pallidum*. *Infect. Immun.* 18:857-859 (1977).
46. J. C. Nichols and J. B. Baseman. Ribosomal ribonucleic acid synthesis by virulent *Treponema pallidum*. *Infect. Immun.* 19: 854-860 (1978).
47. J. E. M. Midgley. Effects of different extraction procedures on the molecular characteristics of bacterial ribosomal ribonucleic acid. *Biochim. Biophys. Acta* 95:232-243 (1965).
48. S. J. Norris, J. N. Miller, and J. A. Sykes. Long-term incorporation of tritiated adenine into deoxyribonucleic acid and ribonucleic acid by *Treponema pallidum* (Nichols strain). *Infect. Immun.* 29:1040-1049 (1980).
49. J. B. Baseman, J. C. Nichols, and S. Mogerley. Capacity of virulent *Treponema pallidum* (Nichols) for deoxyribonucleic acid synthesis. *Infect. Immun.* 23:392-397 (1979).
50. J. T. Barbieri and C. D. Cox. Glucose incorporation by *Treponema pallidum*. *Infect. Immun.* 24:291-293 (1979).

51. M. C. Cumberland and T. B. Turner. The rate of multiplication of *T. pallidum* in normal and immune rabbits. *Am. J. Syph. Gonorrhea Vener. Dis. 33*:201-212 (1949).
52. H. J. Magnuson, H. Eagle, and R. Fleischman. The minimal infectious inoculum of *Spirochaeta pallida* (Nichols strain) and a consideration of its rate of multiplication in vivo. *Am. J. Syph. Gonorrhea Vener. Dis. 32*:1-18 (1948).
53. B. D. Davis. Bacterial nutrition and growth. In *Microbiology* (B. D. Davis, R. Dulbecco, H. N. Eisen, H. S. Ginsberg, and W. B. Wood, Eds.), Harper and Row, New York, 1973, pp. 90-104.
54. P. H. Hardy Jr., and E. E. Nell. Isolation and purification of *Treponema pallidum* from syphilitic lesions in rabbits. *Infect. Immun. 11*:1296-1299 (1975).
55. H. M. Matthews, T. K. Yang, and H. M. Jenkin. Unique lipid composition of *Treponema pallidum* (Nichols virulent strain). *Infect. Immun. 24*:713-719 (1979).
56. S. L. Allen, R. C. Johnson, and D. Peterson. Metabolism of common substrates by the Reiter strain of *Treponema pallidum*. *Infect. Immun. 3*:727-734 (1971).
57. Joseph T. Barbieri, and C. D. Cox. Influence of Oxygen on respiration and glucose catabolism by *Treponema pallidum*. *Infect. Immun. 31*:992-997 (1981).
58. Joseph T. Barbieri, Faye E. Austin, and C. D. Cox. Distribution of glucose incorporated into macromolecular material by *Treponema pallidum*. *Infect. Immun. 31*:1071-1077 (1981).
59. Faye E. Austin, Joseph T. Barbieri, Robert E. Corin, Kathryn E. Grigas, and C. D. Cox. Distribution of superoxide dismutase, catalase, and peroxidase activities among *Treponema pallidum* and other spirochetes. *Infect. Immun. 33*:372-379 (1981).
60. J. F. Alderete and J. B. Baseman. Surface-associated host proteins on virulent *Treponema pallidum*. *Infect. Immun. 26*:1048-1056 (1979).

5
In Vitro Cultivation of *Treponema pallidum*

HOWARD M. JENKIN
The Hormel Institute
University of Minnesota
Austin, Minnesota

PAUL L. SANDOK
University of North Carolina
at Charlotte
Charlotte, North Carolina

Passage and Harvest of *Treponema pallidum* in Rabbits 72
Estimation of Treponemal Numbers in Culture 73
Preparation and Constituents of Media 75
Oxygen Requirements 80
Mammalian Cell-Treponeme Coincubation 80
Cell-Free Systems of Incubation for *Treponema pallidum* In Vitro 85
Miscellaneous Observations 86
References 94

In vitro cultivation of treponemes which cause human disease has eluded investigators since the first attempts in 1905, by Schereschewsky, who published his observations in 1908 (1), and in 1906, by Volpino and Fontana (2). These investigators relied heavily on living fragments of tissue, derived from human or rabbit sources, to condition the medium ostensibly to make it suitable for treponemal survival or growth. An early attempt to cultivate *Treponema pallidum* in vitro was performed by Steinhardt (3), using explanted tissue infected with *T. pallidum* which was embedded in rabbit plasma. Cells grew out of the explant, and 25 days after incubation many motile short treponemes were observed which were thought to have resulted from multiplication; however, these organisms proved to be avirulent. Attempts to cultivate *T. pallidum* in vitro using infected rabbit fragments and subsequent serial passage of the organisms three times showed motile treponemes only in the first passage. A number of investigators, from Levaditi in 1920 (4) to Wright in 1962 (5), were able to increase the time during which treponemes retained motility in vitro, but serial cultivation and long-term maintenance of virulence of the organism was not observed. Attempts to cultivate virulent treponemes during the last decade followed similar approaches to the problem, except that cell monolayers and culture media, supplemented with different animal sera and a variety of reducing agents with and without the presence of oxygen, were used instead of simply employing tissue fragments incubated in by-products of horse serum.

For the most part, the following review will be limited to reports published from 1975 through the middle of 1981, as well as to some previously unpublished data from our laboratory dealing with attempts to serially cultivate *T. pallidum* in vitro. Bibliographic compendiums, reviews, and published summaries of NIH-sponsored workshops partly or completely concerned with earlier work on treponemal cultivation have been written by Turner and Hollander (6), Willcox and Guthe (7), Krause (8), Johnson, (9,10), Baseman (11), and Canale-Parola (12).

Passage and Harvest of *Treponema pallidum* in Rabbits

Treponemes were in general propagated in the testes of white New Zealand and occasionally Dutchbelt rabbits free of treponemal reaginic antibody, and testicular extracts containing treponemes were used for in vitro culture studies. Testes from rabbits having a palpable orchitis were used as early as 8 days and as late as 43 days after inoculation (13,14). Some investigators used corticosteroids such as cortisone acetate or triamcinolone (15-17), as described by Hardy and Nell (18), to improve consistency in obtaining large numbers of treponemes from one rabbit to the next, as well as organisms relatively free from cell debris. Usually, harvests resulting in 10^8 to 10^{10} treponemes per milliliter were used for subsequent subculturing attempts.

The microorganisms were eluted by mincing infected testicular tissue in a physiologic solution, usually the medium used subsequently for in vitro culture. Most investigators harvested the treponemes under ordinary atmospheric conditions, although in some reports the elutions were performed under strict anaerobiosis (19). Imposition of deoxygenated gases upon culture fluids containing suspended treponemes during harvest and subsequent incubation inhibited increases in treponemal numbers (20) and negated treponemal protein synthesis (19). Clumping of the microorganisms during the harvesting procedure was due to the formation of fibrinous clots, which was minimized by constant agitation of the testicular mincings (21), by use of heparin in the harvest medium (16), or by discarding the first two or three

5. In Vitro Cultivation

rinsings from the testicular fragments prior to collecting the elutions to be used for culture (13,20,22). When necessary, large testicular particulate debris and spermatozoa were removed from freshly harvested treponemal suspensions by using low-speed sedimentation at 250 to 1000 g (15,16,23,24). Further steps in obtaining highly purified microorganisms for special studies to identify molecular constituents or examine the metabolic potential of the microorganism are summarized elsewhere in this volume. Treponemes were generally inoculated into experimental media within 30 to 45 min after animals were sacrificed.

Estimation of Treponemal Numbers in Culture

Direct counting of treponemes and retention of motility and virulence are critical criteria in determining whether serial passage of virulent human treponemes has been achieved. The following section is a review of pertinent past and present methods employed for estimating the number of virulent cell-free and cell-associated treponemes in vitro as related to attempts to cultivate these organisms.

Much effort has been spent by a number of investigators to increase the duration of motility and virulence retention by *T. pallidum* (13,20, 23-27) in attempts to cultivate the virulent spirochete. Direct counts of wet mount preparations under cover slips using phase-contrast or dark-field microscopy remain the most useful method of estimating numbers of treponemes in suspension or attached to cells. This technique was described for cell-free cultures by Morgan and Vryonis (28), and its accuracy extensively analyzed by Artley and Clark (29), With the single exception of Sandok et al. (20), recent investigators did not publish established limits within which the accuracy of their counting procedures would fall. Differences of at least 50% in the numbers of microorganisms were detectable with 95% confidence in cultures containing at least 2.7×10^6 but no more than 10×10^6 treponemes per milliliter (20). At least 250 microorganisms were counted per treatment, employing two to four cultures and counting four to eight individual slide preparations, respectively. Although small increases (two- to fivefold) in the numbers of microorganisms were detected using this procedure for counting treponemes, the biological significance of less than sustained microbial growth after serial passage will remain controversial (24).

Quantitation of numbers of microorganisms attached to cells has proven to be more difficult than estimating numbers of microorganisms in fluid suspension. It has been observed in wet mounts, under phase and/or dark-field microscopy, that microorganisms attach to cells in a nonrandom fashion, making estimates of the numbers of microorganisms per cell difficult to interpret (15,20,30,31). Depending upon the techniques and media used to incubate treponemes with cultured cells, as few as 5% to as many as 75% of the microorganisms attached to cells (20,23). The numbers of fields or the numbers of cells examined for attached treponemes, upon which estimates of numbers of treponemes were based, varied between laboratories, as did the accuracy of such estimates. Fieldsteel et al. (17) removed the cell monolayers with attached treponemes using trypsin, dislodged the treponemes by re-pipetting, and counted the resulting suspension using dark-field microscopy.

Retention of motility by treponemes was used by many investigators as a parameter to examine the suitability of a variety of conditions for culturing *T. pallidum* in vitro. Estimates of motility were made on the basis of data from direct counts differentiating between rapidly flexing and motionless microorganisms. In our experience, the major shortcoming of expressing treponemal survival solely in terms of the retention of motility is that fluctuations in the ratio of motile to nonmotile microorganisms may not correspond to major changes in the numbers of motile, nonmotile, or total microorganisms (20). Thus cultures losing up to 90% of the initial treponemal numbers may exhibit 70 to 90% motility after 6 days in the remaining 10% of the original inoculum (20).

Treponemal translational motility has been observed in cell cultures, in testicular fluids, and in 0.1 to 0.4% methyl cellulose (24,32). To date, this type of motility has not been used as a parameter to measure the survival of *T. pallidum* in vitro.

The rabbit skin lesion test, described by Magnuson et al. (33), has been used to evaluate the virulence of *T. pallidum* after culture in vitro. Most investigators developed their own standard curve to correlate the numbers of freshly harvested microorganisms inoculated per site with a mean date of lesion appearance at a number of sites on several animals receiving identically diluted treponemal inocula. Estimates of the numbers of virulent microorganisms based on standard dilution curves generally have inherent errors, with values obtained as much as 1.4 $\log_{10}$ higher than the actual number of organisms (20). Additional difficulties arise because the standard curve is established using cell-free treponemal suspensions and the samples to be counted contain treponemes attached to cells. The cells themselves may cause induration similar to early syphilitic lesions (32), and it is necessary to examine exudates of rabbit lesions for motile microorganisms to avoid false positive results. The cells could also protect, retain, or modify the parasitic treponemes in situ in a manner resulting in the early or late appearance of lesions, or their absence altogether. Such cellular influence on *T. pallidum* may be suspected when no change in virulence is observed after several days of incubation in vitro without treponemal multiplication (30), or when virulence undergoes apparent eclipses and reappearances during culture (14).

5. In Vitro Cultivation

Preparation and Constituents of Media

Treponemal media devised by most investigators were adequate for the cultivation of mammalian cells. Starting with Eagle's medium in Earle's balanced salt solution (34), Fieldsteel et al. (16,17,31) added 2 mM glutamine, fetal bovine serum (10%), and freshly prepared reducing agents (100 mg/liter dithiothreitol, 200 mg/liter DL-cysteine HCl, and 400 mg/liter reduced glutathione). The pH of the medium was stabilized at 7.3 using 25 mM N-2-hydroxyethyl piperazine-N^1-2-ethanesulfonic acid (HEPES) buffer. Fieldsteel's group found it essential to screen commercially obtained Eagle's medium and fetal bovine serum for toxicity to treponemes prior to use in their experiments. Heparin (1000 units/liter) and the redox dye resazurin (0.0001%) were also incorporated into Fieldsteel's medium. All sterilization was performed by filtration (17).

Fitzgerald et al. (30) and Norris et al. (35) used Eagle's medium supplemented with one or two times concentrated Eagle's amino acids, vitamins, 4 mM sodium bicarbonate, and 20 or 30 mM HEPES buffer at pH 7.2 to 7.3. These investigators used reduced glutathione (1200 mg/liter), cysteine (120 mg/liter), or 1 to 2 mM dithiothreitol, which was dissolved and filter sterilized as concentrated solution immediately prior to supplementing the medium. This medium was further supplemented with fetal calf serum (5 to 30%), which permitted better survival of *T. pallidum* than the same medium without reducing agents (30,35). In cell-free cultures, physiological saline with supplemental reducing agents plus fetal bovine serum (50%) maintained the motility of the microorganisms under 3% oxygen as well as the complete medium (35).

Hayes et al. (15) used Dulbecco modified minimum essential medium (MEM) supplemented with 0.35% glucose, 10% tryptose phosphate, and 10% fetal calf serum. As a buffer, 10 mM TES was used to obtain pH 7.4. The redox potential of the medium was reduced using a filter-sterilized concentrate containing 800 mg/liter cysteine and 700 mg/liter sodium thioglycollate.

Sandok et al. (24) devised a complex medium based on earlier formulations of Eagle (34) and Richter et al. (36) supplemented with 10% newborn calf serum as shown in Table 1 (24). All components were filter sterilized except for Hanks' balanced salt solution (HBSS) containing 20 times concentrated reduced glutathione. Hanks' balanced salt solution was deoxygenated and anaerobically sterilized under N_2 in an autoclave in pressure-sealed tubes. Incorporation of the resulting sterile solution into unreduced medium caused the redox potential of the medium to drop to levels optimal for treponemal survival (E_{cal} = -240 to -330 mV), as described by Graves et al. (13). The same concentration of filter-sterilized but not steam-sterilized glutathione, 307 mg/liter, in unreduced medium resulted in a less dramatic (E_{cal} = -150 mV) lowering of the redox potential. Further details on the preparation and components of this medium are given in Table 1.

Jones et al. (14), using a baby hamster kidney cell strain, devised a medium which was reported to permit growth of *T. pallidum*. Earle's salt solution was supplemented with vitamin B_{12}, biotin, cobalt chloride, sodium bicarbonate, and a delipidized bovine serum albumin complexed with sodium oleate and sodium stearate (TCM-1). This medium differed from other media conventionally used in that it lacked reducing agents and serum. Jones' group, utilizing a statistically questionable procedure for the enumeration of *T. pallidum* in which too few organisms were counted, observed what appeared to be growing motile treponemes for 9 days in cell culture employing aerobic conditions (14). Unfortunately, these results could not be reproduced by several independent laboratories, including that of Foster et al. (37). The rabbit virulence tests, using samples obtained during the course of the experiment, gave variable results which could not plausibly be explained (14). As Turner (38) succinctly stated, "failure to confirm previous reports is not in itself cause for undue pessimism, but when linked with many other unsuccessful attempts the burden of proof shifts back to the original proponents of the method." Horvath et al. (39) used a balanced salt solution supplemented with the reducing

Table 1 Preparation of 0.5 liter of Prereduced Medium ($PRNF_{10}^-B$)[a]

Component[b]	Concentration of stock solution (g/liter)	Amount of stock solution (ml)
Double glass-distilled water		260.5
Mixture of		
NaCl (1)	85.00	
KCl (6)	4.06	
$MgSO_4$ anhydrous (2)	1.50	30.0
KH_2PO_4 (2)	1.85	
Glucose (2)	25.00	
Phenol red (9)	0.02	
$NaHCO_2$ (8)	88.00	13.3
$CaCl_2$ anhydrous (1)	10.00	10.4
HEPES (7)[c]	477.00	4.8
Newborn calf serum (11,13)[d]	Undiluted	50.0
Mixture of		
Choline chloride (4)	10.00	
Ethanolamine (4)	10.00	4.0
Inositol (3)	10.00	

Table 1 (Continued)

Component[b]	Concentration of stock solution (g/liter)	Amount of stock solution (ml)
L-Serine (4)	2.10	4.0
DL-Ornithine (3)[e]	2.00	4.0
Eagle minimum essential amino acids (50× concentrate) (11,13)[f]		
Mixture of		
$CoCl_2 \cdot 6H_2O$ (1)	0.0005	
$MnCl_2 \cdot 4H_2O$ (1)	0.0010	
$ZnSO_4 \cdot 7H_2O$ (2)	0.0140	4.0
$Fe(NO_3)_3 \cdot 9H_2O$ (2)	0.0810	
$(NH_4)_6Mo_7O_{24} \cdot 4H_2O$ (1)	0.5000	
$(NH_4)_2SO_4$ (10)	9.6	4.0
Mixture of		
Adenine (4)	1.5	4.0
Uracil (4)	1.5	
Oleic acid (14)[g]	0.4	4.0
Palmitic acid (14)[h]	0.4	4.0
FAF-BSA (15)	200.0	8.0
Ox serum ultrafiltrate (12)	Undiluted	17.0
Galactose (7)	190.8	4.0
L-Tryptophan (3)	4.0	4.0
Sodium pyruvate (100× concentrate) (13)		
L-Glutamine grade B (4)	2.92	4.0
Mixture of		
DL-Alanine (5)	1.78	
L-Asparagine (3)	3.00	
L-Aspartic acid (3)	2.66	8.0
L-Glutamic acid (3)	2.94	
Glycine (4)	1.50	
L-Proline (3)	2.30	
Eagle vitamins (100× concentrate) (11,13)[f]		4.0

Table 1 (Continued)

Component[b]	Concentration of stock solution (g/liter)	Amount of stock solution (ml)
Mixture of additional cofactors/vitamins[i]		
NADP (4)	0.4	
Pyridoxal PO$_4$ (4)	0.1	
α-Lipoate (4)[f]	0.1	
CoA (7)	0.25	
B$_{12}$ (7)	0.125	4.0
Thiamine pyrophosphate chloride (7)	0.25	
Biotin (3)	0.01	
NADH (4)	0.70	
Folinic acid (16)	0.10	
Mixture of		
Reduced glutathione (4)[k]	12.3	
NaCl (1)	6.8	
KCl (6)	0.4	
MgSO$_4$·7H$_2$O (2)	0.2	
KH$_2$PO$_4$ (2)	0.06	25.0
Na$_2$HPO$_4$ (2)	0.06	
Glucose (2)	1.00	
CaCl$_2$·2H$_2$O (1)	0.14	
Resazurin (1)	0.0025	
Sodium ascorbate (4)[l]	5.0	5.0

[a] A total of 10 ml of the completed prereduced medium was withdrawn from the vessel and placed into an anaerobic culture tube under 100% N$_2$. The redox potential [(-275 ± 25) mV E$_{cal}$] and pH (7.3 ± 0.1) of the completed medium were measured by using a saturated KCl calomel electrode and a pH probe as described previously.

[b] All stock solutions were sterilized by using a prerinsed 0.45-μm membrane filter (Millipore Corp.), except as noted below. Components were added to the medium in the sequence shown in the table. The number in parentheses following each component corresponds to the vendors of each reagent: (1) Fisher Scientific Company, Fairlawn, N.J.; (2) Mallinckrodt Chemical Works, St. Louis, Mo.; (3) Nutritional Biochemicals Corp., Cleveland, Ohio; (4) Calbiochem, Los Angeles, Calif.; (5) Eastman Kodak Co., Rochester, N.Y.; (6) Merck & Co., Inc., Rahway, N.J.; (7) Sigma Chemical Co., St. Louis,

5. In Vitro Cultivation

Table 1 (Continued)

Mo.; (8) Matheson Coleman and Bell, Norwood, Ohio; (9) J. T. Baker Chemical Co., Phillipsburg, N.J.; (10) Schwarz/Mann, Orangeburg, N.J.; (11) International Scientific Industries, Cary, Ill.; (12) Colorado Serum Co., Denver; (13) Grand Island Biological Co., Grand Island, N.Y.; (14) Nu-Check-Prep, Inc., Elysian, Minn.; (15) Miles Lab, Inc., Elkhart, Ind.; (16) ICN and K & K Laboratories, Inc., Plainview, N.Y.

[c]Stock HEPES (N-2-hydroxyethyl piperazine-N-2-ethanesulfonic acid) solution was adjusted to pH 7.3 with NaOH and autoclaved before use.

[d]Newborn calf serum was heat inactivated at 56°C for 30 min.

[e]DL-Ornithine (200 mg) was dissolved in 10 ml of 1 N HCl and then diluted to 100 ml with glass-distilled water before filtration.

[f]See Ref. 8.

[g]Sterile oleic acid (100 mg) was combined with 3.9 ml of sterile 0.1 N NaOH and rapidly heated to 75°C until dissolved. The warm solution was immediately diluted with 15.7 ml of calcium- and magnesium-free saline (20). The sodium oleate solution (0.8 ml) was complexed to 9.2 ml of 20% fatty acid-free bovine serum albumin (FAF-BSA). The BSA-oleate complex was directly incorporated into the medium. Excess BSA-oleate was stored at 4°C.

[h]Sterile palmitic acid (16 mg) was combined with 1 ml of 0.1 N NaOH and heated rapidly to 75°C until dissolved. The resulting solution was immediately complexed to 9 ml of warm (48 to 50°C) 20% FAF-BSA. The BSA-palmitate complex was diluted with 30 ml of 20% FAF-BSA at 37°C, and the final solution was directly incorporated into the medium. Excess BSA-palmitate was stored at 4°C.

[i]NADP, Nicotinamide adenine dinucleotide phosphate; CoA, coenzyme A; NADH, reduced nicotinamide adenine dinucleotide.

[j]α-Lipoate (100 mg) was dissolved in 1 ml of 0.2 N NaOH and the volume was adjusted to 10 ml with glass-distilled water before incorporation into the concentrated solution.

[k]The prereduced solution was made in 50- or 100-ml volumes. Powdered reduced glutathione was dissolved in the salts solution after the solution was degassed, using an autoclave at 215 lb/in^2 for 7 min. This mixture was adjusted to pH 6.8 with 10 N NaOH under 100% N_2; the vessel was stoppered and autoclaved for 25 min at 15 lb/in^2, using an anaerobic tube press (Bellco, Vineland, N.J.). The autoclaved solution was added to the unreduced medium under a constant flow of 100% N_2. If necessary, the unreduced medium was adjusted to pH 7.3 with 0.2 N NaOH before solution of the prereduced, anaerobically sterilized salts solution.

[l]The sodium ascorbate was dissolved in glass-distilled water, filter sterilized, and added to the completed medium immediately.

Source: Reference 24.

agents cysteine, thioglycollate, and glutathione and 10% fetal calf serum. As long as precautions were made to prepare and distribute the medium under strictly anaerobic conditions (85% N_2 + 10% H_2 + 5% CO_2), the treponemes appeared to retain their motility at least for 168 hr in vitro. The most recent published formulation of medium of Fieldsteel's group, in which a 50- to 100-fold increase of organisms was observed when coincubated with Sf_1Ep cells, is shown in Table 2 (17). The combinations of components of this medium are unlike most preparations previously employed in attempts to grow *T. pallidum*.

Oxygen Requirements

Cox and Barber in 1974 (40) reported that virulent *T. pallidum* appeared to have a requirement for oxygen, whereas this organism had previously been considered a strict anaerobe. Subsequently, Lysko and Cox in 1977 (41) showed that *T. pallidum* has a flavoprotein-cytochrome electron transport system that may function in aerobic respiration. Baseman et al. in 1976 (42) observed that 10 to 20% O_2 in the presence of CO_2, N_2, and H_2 can stimulate the incorporation of some amino acids into *T. pallidum* as well alter carbohydrate metabolism. A number of other investigators reexamined the role of O_2 in vitro and in vivo in an effort to confirm earlier data and/or tried to grow *T. pallidum* in vitro (17,24,30,31,35,39,43-47). The optimum amount of O_2 used in recent studies was 1.5% in attempts to grow *T. pallidum* in cell-free and cell-associated systems (17,24,30,31,35). In contrast, Horvath et al. (39) observed dramatic decreases in the motility of the microorganism under 3.5% O_2.

Mammalian Cell-Treponeme Coincubation

Among the earliest workers to screen a variety of cell monolayers was Wright (5), who examined the effects of *T. pallidum* and *Treponema pertenue* on cells derived from rabbit testes, liver, and kidney, as well as on human amnionic and embryonic cells and HeLa cells. The cell cultures were removed from an aerobic environment to a deoxygenated one and incubated with treponemes. Medium 199 with Earle's salts, supplemented with 5% calf serum, did not support treponemal growth in these cell cultures.

Early in 1974 several additional workers began to investigate the possibility that *T. pallidum* could be cultivated in the presence of living mammalian cell monolayers. An observation common to all investigations was that virulent treponemes attached to many types of cells examined.

Fitzgerald et al. (23) derived primary cultures from testicular fragments of normal rabbits to prepare secondary cultures for coincubation

5. In Vitro Cultivation

with *T. pallidum*. These workers also used an epithelial cell line, ME-180, from a human cervical carcinoma. Both cell cultures extended treponemal survival and retention of treponemal virulence under aerobic conditions for 5 hr longer than cultures without cells. Numbers of motile treponemes disappeared after 10 hr incubation in vitro.

Sandok et al. (20) used a rat glial cell line to prepare cell cultures using Leighton tubes. Rat glial cells, RGC-6, at an initial inoculum of 2×10^5 cells per culture, supported 100% treponemal motility retention by attached microorganisms under a deoxygenated atmosphere for 24 hr in prereduced Eagle's medium (22). Supernatant fluids from aerobically cultivated rat cell cultures sustained motility of 50% of the

Table 2 Preparation of Fieldsteel et al. Medium (17) to Cocultivate *Treponema pallidum* with Cottontail Rabbit Epithelium Cells (Sf_1Ep)

Basal medium-Eagle's MEM (34)	
Rabbit infected testes extract (Ref. 17, p. 909, 1:30 dilution)	
Earle's balanced salt solution (10×) (no phenol red and $NaHCO_3$)	10 ml
Eagle's MEM amino acids (50×)	2 ml
Eagle's MEM nonessential amino acids (100×)	1 ml
Eagle's MEM vitamins (100×)	1 ml
L-Glutamine, 200 mM	1 ml
Sodium heparin, 100 units/ml gas above solution briefly with CO_2	
Add	
$NaHCO_3$ (7.5%)	3.38 ml
HEPES buffer, 1 M	3.13 ml
Resazurin (20 mg/100 ml)	0.63 ml
Sodium pyruvate	10 mg
Dithiothreitol	10 mg
Glucose	150 mg

Make up to 100 ml, filter sterilize, and add 25 ml of heat-inactivated fetal calf serum (final amount of serum 20%) to make 125 ml of the solution. The modified basal medium is flushed with 5% CO_2 and 95% nitrogen three times and the medium stored overnight before use.

Source: Reference 17.

treponemes for a little over 2 days, compared to 18 hr in freshly prepared medium. Subsequently Sandok et al. (20,22) added several supplemental nutrients to their basal medium and replaced rat glial cells with primary human prepuce cells, and observed up to five-fold increases in the numbers of treponemes in the supernatant fluids of cell cultures. Counts of treponemes attached to cells were separately made, but estimates were crude and did not significantly affect the total count per culture. Cells and treponemes survived optimally at 34°C using a pH of 7.4 in an atmosphere of 3% oxygen plus 5% CO_2 combined with 20% H_2, 5% CO_2, and 75% N_2 (24). No coincident increases in the numbers of virulent microorganisms were observed with increases in the numbers of treponemes. Virulent organisms were detected up to 6 days in vitro.

Baby hamster kidney cells (BHK-21) subcultured in Eagle's medium plus 2% fetal calf serum were established in multidish tissue culture plates containing 10^5 tissue cells by Jones et al. (14) to cultivate *T. pallidum*. Prior to inoculation with treponemes, the cultures were rinsed free of serum and preincubated for 24 hr in TCM-1, a culture medium described earlier (14). In order to assure continued cultivation of the treponemes, it was necessary to harvest and transfer the microorganisms from old cultures to new ones every 24 hr. A temperature of 33°C and an atmosphere of 7% CO_2 in air was maintained during incubation.

Kiraly and Horvath (46) used HeLa, Detroit-6, HEP 2, and KB cell lines, as well as primary cultures prepared from human amnion, human embryo, and pig kidney. They used equal parts of Nelson's medium (25) and medium 199 plus HBSS to incubate the cells in air 5 days prior to use. After inoculation with 1.0×10^7 to 1.5×10^7 treponemes per milliliter the cultures were incubated at 30°C under 7 mmHg O_2, 40 mmHg CO_2, and 600 mmHg N_2. Half of the microorganisms remained motile for about 3 days in the cell culture. All cell types equally maintained treponemal survival.

After reducing the oxygen level to 3% and supplementing the medium with reducing agents, Fitzgerald et al. (30) observed a marked improvement in the maintenance of treponemal motility and the retention of virulence in cell-treponeme coincubation cultures. Fitzgerald et al. (30) coincubated *T. pallidum* with tumor-derived rat glial cells (C6), rabbit kidney (TRK-1 simian virus transformed cell), rabbit kidney cell (LLC-RK$_1$), rabbit epidermis (Sf$_1$Ep-NBL-11), normal rabbit testes (NRT), and human skin epithelium (HSE). The experiments were performed using confluent monolayers in T-30 flasks and 15 ml medium containing 5×10^7 suspended *T. pallidum* per milliliter. Cultures containing Sf$_1$Ep-NBL-11 cells maintained virulent microorganisms for at least 7 days in vitro and were superior in this function to all the other cell types examined.

Fieldsteel et al. (17,31) used cells derived from adult rabbit testes, adult human foreskin, human fetal lung, human fetal kidney, rat peritoneal macrophages, rat nose, rat footpad, mouse sarcoma, dog kidney, cottontail rabbit epithelium (Sf$_1$Ep), rabbit embryonic skin, rabbit cornea, and nude mouse ear fibroblasts. The cells were added to culture vessels (Leighton tubes or shell vials) with cover slips, sealed with silicone rubber stoppers, and incubated aerobically at 33°C for 2 to 3 days before use. Approximately 5×10^6 treponemes suspended in 1 ml medium were coincubated with cultured cells in vitro. The air was displaced with 5% CO_2 in H_2, sealed with a silicone rubber stopper, and incubated at 33°C. Cultures incubated in a horizontal position permitted treponemal survival (50% retention of motility) for 1 to at least 8 days, depending on the cell type. Cells derived from rabbit epithelium (Sf$_1$Ep) were superior to all other cell types examined. When the coincubation cultures containing Sf$_1$Ep cells and *T. pallidum* were incubated in a vertical position with enough medium to fill at least the lower 125 mm of the Leighton tubes, an oxygen and redox gradient was established to sustain treponemal motility and retention of virulence for up to 21 days (16). Further investigation using a more recent isolate of *T. pallidum* (strain KKJ, isolated in 1973) revealed no significant difference in the activity of this microorganism in the presence of Sf$_1$Ep cells compared to that observed for *T. pallidum* (Nichols virulent strain) (31). Survival of *T. pertenue* was enhanced in the gradient using the same type of coincubation system described above after examining a broad spectrum of diploid and heteroploid cells in vitro. *Treponema pertenue* maintained motility and virulence. An increase in the number of treponemes was observed to about the same extent with all the mammalian cell types employed (31).

Based on estimates of the numbers of attached microorganisms, Fieldsteel et al. (31) observed three- to five-fold increases in the numbers of motile microorganisms for at least 12 days in vitro. Modification of the cell culture system for incubation by utilizing 1.5% oxygen at 33°C permitted an 8- to 25.9-fold increase in the number of treponemes after 5 days of incubation (17). After 9 to 12 days, the numbers of treponemes increased 50-fold on the average and 100-fold maximally, starting with an original inoculum of 10^6 *T. pallidum* (17, see Table 3). There was no direct evidence that these increases were due to treponemal redistribution by translational motility. There was excellent correlation between assays for deoxyribonucleic acid and the estimates based on direct counts which further verified that *T. pallidum* had multiplied. Samples withdrawn from cell cultures after a 7-day incubation at 33°C were diluted to obtain as few as an average of 6.59 treponemes which retained virulence for the rabbit skin (17, Table 3). Serial cultivation of the treponemes using the shell vial system has not been achieved for any length of time (H. Fieldsteel, personal communications).

Table 3 Growth of *T. pallidum* in Tissue Cultures of Sf_1Ep [a]

Inoculum	Day of observation	Average number of treponemes × 10^7 per flask (range)	Average fold increase (range)	Motility (%) (range)	Micrograms of DNA per flask (mean ± SD)	DNA per treponeme × 10^{-14} g (mean ± SD)
10^6	5	1.59 (0.80-2.59)	15.9 (8.0-25.9)	90.5 (86.5-97.2)	0.64 ± 0.25	3.76 ± 0.70
	7[b]	3.27 (1.44-6.92)	32.7 (14.4-69.2)	87.8 (78.2-93.2)	0.99 ± 0.38	3.25 ± 0.97
	9	4.93 (2.29-9.69)	49.3 (22.9-96.9)	72.2 (38.1-89.1)	1.62 ± 0.54	3.43 ± 0.74
	12	4.91 (1.52-10.00)	49.1 (15.2-100.0)	30.6 (7.8-59.9)	ND[c]	ND
2.5×10^6	5	2.57 (1.81-3.99)	10.3 (7.2-16.0)	90.5 (86.3-94.3)	1.06 ± 0.31	3.91 ± 0.66
	7	4.97 (3.09-8.30)	19.9 (12.4-33.2)	89.2 (85.8-95.1)	1.60 ± 0.33	3.31 ± 0.50
	9	6.88 (4.00-10.0)	27.5 (16.0-40.0)	73.7 (59.9-91.8)	1.99 ± 0.53	2.96 ± 0.49
	12	6.06 (2.82-12.50)	24.3 (11.3-50.0)	28.4 (4.8-55.2)	ND	ND
10^7	1	1.00		ND	0.33 ± 0.04	3.30 ± 0.34
	5	4.95 (3.87-6.00)	5.0 (3.9-6.0)	88.2 (90.1-86.3)	1.51 ± 0.33	3.10 ± 0.80
	7	9.03 (8.10-11.30)	9.0 (8.1-11.3)	89.6 (85.1-93.8)	2.16 ± 0.24	2.41 ± 0.32
	9	11.76 (7.75-15.20)	11.8 (7.8-15.30)	71.8 (54.2-90.8)	2.56 ± 0.85	2.32 ± 0.18
	12	10.04 (6.57-13.50)	10.0 (6.6-13.5)	16.0 (5.3-35.6)	ND	ND
10^8	1	10.0		ND	2.02 ± 0.23	2.02 ± 0.23
	5	16.04 (13.80-21.00)	1.6 (1.4-2.1)	82.4-(75.2-87.5)	2.89 ± 0.75	1.66 ± 0.30
	7	17.48 (12.10-23.7)	1.7 (1.2-2.4)	76.6 (68.2-89.4)	2.93 ± 0.26	1.76 ± 0.46
	9	16.80 (14.50-18.60)	1.7 (1.5-1.9)	66.9 (60.4-72.9)	3.07 ± 0.55	1.83 ± 0.20
	12	13.41 (8.02-20.0)	1.3 (0.8-2.0)	13.7 (2.6-36.2)	ND	ND

[a]Combined data from seven separate experiments. SD, standard deviation.
[b]In each experiment, organisms taken at this time produced treponeme-containing lesions in rabbits. An average of 6.59 treponemes (range, 1.52 to 18.5) was required to produce a lesion.
[c]ND, not done.
Source: Reference 17.

Cell-Free Systems of Incubation for *Treponema pallidum* In Vitro

Investigators devising media for cell-treponeme cocultivation almost always reported having obtained results when treponemes were incubated in medium without cells. The most frequent observation was that the medium alone could not support treponemal survival as well as in the presence of cells. Exceptions to these observations were reported by Kiraly and Horvath (46), Horvath et al. (39), and Sandok et al. (20,24). Kiraly and Horvath (46) observed that their medium used under 7 mmHg O_2 permitted a more prolonged retention of motility by *T. pallidum* than cultures containing medium together with cells. Recently Horvath et al. (39) reported that all O_2 levels were detrimental to *T. pallidum*. Increases in treponemal floccules, which they believed to be growing treponemes, occurred less frequently or not al all under O_2 as opposed to under anaerobic conditions in their special medium. Sandok et al. (22) found that Eagle's MEM (34) plus a supplement with reducing agents was unsatisfactory for sustaining motility of the microorganism unless the medium was further enriched with rat glial cell by-products (spent cell culture medium). Subsequent work led to the substitution of spent cell culture medium with new medium containing a variety of supplemental nutrients, as shown in Table 1. The medium permitted maintainance of treponemal motility, virulence, and numbers (4 to 5 days) just as well as mammalian cell-treponeme cultures under similar conditions of incubation.

Norris et al. (35), using cell-free cultures, reevaluated a medium similar to that described by Fitzgerald et al. (23,30), who coincubated *T. pallidum* with a variety of cells. Normal rabbit serum (50%) appeared to protect the microorganism from deleterious effects of O_2. Reducing agents, glutathione, dithioerythritol, or dithiothreitol but not cysteine, enhanced treponemal survival under 3% O_2 but had no effect in cultures incubated under deoxygenated gases. Increasing amounts of dithiothreitol (DTT) up to 1.2 mM increased retention of treponemal motility under 3% O_2, but decreased motility retention under anaerobic conditions. Decreased motility retention of treponemes cultured under deoxygenated conditions was observed to be a function of excessively low redox potentials, as shown by Sandok et al. (22), using similar medium but different reducing agents, and by Graves et al. (13) using modified Nelson's medium (25). It is possible that the observations by Norris et al. (35) were due to oxidation of DTT (1 mM) under 3% O_2 resulting in the evolution of an optimal redox potential during the incubation period. Medium further supplemented with glutathione and cysteine was used to attempt to cultivate *T. pallidum* under oxygen. Reduced longevity of treponemal motility was observed compared to unsupplemented cultures of Norris et al. (35). Sandok et al. (22) suggested that DTT (0.324 mM) added to cultures containing glutathione (2 mM) and cysteine (0.206 mM) conferred no additional advantage (Table 4).

Miscellaneous Observations

Reproducibility of data between experiments, within the same laboratory or between laboratories, has always been a problem in treponemal research. Part of the problem may center around variations in treponemal viability as a function of harvests from different animals. Such

Table 4 Increase in Number and Survival of *Treponema pallidum* (Nichols Virulent Strain) In Vitro. Influence of Reduced Glutathione, Cysteine, and Dithiothreitol, Alone or in Combination in Cell-Free Cultures[a].

Incubation (hrs)	Motile *T. pallidum* $\times 10^6$ per milliliter				
	Glut[c]	Glut, DTT	Glut, DTT Cys[c]	Glut, DTT[c]	DTT[c]
0	8.0	7.7	9.0	7.4	9.2
24	10.7	17.1	15.8	15.8	10.4
48	18.0	21.6	23.6	20.2	20.9
72	20.3	20.5	20.2	12.0	21.8
192	0.0	ND[d]	ND[d]	0.0	7.9
216	0.0	4.4	7.1	0.0	ND[d]
240	0.0	ND[d]	ND[d]	0.0	2.0

[a]The treponemes were incubated in our new formula medium, $PRNF_{10}\text{-}B$, supplemented with 22.8 mg/liter glucuronic acid and 500 mg/liter fructose. Each culture tube containing 4.5 ml medium was inoculated with 0.5 ml suspension of approximately 8.0×10^7 *T. pallidum* per milliliter. The cultures were prepared under a constant flow of the gas combination of 95% O_2 + 5% CO_2 (80 cm^3/min) and 75% N_2 + 20% H_2 + 5% CO_2 (1250 cm^3/min). The tubes were stoppered and incubated at (34.0 ± 0.5)°C. All cultures were counted under dark-field microscopy and regassed at the intervals of time noted in the table.
[b]Estimates were based on counts from four cover slips prepared from two cultures. The standard error of the mean varied between 5 and 15% of the values given in the table.
[c]Glut = 307 mg/liter glutathione (2 mM); DTT = 50 mg/liter dithiothreitol (0.324 mM); Cys = 25 mg/liter cysteine (0.206 mM). The reducing agents were prepared alone or in the combinations given in the table at 50× concentration under deoxygenated nitrogen. The reduced compounds were dissolved in Hanks' balanced salt solution, sterilized at 215°F for 15-20 min, and incorporated into the unreduced medium in a volume to volume ratio of 2 ml reducing agent(s):100 ml medium.
[d]ND = not determined.
Source: Reference 24.

5. In Vitro Cultivation

variations could be due to shifts in the quantity or quality of proteins or mucopolysaccharides attached to the outer surface of the microorganism (44-50). Alternatively, components of cell culture media, whether freshly prepared from individual constituents or purchased partially prepared from reputable vendors, may be toxic for *T. pallidum* (16,31). Sandok's group (unpublished data) incubated *T. pallidum* with sera from a number of commercial sources in different systems of cultivation. As shown in Table 5, the time during incubation when peak increases in treponemal numbers were observed varied unpredictably. The influence of sera on peak numbers of microorganisms varied as a function of the system of incubation using only two of the four sera from different vendors of fetal or newborn calf serum. In the presence of sera from suppliers C and D, two-fold increases in the number of microorganisms did not occur 24 hr in vitro in the cell-treponeme coincubation system. Regardless of the source of the sera or condition of incubation, peak increases in the numbers of motile microorganisms were not significantly different from each other ($P \leq 0.05$, Student's t-test). Peak numbers of microorganisms were observed in cultures where the motile treponemes consisted of 83% of the population. The actual increases in treponemal numbers (motile plus nonmotile) exceeded by 5 to 17% the data shown in Table 5. These increases were not significant.

Fieldsteel et al. (51) tested the survival of *T. pallidum* coincubated with rabbit epithelial cells (Sf_1Ep) in their gradient culture system, using various lots of fetal calf serum as well as cell media from different commercial sources. Variable results were obtained from different vendors of sera and media. This means that components of the medium should be screened carefully against components known to support the motility, survival, and multiplication of *T. pallidum*.

In a cell-free system of cultivation, the effect of the serial transfer of medium every 24 hr was explored to determine when increases of numbers of *T. pallidum* might occur. Table 6 illustrates the results of such studies. The largest decreases in the numbers of motile microorganisms occurred after 72 to 96 hr in the same culture tube during the first four daily dilution transfers. Motile microorganisms were observed at least 3 days longer in cultures transferred three to seven times on a daily schedule. Several questions arose out of this study: Was something present in the original treponemal extract which was gradually removed by serial dilution during the course of the 24-hr serial transfers? Did toxic by-products of metabolism accumulate more rapidly than they could be diluted by transfer? Was there a basic growth factor missing or present in a nonoptimal concentration? For this particular experimental system, were the appropriate gas ratios present? Any one variable or combination of variables may be the key to the question of how to continuously grow *T. pallidum*.

As noted above, the serum used in medium is an additional uncontrollable variable in treponemal research. We performed several

Table 5 Influence of Sera from Different Vendors and Dithiothreitol on the Peak Time of Increase in Numbers of T. pallidum

System of incubation	Source of serum[a]							
	A		B		C		D	
	Increase[b]	Hours[c]	Increase	Hours	Increase	Hours	Increase	Hours
Coincubation[d]	2.9	72	2.8	144	1.5	48	1.7	48
Cell-free[e]	2.6	24	2.9	24	2.3	48	2.7	96
Cell free + DTT[f]	2.2	72	2.1	72	2.4	48	2.0	72
Cell-free transfers[g]	2.9	48	2.9	24	2.5	48	2.4	96

[a] Newborn calf sera were obtained from the following vendors: (A) Kansas City Biological Inc., Lexana, Kans.; (B) Grand Island Biological Co., Grand Island, N.Y.; and (C) Biologos, Inc., Naperville, Ill. The fetal calf serum was obtained from (D) Sterile Systems, Inc., Logan, Utah. The medium, PRNF$_{10}$-B, was prepared as described by Sandok (24) and supplemented with 10% serum.
[b] Increase = (peak numbers/ml)/(numbers/ml at t_0), where the inoculum at the beginning of the experiment (t_0) was at least 4.5×10^6 T. pallidum/per milliliter (8 to 9 T. pallidum per microscopic field at 400× magnification).
[c] Hours = time in hours during incubation when peak numbers were observed.
[d] Coincubation cultures contained human prepuce cells incubated with T. pallidum, incubated at 34°C under 3.8% O_2 + 5% CO_2 + 20% H_2 in nitrogen.
[e] Stoppered culture tubes containing 5 ml medium with suspended treponemes had 15-ml head space with 6% O_2 + 5% CO_2 + 20% H_2 in nitrogen.
[f] Cultures as described in (e) were prepared using medium supplemented with dithiothreitol; final concentration; 100 mg/liter.
[g] Cultures prepared as described in (e) were diluted 1:2 using fresh medium and transferred to new culture tubes after 24 and 48 hr.

Table 6 Multiplication and Survival of *Treponema pallidum* (Nichols Virulent Strain) In Vitro—Maintenance of *T. pallidum* after Dilution and Transfer of the Cultures Using Fresh Medium[a]

Incubation (hrs)	Motile *T. pallidum* × 10^6 per milliliter[b]								
	None[c]	1:2/1[c,d]	1:4/2	1:8/3	1:16/4	1:32/5	1:64/6	1:128/7	1:128/7
0	8.6	8.8							
24	11.7	12.7	10.8[e]						
48	24.2	23.0	22.4	23.7[e]					
72	18.9	21.5	19.0	12.6	12.5[e]				
96	16.7	22.0	18.9	24.8	20.3	14.4[e]			
120	0.6	6.7	13.4	19.3	15.5	11.2	11.0[e]		
144	0.0	0.7	4.2	10.6	11.0	7.6	8.0	5.1[e]	
168	0.0	0.0	0.7	8.0	5.9	8.9	5.5	5.1	3.4
192	0.0	0.0	0.0	3.0	1.3	2.1	3.4	3.4	1.7

[a] The treponemes were incubated in a new formula medium, PRNF10-B (24), supplemented with 22.8 mg/liter glucuronic acid and 500 mg/liter fructose. The electronegative potential of the medium was lowered using reduced dithiothreitol (86.4 mg/liter), cysteine (14.0 mg/liter), and glutathione (17.8 mg/liter). Each culture tube containing 4.5 ml medium was inoculated with 0.5 ml suspension containing approximately 8.7 v 10^7 *T. pallidum* per milliliter. The cultures were prepared under a constant flow of the gas combination 95% O_2 + 5% CO_2 (80 cm^3/min) and 75% N_2 + 20% H_2 + 5% CO_2 (1250 cm^3/min). The tubes were stoppered and incubated at $(34.0 \pm 0.5)°C$. All cultures were counted under dark-field microscopy every 24 hr. Two cultures were diluted 1:2 (volume to volume) every 24 hr using fresh medium to obtain four cultures having the same progressively higher dilution factor as the previous transfer. Two of the four cultures were retained undiluted, regassed, and counted every 24 hr thereafter.

[b] The standard error of the mean varied as a function of the decreasing numbers of microorganisms, from 5 to 10% for the highest counts to ±30% for the lowest. Estimates are based on two or four cultures, as described in (c) and (e). All estimates in the table are corrected for dilution.

[c] All estimates in the column are based on counts from eight cover slips prepared from four cultures.

[d] The volume to volume dilution expressed as a ratio a:x/number of times the cultures were transferred.

[e] Estimates were based on counts obtained from four cover slips prepared from two cultures after dilution and transfer at the interval of time given in the left column.

experiments to gauge the response of treponemes to serum-free medium. Some of this work was reported by Matthews et al. (52). Under deoxygenated gas, serum-free medium was supplemented with the sodium salts of fatty acids complexed to fatty acid-free bovine serum albumin (FAF-BSA). These media did not sustain the microorganisms as well as medium containing 10% serum. The effect of fatty acids was used under the usual mixture of gases with 6% O_2 (Table 7). When saturated or cis unsaturated fatty acids were excluded from the serum-free medium, the treponemes were rapidly killed. Paradoxically, the microorganism could tolerate molar ratios of saturated to cis unsaturated fatty acids of 1:1 complexed to FAF-BSA. In contrast, the trans isomer of oleic acid and elaidic acid, were nontoxic to *T. pallidum* when incubated as the sole fatty acid supplement. Mixtures of palmitic and oleic acids up to 80 µg/ml each were the least toxic combinations of fatty acids examined when complexed with 15 mg/ml FAF-BSA. Tween 40, Tween 60, and Tween 80 (fatty acid esters of polyoxyethylene

Table 7 Multiplication and Survival of *Treponema pallidum* (Nichols Virulent Strain) In Vitro—Influence of Supplementary Palmitic and Oleic Acids in Cell-Free Cultures[a]

Incubation (hr)	Motile *T. pallidum* × 10^6 per milliliter[b]	
	With fatty acids[c]	No fatty acids
0	8.1	7.4
24	11.2	11.0
48	16.5	19.7
72	21.2	17.0
96	19.4	12.8

[a]The treponemes were incubated in a new formula medium, $PRNF_{10}$-B, supplemented with 22.8 mg/liter glucuronic acid. Each culture tube containing 4.5 ml medium was inoculated with 0.5 ml suspension of approximately 7.5 × 10^7 *T. pallidum* per milliliter. The cultures were prepared under a constant flow of the gas combination 95% O_2 + 5% CO_2 (80 cm3/min) and 75% N_2 + 20% H_2 + 5% CO_2 (1250 cm3/min). The tubes were stoppered and incubated at (34 ± 0.5)°C. Cultures were counted under dark-field microscopy and regassed every 24 hr.
[b]Estimates were based on counts from four cover slips prepared from two cultures. The standard error of the mean varied between 5 to 15% of the values given in the table.
[c]Fatty acids, palmitic acid, and oleic acid were supplemented in the medium using 10 mg/liter each. The additions were made as the sodium salts of the fatty acids complexed with fatty acid-free bovine serum albumin, as described in Sandok et al. (24).
Source: Reference 52.

5. In Vitro Cultivation

sorbitan) were toxic. Auto-oxidized oleic acid lost its toxicity for treponemes, while at the same time it became toxic for baby hamster kidney cells (BHK-21). Since lipids in general play an important role in spirochetal growth, further work is required in this area to more definitively supplement the medium with appropriately solubilized lipids.

It is difficult to establish the nutrient requirements for *T. pallidum* when unknown nutrients are present in testicular tissue or fluid. H. M. Matthews, in our laboratory, devised a system of purification of the organism based on a series of sedimentations and resuspensions of treponemes resulting in the dilution of testicular fluids in excess of 1:63,000 (52, Table 8). This system of purification may be useful in identifying nutrients for *T. pallidum* without interference from testicular nutrients. Low-speed centrifugation, 250 g, of treponemal harvests sediments spermatozoa and large particulate debris, while the treponemes remain in the supernatant fluid [low-speed supernatant (LSS)] along with soluble testicular materials. The LSS was treated with a solution containing 40 mM glutathione to obtain 2 mM glutathione under deoxygenated gas. Tubes containing suspended treponemes were capped and centrifuged for 15 min at 15°C at 15,000 g. The microorganisms were pelleted by high-speed centrifugation to obtain the high-speed pellet (HSP) and the high-speed supernatant (HSS) fluid, enriched with dissolved testicular nutrients which were discarded. The pellets were resuspended in serum-free medium and treponemes derived from this treatment retained 90 to 95% motility for as long as 72 to 96 hr under 5% CO_2. The balance of the gases were 20% H_2 in N_2. This motility was similar to that of treponemes incubated in solutions with high amounts of testicular nutrients such as the LSS, or treponemes from the HSP resuspended in the HSS (Table 8).

When medium used for the incubation of treponemes obtained from the HSP was modified by deleting amino acids, ox serum ultrafiltrate, glutamine, and nonessential amino acids, the numbers of motile microorganisms decreased by 80 to 90% within 24 hr and disappeared by 72 hr [$PRNF_0$-B(M)] (Table 8).

There were unexplained variations between harvests using washed microorganisms. Sometimes when medium was used without serum for suspending and incubating the HSP microorganisms, we observed maintenance of treponemal motility equivalent to that of treponemes incubated in the LSS or HSS. At other times, treponemes derived from the HSP decreased in motility rapidly when incubated in the same medium (compare HSP under $PRNF_0$-B experiments 2 and 3, Table 8).

In summary, virulent treponemes which cause human disease have not yet been serially cultivated in a reproducible and continuous manner in vitro. Results obtained in the last decade permit some optimism that virulent *T. pallidum* will be serially cultivated. To date, a number

Table 8 Effect of Washing on Motility Retention by *T. pallidum* Incubated under an Atmosphere of 6% Oxygen in Medium Containing Serum and in Serum-Free Medium with and without Amino Acids[a]

Hours of incubation	Experiment 1[b] PRNF₀-B[d] Not washed			Washed + serum			Experiment 2[c] PRNF₀-B(M)[e] Not washed			Washed − serum			PRNF₀-B Not washed			Washed − serum			Experiment 3[c] PRNF₀-B(M) Not washed			Washed − serum			PRNF₀-B Not washed			Washed − serum			PRNF₁₀-B[d] Not washed			Washed − serum		
	LSS	HSP	HSS	LSS	HSP + HSP	HSS + HSS	LSS	HSP	HSS	LSS	HSP + HSP	HSS + HSS	LSS	HSP	HSS	LSS	HSP + HSP	HSS + HSS	LSS	HSP	HSS	LSS	HSP + HSP	HSS + HSS	LSS	HSP	HSS	LSS	HSP + HSP	HSS + HSS	LSS	HSP	HSS	LSS	HSP + HSP	HSS + HSS
0	59.5[f]	55.8	55.8	41.0	55.8	41.0	57.0	57.0	57.0	57.0	5.5	66.0	57.0	57.0	57.0	57.0	56.2	45.0	76.0	76.0	76.0	55.5	8.1	60.0	76.0	76.0	76.0	55.5	63.0	60.0	76.0	80.8	97.8	55.5	69.8	62.0
24	50.3	52.0	48.0	34.0	48.0	40.0	54.8	56.0	NC	5.5	NC	56.3	51.2	48.5	52.5	56.2	45.0	57.0	83.6	30.0	10.4	55.5	70.4	51.6	80.2	86.8	86.8	63.0	32.8	5.0	80.8	97.8	83.0	69.8	54.4	55.3
48	58.0	51.3	50.4	32.5	NC	37.5	56.0	NC	NC	NC	NC	NC	48.5	50.5	45.8	56.2	45.0	38.6	30.0	10.4	NC	5.3	14.8	NC	86.8	86.8	NC	32.8	5.0	NC	97.8	83.0	NC	54.4	55.3	NC
72	60.0	59.3	52.8	30.8	NC	37.4	40.8	NC	NC	58.3	NC	NC	50.5	22.3	49.2	45.8	38.6	NC	10.4	NC	NC	14.8	NC	NC	86.8	NC	NC	5.0	NC	NC	83.0	NC	NC	55.3	NC	55.6
96	NC[g]	NC	NC	NC	NC	NC	14.2	NC	NC	25.2	NC	NC	22.3	21.6	38.6	NC	NC	NC	NC	NC	NC	NC	NC	NC	NC	NC	NC	NC	NC	NC	NC	NC	NC	NC	NC	NC

[a] *Treponema pallidum* was extracted aerobically from infected rabbit testes by sequentially mincing the testicular tissue 8 to 12 times. The eluates (24 to 36 ml) were combined with prereduced balanced salt solution containing glutathione and centrifuged at 500 g for 10 min at 21°C. A portion of the low-speed supernatant (LSS) containing unwashed *T. pallidum* was inoculated into medium for incubation. A second portion of the LSS was centrifuged at 18,800 g for 15 min at 15°C to sediment *T. pallidum*. The high-speed supernatant (HSS) was removed from the high-speed pellet (HSP) of treponemes and saved. The HSP (= *T. pallidum*) was washed either one or two times by being suspended in 20 ml of reduced extraction medium followed by high-speed centrifugation as before. The final high-speed pellet of washed *T. pallidum* was suspended in 10 to 20 ml of reduced extraction medium and centrifuged at low speed as before to sediment aggregated tissue debris resulting from high-speed centrifugation. The resulting supernatant was used as the inoculum of washed *T. pallidum* designated as HSP. Some cultures in addition to being inoculated with washed HSP treponemes also received HSS material from the first centrifugation at 18,800 g. The HSS contained soluble and small particulate testicular material.

[b] In experiment 1, organisms were extracted in unreduced $PRNF_0$-B medium without serum. One-half of the extracted treponemes were washed one time with reduced $PRNF_0$-B medium, and the other half was washed with the same medium containing 10% calf serum. The washed pellets were then suspended in 8 ml of serum-free medium and further diluted 1:6 with the same medium before being inoculated into medium for the experiment. This procedure resulted in about 0.01% serum in cultures that had been washed with serum. Minimum tissue dilution in the final cultures was 1:63,000.

[c] In experiments 2 and 3, organisms were extracted in unreduced $PRNF_0$-B(M) medium without serum and washed two times in the same medium that had been reduced. Minimum tissue dilution in the final cultures was $1:1.4 \times 10^6$ in experiments 2 and 3, respectively.

[d] $PRNF_0$-B medium (24); serum free. $PRNF_{10}$-B medium contains 10% calf serum.

[e] $PRNF_0$-B(M) is modified serum-free $PRNF_0$-B medium lacking MEM essential amino acids, ox serum ultrafiltrate, glutamine, and nonessential amino acids.

[f] Motile *T. pallidum* $\times 10^5$ per milliliter.

[g] NC = not counted.

Source: Reference 52.

of investigators have exploited cell culture techniques resulting in increases of at least five times the initial numbers of treponemes with and without limited serial transfer (24,31). Particularly exciting is the recently reported work of Fieldsteel et al. (17), who observed up to a 100-fold increase of *T. pallidum* numbers with retention of virulence for at least 7 days but could not serially cultivate *T. pallidum*. Increases in numbers of *T. pallidum* seem to be most dependent on a delicate, undefined balance between oxygenation of the medium, the appropriate combination of reducing agents, oxidation products, and electronegative potential. Culture systems have been devised to permit treponemal synthesis of glycosominoglycans in vitro which may prove to be virulence factors of pathogenic *T. pallidum* (48,53).

Systems of purifying treponemes devised during the last decade will be useful for the further detection and identification of nutrients required by *T. pallidum*. It would seem at this time that a fruitful approach to cultivation of the microorganism would be to devise a system of incubation in which the temperature, pH, oxygenation, maintenance of electronegative potential, replenishment of used nutrients, and removal of toxic by-products will be controlled automatically using a chemostat system. Sandok and Jenkin (unpublished data) have developed such a model system and have obtained preliminary results suggesting that it can be used to attempt to grow *T. pallidum* with simultaneous control of these five variables. In the first crude experiments, motility of *T. pallidum* could be maintained for only 24 hr with no increase of organisms noted. Much manipulation of the variables will be necessary to make the quantum leap to grow virulent *T. pallidum* in a continuous passage flow-through system of cultivation.

Acknowledgments

This work was supported in part by Public Health Service research grant HL 08214 from the Program Project Branch, Extramural Programs, National Heart, Lung and Blood Institute; by U. S. Army Medical Research and Development Command contract #DAMD-17-81-C 1029; and by The Hormel Foundation.

References

1. J. Schereschewsky. Experimentelle Beitrage zum Studium der Syphilis. *Zentralbl. Bakteriol.* 47:41 (1908).
2. G. Volpino and A. Fontana. Einige Voruntersuchungen über kunstliche Kultivierung die Spirochaete pallida (Schaudinn). *Zentralbl. Bakteriol. I Abt. Orig.* 42:666-669 (1906).
3. E. Steinhardt. A preliminary note on *Spirochaeta pallida* and living tissue cells *in vitro*. *J. Am. Med. Assoc.* 61:1810 (1913).

4. C. Levaditi. Tentative de culture du tréponéme pâle en symbiose avec les éléments cellulaires. *C. R. Acad. Sci. 171*: 410 (1920).
5. M. I. Wright. Exploratory studies in tissue culture of *T. pallidum*. In *Proceedings of the XIIth International Congress on Dermatology*, Vol. 2 (D. M. Pillsbury and C. S. Livingwood, eds.), Excerpta Medica Foundation, Amsterdam, 1962, pp. 884-887.
6. T. B. Turner and D. H. Hollander. *Biology of the Treponematoses*. World Health Organization, Geneva, 1957.
7. R. R. Willcox and T. Guthe. *Treponema pallidum*: A bibliographical review of the morphology, culture and survival of *T. pallidum* and associated organisms. *Bull. WHO* 35:1-169 (1966).
8. R. M. Krause. Workshop on the biology of the treponemes. *J. Infect. Dis.* 125:332-336 (1972).
9. R. C. Johnson. *The Biology of the Parasitic Spirochetes*, Academic, New York, 1976.
10. R. C. Johnson. The spirochetes. *Annu. Rev. Microbiol.* 31:89-106 (1977).
11. J. B. Baseman. Summary of the workshop on the biology of *Treponema pallidum*: Cultivation and vaccine development. *J. Infect. Dis.* 136:308-311 (1977).
12. E. Canale-Parola. Physiology and evolution of spirochetes. *Bacteriol. Rev.* 41:181-204 (1977).
13. S. R. Graves, P. L. Sandok, H. M. Jenkin, and R. C. Johnson. Retention of motility and virulence of *Treponema pallidum* (Nichols strain) in vitro. *Infect. Immun.* 12:1116-1120 (1975).
14. R. H. Jones, M. A. Finn, J. J. Thomas, and C. Folger. Growth and subculture of pathogenic *T. pallidum* (Nichols strain) in BHK-21 cultured tissue cell. *Br. J. Vener. Dis.* 52:18-23 (1976).
15. N. S. Hayes, K. E. Muse, A. M. Collier, and J. B. Baseman. Parasitism by virulent *Treponema pallidum* of host cell surfaces. *Infect. Immun.* 17:174-186 (1977).
16. A. H. Fieldsteel, F. A. Becker, and J. G. Stout. Prolonged survival of virulent *Treponema pallidum* (Nichols strain) in cell-free and tissue culture systems. *Infect. Immun.* 18:173-182 (1977).
17. A. H. Fieldsteel, D. L. Cox, and R. A. Moechli. Cultivation of virulent *Treponema pallidum* in tissue culture. *Infect. Immun.* 32:908-915 (1981).
18. P. H. Hardy and E. E. Nell. Specific agglutination of *Treponema pallidum* by sera from rabbits and human beings with treponemal infections. *J. Exp. Med.* 101:367-382 (1955).
19. J. B. Baseman and N. S. Hayes. Anabolic potential of virulent *Treponema pallidum*. *Infect. Immun.* 18:857-859 (1977).

20. P. L. Sandok, H. M. Jenkin, S. R. Graves, and S. T. Knight. Retention of motility of *Treponema pallidum* (Nichols virulent strain) in an anaerobic cell culture system and in a cell-free system. *J. Clin. Microbiol.* 3:72-74 (1976).
21. J. C. Nichols and J. B. Baseman. Carbon sources utilized by virulent *Treponema pallidum*. *Infect. Immun.* 12:1044-1050 (1975).
22. P. L. Sandok, S. T. Knight, and H. M. Jenkin. Examination of various cell culture techniques for coincubation of virulent *Treponema pallidum* (Nichols I strain) under anaerobic conditions. *J. Clin. Microbiol.* 4:360-371 (1976).
23. T. J. Fitzgerald, J. N. Miller, and J. A. Sykes. *Treponema pallidum* (Nichols strain) in tissue cultures: Cellular attachment, entry, and survival. *Infect. Immun.* 11:1133-1140 (1975).
24. P. L. Sandok, H. M. Jenkin, H. M. Matthews, and M. S. Roberts. Unsustained multiplication of *Treponema pallidum* (Nichols virulent strain) in vitro in the presence of oxygen. *Infect. Immun.* 19:421-429 (1978).
25. R. A. Nelson, Jr., and J. A. Diesendruck. Studies on treponemal immobilizing antibodies in syphilis. *J. Immunol.* 66:667-685 (1951).
26. G. E. Kimm, R. H. Allen, H. J. Morton, and J. F. Morgan. Enhancement of survival in vitro of *Treponema pallidum* by addition of glucose and magnesium. *J. Bacteriol.* 80:726-727 (1960).
27. M. D. Weber. Factors influencing survival of *Treponema pallidum*. *Am. J. Hyg.* 71:401-417 (1960).
28. H. J. Morgan and G. P. Vryonis. A method for the quantitation of inocula in experimental syphilis. *Am. J. Syph. Gonorrhea Vener. Dis.* 22:462-469 (1938).
29. C. W. Artley and J. W. Clark, Jr. Statistical approach to evaluating the method of Morgan and Vryonis for enumerating *Treponema pallidum*. *Appl. Microbiol.* 17:665-670 (1969).
30. T. J. Fitzgerald, R. C. Johnson, J. A. Sykes, and J. N. Miller. Interaction of *Treponema pallidum* (Nichols strain) with cultured mammalian cells: Effects of oxygen, reducing agents, serum supplements, and different cell types. *Infect. Immun.* 15:444-452 (1977).
31. A. H. Fieldsteel, J. G. Stout, and F. A. Becker. Comparative behavior of virulent strains of *Treponema pallidum* and *Treponema pertenue* in gradient cultures of various mammalian cells. *Infect. Immun.* 24:337-345 (1979).
32. T. J. Fitzgerald, R. C. Johnson, and D. M. Ritzi. Relationship of *Treponema pallidum* to acidic mucopolysaccharides. *Infect. Immun.* 24:252-260 (1979).
33. H. J. Magnuson, H. Eagle, and R. Fleischman. The minimum infectious inoculum of *Spirochaeta pallida* (Nichols strain) and a

consideration of its rate of multiplication *in vivo*. *Am. J. Syph. Gonnorrhea Vener. Dis.* 32:1-8 (1948).
34. H. Eagle. Amino acid metabolism in mammalian cell cultures. *Science* 130:432-437 (1959).
35. S. J. Norris, J. N. Miller, J. A. Sykes, and T. J. Fitzgerald. Influence of oxygen tension, sulfhydryl compounds, and serum on the motility and virulence of *Treponema pallidum* (Nichols strain) in a cell-free system. *Infect. Immun.* 22:689-697 (1978).
36. A. Richter, K. K. Sanford, and V. J. Evans. Influence of oxygen and culture media on plating efficiency of some mammalian tissue cells. *J. Nat. Cancer Inst.* 49:1705-1712 (1972).
37. J. W. Foster, D. S. Kellog, J. W. Clark, and A. Balows. The *in vitro* cultivation of *Treponema pallidum* corroborative studies. *Br. J. Vener. Dis.* 53:338-339 (1977).
38. T. R. Turner. Cultivation of *Treponema pallidum*. *Br. J. Vener. Dis.* 53:337 (1977).
39. I. Horvath, W. P. Duncan, and J. C. Bullard. Cultivation of pathogenic *Treponema pallidum* in vitro. *Acta Microbiol. Acad. Sci. Hung.* 28:7-24 (1981).
40. C. D. Cox and M. K. Barber. Oxygen uptake by *Treponema pallidum*. *Infect. Immun.* 10:123-127 (1974).
41. P. G. Lysko and C. D. Cox. Terminal electron transport in *Treponema pallidum*. *Infect. Immun.* 16:885-890 (1977).
42. J. B. Baseman, J. C. Nichols, and N. S. Hayes. Virulent *Treponema pallidum* aerobe or anaerobe? *Infect. Immun.* 13:704-711 (1976).
43. E. I. Grin, M. Nadozdin, and M. Svob. Effects of hyperbaric oxygen on experimental syphilis in the rabbit. *Br. J. Vener. Dis.* 49:405-407 (1973).
44. I. Horvath, R. J. Arko, and J. C. Bullard. Effects of oxygen and nitrogen on the character of *T. pallidum* in subcutaneous chambers in mice. *Br. J. Exp. Vener. Dis.* 51:301-304 (1975).
45. T. Rathlev. Investigations on *in vitro* survival and virulence of *T. pallidum* under aerobiosis. *Br. J. Vener. Dis.* 51:296-300 (1975).
46. K. Kiraly and I. Horvath. Survival of *T. pallidum* under microaerobic conditions in cell and tissue cultures. *Zentralbl. Bakteriol. Hyg. I Abt. Orig. A.* 235:500-505 (1976).
47. S. Graves and T. Billington. Optimum concentrations of dissolved oxygen for the survival of virulent *Treponema pallidum* under conditions of low oxidation-reduction potential. *Br. J. Vener. Dis.* 55:387-893 (1979).
48. J. A. Ziegler, A. M. Jones, R. H. Jones, and K. M. Kubica. Demonstration of extracellular material at the surface of pathogenic *T. pallidum* cells. *Br. J. Vener. Dis.* 52:1-8 (1976).

49. J. F. Alderete and J. B. Baseman. Surface-associated host proteins on virulent *Treponema pallidum*. *Infect. Immun.* 26:1048-1056 (1979).
50. T. J. Fitzgerald and R. C. Johnson. Mucopolysaccharides of *Treponema pallidum*. *Infect. Immun.* 24:261-268 (1979).
51. A. H. Fieldsteel, J. G. Stout, and F. A. Becker. Role of serum in survival of *Treponema pallidum* in tissue culture. *In Vitro* 17:28-32 (1981).
52. H. M. Matthews, H. M. Jenkin, K. Crilly, and P. L. Sandok. Effects of fatty acids on motility retention by *Treponema pallidum* in vitro. *Infect. Immun.* 19:814-821 (1978).
53. T. J. Fitzgerald, R. C. Johnson, and E. T. Wolff. Mucopolysaccharide material resulting from the interaction of *Treponema pallidum* (Nichols strain) with cultured mammalian cells. *Infect. Immun.* 22:575-584 (1978).

Part II
Treponemal Infections

6
Syphilis and Yaws

DANIEL M. MUSHER
Baylor College of Medicine and Veterans Administration Medical Center
Houston, Texas

JOHN M. KNOX
Baylor College of Medicine
Houston, Texas

Syphilis 101
Yaws 114
References 115

Syphilis

Treponema pallidum is not found in the environment and is a natural pathogen only for man. As a result, with the extraordinarily rare exception of infection due to blood transfusion (1) or contact with infected laboratory animals (2), syphilis is acquired from an infected human being through intimate, usually sexual or venereal contact. An obvious exception is congenital syphilis, in which the fetus becomes infected by transplacental passage of *T. pallidum*. The infecting organism usually enters the body through abraded areas of the skin; although penetration through intact mucosal membranes has been postulated, the presence of inapparent breaks in these surfaces may still be responsible.

Once the organism has entered the tissues, two kinds of events occur simultaneously: (1) local replication and (2) escape from the local site with dissemination via lymphatics. The dividing time of *T. pallidum* has been estimated at 30-33 hr by measuring the number of treponemes in evolving syphilitic lesions (3); the actual dividing time is probably somewhat shorter, since this estimate did not consider the possibility of continued migration of treponemes out of the infected area. Organisms which escape from the initial site of infection may be trapped by regional lymph nodes or spread hematogenously throughout the body, setting the stage for secondary (disseminated) syphilis.

Primary Syphilis

Fourteen to twenty-one days after the initial infection, a red, painless papule 0.5 to 2 cm in diameter appears at the site of inoculation. The usual 2- to 3-week incubation period is supported by clinical and epidemiologic observations and by experimental studies in human subjects (4) or rabbits (3). A shorter incubation may be seen in the case of a particularly large inoculum of *T. pallidum*, and a longer one might reflect a small inoculum, an intense immune response in the lesion from which infection was acquired (3), partial immunity of the host due to earlier syphilitic infection (4), or other poorly defined host conditions.

Histologic examination of the papule reveals a relatively avascular center which contains large amounts of mucopolysaccharide and a few inflammatory cells, and a more peripheral infiltrated area containing polymorphonuclear leukoctyes, lymphocytes, and macrophages. Within a few days, the papule ulcerates, producing the typical chancre of primary syphilis, a dull-red ulcerated area sometimes covered by a slight yellowish or grayish exudate and usually surrounded by an indurated margin (Fig. 1). The chancre usually does not cause pain to the patient, but it may be somewhat tender when examined by the physician. Chancres may be round of elongated, following tissue lines. Enlargement of inguinal lymph nodes, frequently bilaterally, is observed in 80% of patients with a syphilitic chancre (5). As the papule evolves

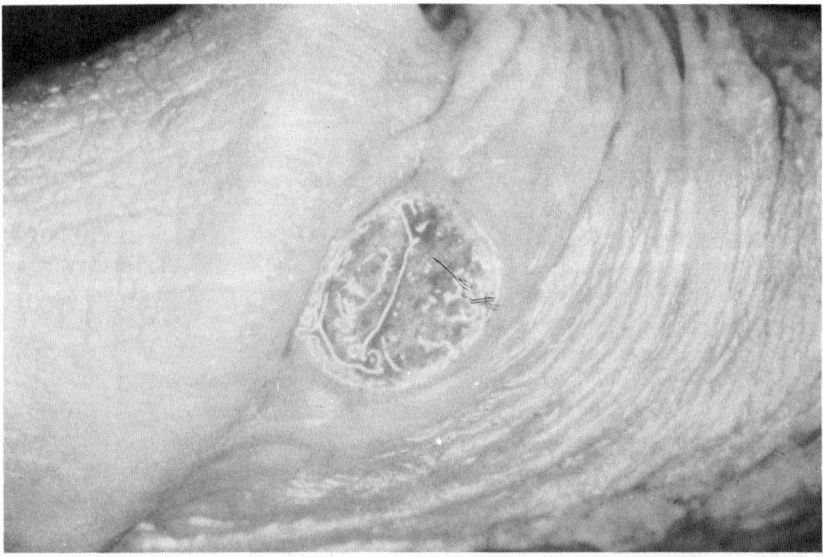

Figure 1 Solitary ("typical") syphiltic chancre.

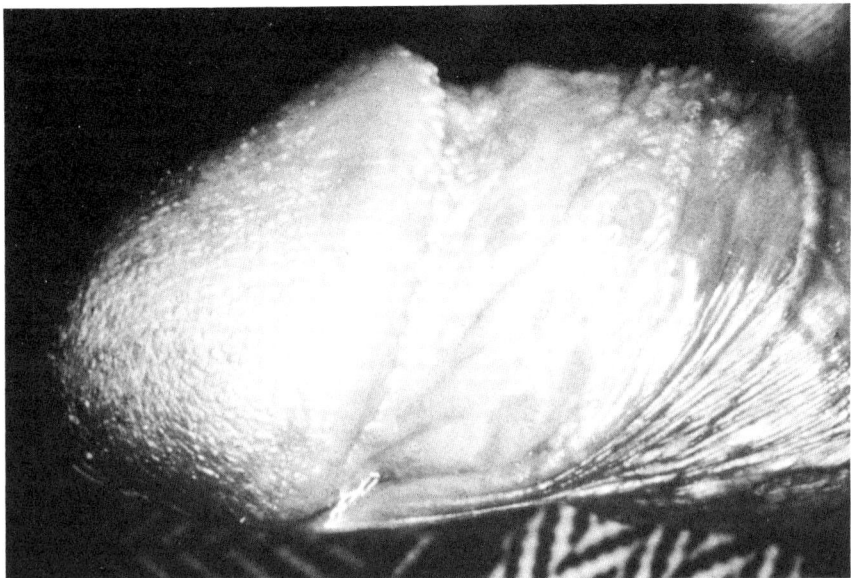

Figure 2 Multiple syphilitic chancres; diagnosis proven by dark-field examination.

into a chancre, the central area necroses and plasma cells and macrophages come to predominate at the periphery. Endothelial proliferation and perivascular infiltration by lymphocytes and plasma cells are characteristically present.

Because of their venereal origin, primary syphilitic chancres most frequently occur in the genital, perineal, or anal areas, or in and around the mouth; however, any part of the body may be affected. Although solitary lesions were once said to be characteristic, multiple lesions occur almost as often as solitary ones (Fig. 2) (5,6). Most chancres in men occur on the penis, and those in women on the labia, fourchette, and cervix. Chancres in the anus are particularly common in homosexual men; because they may cause pain on defecation and rectal bleeding, they can be confused with hemorrhoids or neoplasm (7,8). However, chancres are usually not painful when they occur on the labia or cervix or in the anus, and they often go unnoticed, in which case the diagnosis of primary infection is not made at all. In fact, the diagnosis of active syphilis in women or in homosexual men is usually not made in the primary stage.

Antibody to cardiolipin detected by the Veneral Disease Research Laboratories (VDRL) or rapid plasma reagin (RPR) reaction is present in 70-80% of patients at the time they seek attention for primary syphilis (9); antibody to treponemal antigen detected by the fluorescent treponemal antibody postabsorption with *Treponema phagedenis* (FTA-ABS) test is said to be present in up to 90% of patients with primary syphilis, although lower percentages have sometimes been reported (10-13). The VDRL reaction is conventionally reported with a titer; the titer is often low in primary infection. This antibody also appears in low titer in a variety of infectious and autoimmune states (14). The FTA-ABS and the more recently described hemagglutination tests (microtreponemal hemagglutination or MHA-TP test) are only rarely positive in the absence of syphilis (14). Once the FTA-ABS test becomes positive, it persists for many years, often throughout life; hemagglutinating antibody may become undetectable over a prolonged period after treatment. Because the VDRL reaction is only 80% sensitive and somewhat nonspecific, and the FTA-ABS or treponemal hemagglutination (TPHA) test, although highly sensitive, is not specific for an individual bout of syphilis (a positive test may indicate syphilitic infection any time in the past), the diagnosis of primary syphilis in an individual case is made definitively when treponemes are demonstrated by dark-field examination, a test which, when done properly, is very sensitive and nearly 100% specific.

The response of primary syphilitic lesions to treatment with penicillin is dramatic. Within a few hours treponemes disappear from the primary lesion, and over the next several days the chancre undergoes rapid involution. The VDRL reaction becomes negative within 3-6 months (15), although the FTA and TPHA tests remain positive, usually for life. Within 3-4 hr after treatment the Jarisch-Herxheimer reaction begins, characterized by fever up to 105°F, shaking chills, malaise, and transient hyperemia of the lesions. Fever reaches its peak at 4-8 hr and subsides by the end of 16 hr. If patients are monitored carefully, some form of this reaction is detectable in up to 50% of patients with primary syphilis and 90% of those with secondary syphilis (15a); a smaller percentage of patients will actually complain of symptoms. The role of endotoxin (16), an endotoxin-like substance (17), or immune complexes (18) is discussed in Chap. 9.

Secondary (Disseminated) Syphilis

If untreated, syphilitic chancres heal spontaneously within 3 to 8 weeks. The mechanism for healing is obscure; some kind of local immunity is probably responsible, since disseminated (secondary) lesions appear during or after the regression of the primary lesion. Some experimental observations favoring this concept include the following: (1) *Treponema pallidum* from a chancre have a substantially greater minimal infective dose than those from an infected lymph node (3); (2) regression of the lesions is associated with the appearance of T lymphocytes active against *T. pallidum* (19); and (3) systemic activation of acquired cellular resistance does not protect rabbits against chancre development, but local activation does (20-22). The so-called "secondary" lesions of syphilis appear as a result of the dissemination of treponemes from syphilitic chancres, and the term "disseminated syphilis" is probably more appropriate. At least 3 weeks, and often longer, elapse between deposition of T. *pallidum* in the dermis and emergence of these lesions. This delay in development beyond an incubation period of 21 days and the failure of each involved site to develop a lesion that resembles a primary chancre probably reflects a degree of humoral and/or cellular immunity which modifies the evolution of infection. Cases of "malignant" syphilis sometimes occur in which disseminated lesions all resemble primary chancres (23,24), a picture similar to that produced by intravenous injection of T. *pallidum* into nonimmune rabbits; host factors which permit this unusual manifestation of syphilis have not been identified.

The initial finding in disseminated syphilis is said to be an evanescent macular rash which is usually overlooked by the patient, especially if he is dark skinned. A few days later the characteristic widespread symmetric papular eruption is noted. The papules are discrete, and usually 0.5 to 2 cm in size; they may be smooth, follicular, or, rarely, pustular, although a scaly appearance is most common (Fig. 3 and 4). The eruption is red, dusky, or reddish brown. The entire trunk and the extremities including palms and soles are involved; lesions on the palms and soles are usually macular and reddish brown, although they may be hyperkeratotic or pustular (Fig. 5). Vesicles are said not to occur in the generalized lesions of secondary syphilis, although vesiculopustular lesions are seen on rare occasions (25) and may well have been the rule centuries ago when syphilis was called the great pox. Circular (annular) lesions are common in dark-skinned individuals, occurring predominantly on the face (26). Hypo- or hyperpigmentation may be seen (27). Mucosal lesions, either small, superficial ulcerated areas with grayish borders which resemble painless aphthous ulcers or larger gray plaques, also occur commonly (Fig. 6). Erosive gastritis has been documented in a rare instance (28). Condylomata (condyloma lata) are large, whitish confluent lesions which are found in warm, moist areas such as the axilla or groin (Fig. 7). Although classically described as a manifestation of disseminated syphilis, condylomata may be seen in the perineal area before generalized lesions appeared; in either case they are secondary to the local spread of treponemes in a favorable environment, whether from a primary chancre or from disseminated skin lesions.

Secondary lesions have a varied histologic appearance (29,30). Inflammatory cells are regularly seen, but the nature of the inflammation varies considerably from case to case. Some lesions have the so-called classical appearance, with plasma cells being the prominent cells. Frequently, however, a mixed infiltrate is present including lymphocytes, macrophages, and polymorphonuclear leukocytes, and any of these

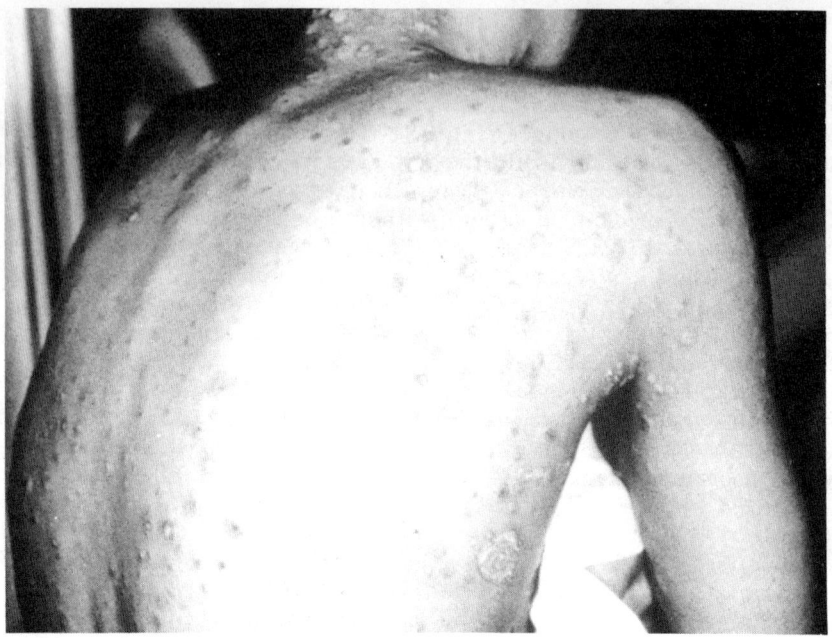

Figure 3 Disseminated syphilis. Scaly lesions resembling psoriasis or pityriasis rosea.

cells may predominate. In one recent study (30), microabscesses were seen in 20% of secondary lesions. In some cases, macrophages predominate, producing a picture suggestive of histiocytosis (30,31). True granulomas with giant cells may also be seen, especially in more chronic lesions, although caseation does not occur. Classically, there is endothelial cell proliferation or swelling with perivascular cuffing in the inflammatory infiltrate. However, there appears to be some difference of opinion on how frequently vascular dilation, the enlargement of vascular endothelial cells, and perivascular inflammation are present (29,30). Follicles and sweat glands are frequently involved and may be the focal point for histologic abnormalities, in which case alopecia may result (Fig. 8).

Disseminated or secondary syphilis is a systemic disease, and interest in the dematologic manifestations should not prevent the physician from recognizing findings such as the malaise, low-grade fever, and diffuse, painless lymph node enlargement which are usually present. The initial manifestation may even be prolonged fever of unknown origin (32). Other symptoms of generalized involvement include a sore

6. Syphilis and Yaws

throat, headache, and arthralgias. Recent studies suggest that pain in the joints may be due to synovitis, and structures resembling treponemes have been detected in synovial tissues (33,34). Bones are commonly involved. Periosteal inflammation was said to be clinically apparent in one-quarter of cases in the pretreatment era (35), with the skull, tibia, sternum and ribs being most frequently involved; a more recent study showed skull roentgenograms to be abnormal in 9% of patients with secondary syphilis (36). Several different kinds of lesions may occur (37), and even in the modern era symptomatic disease is occasionally present (38-40).

Perhaps as many as 10% of patients with secondary syphilis have a subclinical nonspecific hepatitis detectable by laboratory studies and supported by biopsy (41-44). Occasionally a full-blown symptomatic hepatitis results, although it is difficult in an individual case to exclude the coincidental occurrence of viral hepatitis. Histologic examination of the liver has shown focal inflammation with lymphocytes, polymorphonuclear cells, and occasional epithelial cells; true granuomas have not been observed.

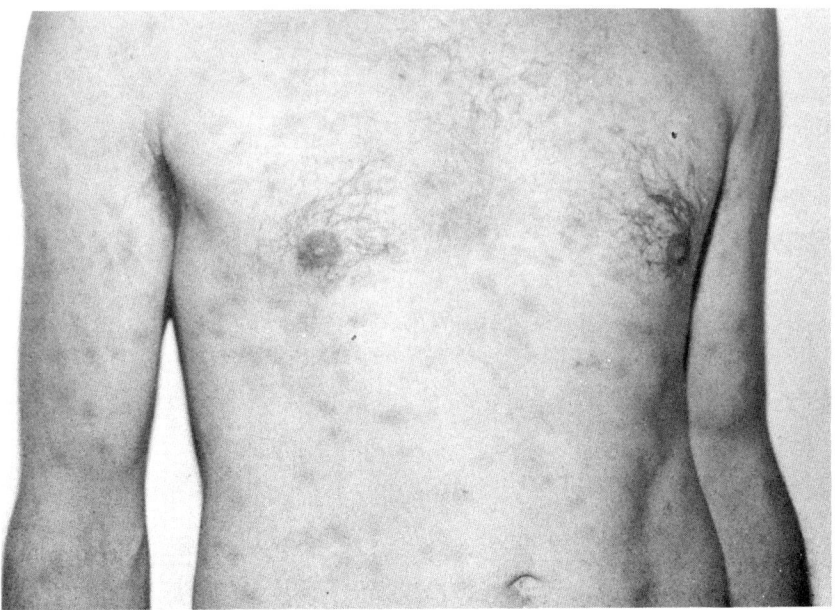

Figure 4 Disseminated lesions of secondary syphilis with a more acutely inflamed, less scaly appearance compared with that shown in Figure 3. (*Source*: courtesy of Dr. Baylor Kurtis, Houston, Texas.)

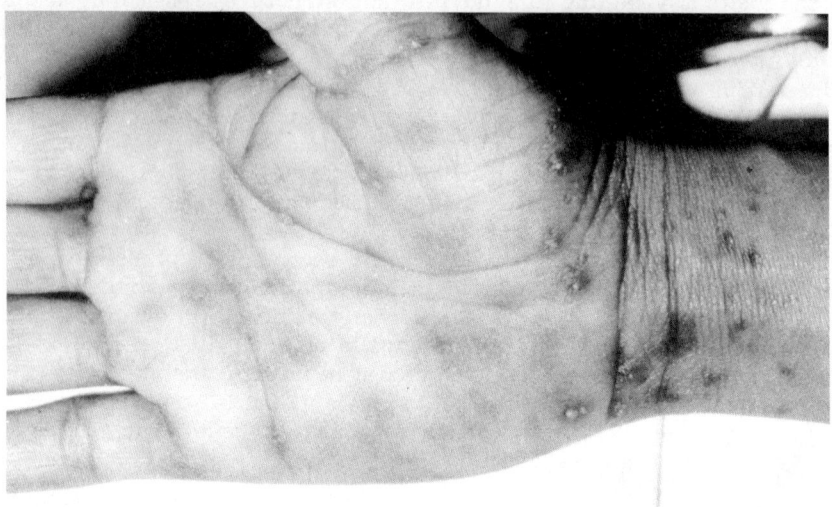

Figure 5 Pustular lesions on palms in disseminated syphilis. (*Source:* courtesy of Dr. Baylor Kurtis, Houston, Texas.)

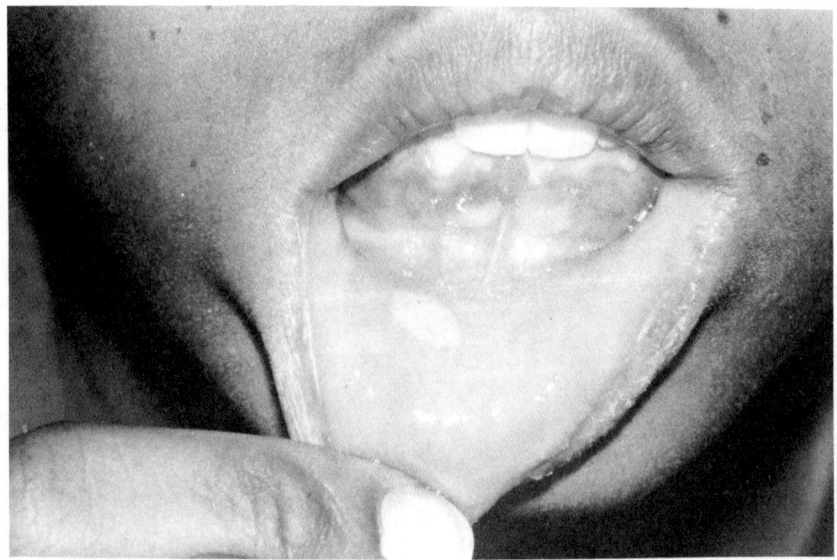

Figure 6 A mucous patch. Mucosal lesion characteristic of seondary syphilis.

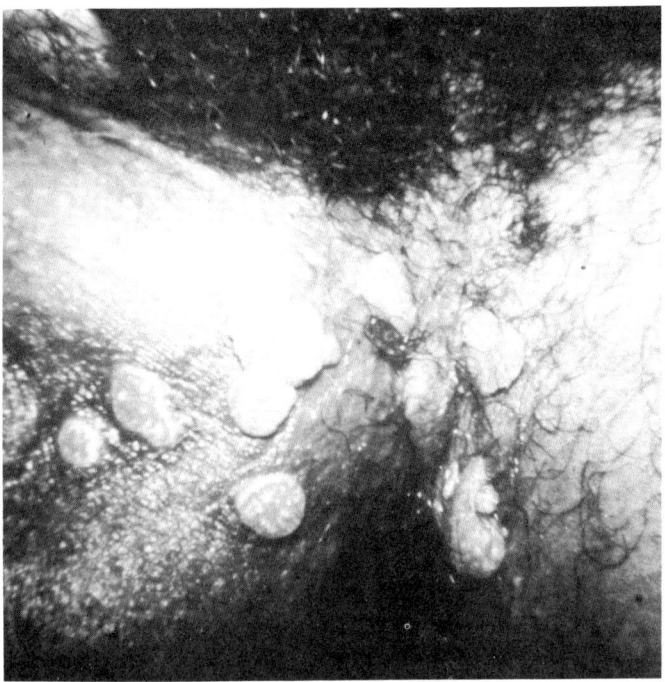

Figure 7 Condylomata observed in the perineal area of a patient who had not yet developed disseminated syphilitic lesions.

Iritis, anterior uveitis, and signs of meningeal inflammation also occur in secondary syphilis. Nephrotic syndrome has been recognized and is presumably due to antigen-antibody deposition in the glomerulus (45-48); a picture more closely resembling that of glomerulitis, both clinically and histologically, may also occur (47). The diagnosis of secondary syphilis is readily supported by laboratory studies. The VDRL and RPR reactions are uniformly positive, usually in high titer ($\geq$ 1:16); the FTA-ABS and TPHA tests are also always positive. A recent report has suggested that the VDRL reaction will be negative in nearly all cases with 2 to 4 years of treatment (49).

Latent Syphilis

The natural history of untreated secondary syphilis is to resolve spontaneously after a period of 3 to 12 weeks, leaving the patient free of lesions and without symptoms. When treatment has not been given, this naturally attained asymptomatic stage is called latency. In the pretreatment era, 20% of patients used to develop relapses, with recurrence of a full-blown picture of secondary syphilis (50). In over 90% of cases, these relapses occurred within 1 year of the onset of latency; accordingly, this period is called early latency. Relapses after this time were very rare; thus after 1 year without a recurrence of disease and before the onset of tertiary syphilis, untreated subjects are said to have entered the late latent period. It has long been recognized that patients with late latent syphilis are immune to reinfection with *T. pallidum* (4).

At the present time, patients are said to have latent syphilis if they have a reactive VDRL in the absence of any apparent signs of disease and if a test for specific antitreponemal antibody is positive. These individuals probably still represent a heterogeneous group in regards

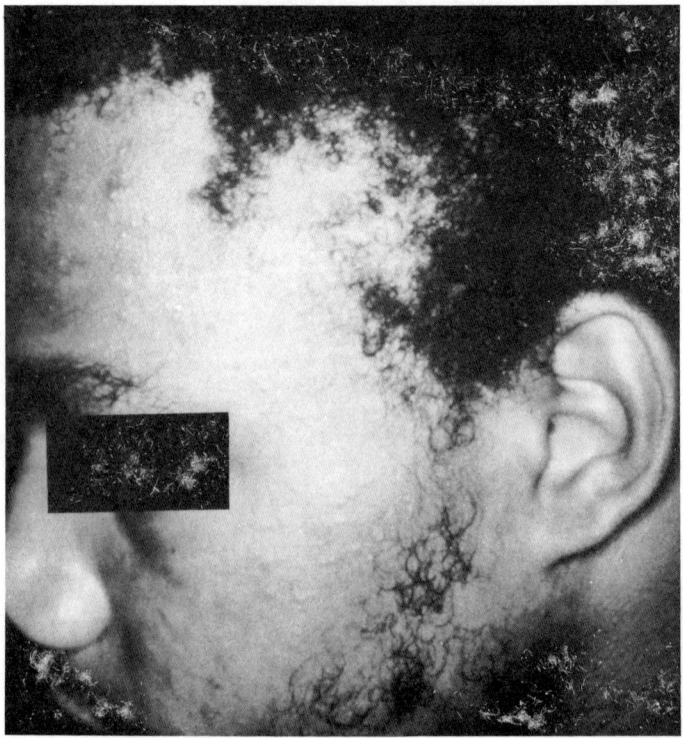

Figure 8 In this patient alopecia was the only manifestation of secondary syphilis. He had a history of venereal exposure to an infected individual, recent development of alopecia, and a VDRL test reactive at 1:256 dilution.

6. Syphilis and Yaws

to their syphilitic infection. Some may have an unrecognized chancre and others may have had resolution of an unrecognized chancre but not yet had the development of disseminated disease. With the widespread availability of antibiotics, other subjects may have persistence of antibodies after having received partial or even adequate antibiotic treatment at a time when syphilis was not recognized (41). Others may retain VDRL antibody despite cure of the infection (a "serofast" state), although some authorities believe that the VDRL reaction always reverts to normal after treatment of primary or secondary syphilis, taking 1 or 2 years, respectively, to do so (15,26). At the present time the majority of patients with a reactive VDRL and FTA-Abs but not signs of syphilitic infection probably do not have true latent infection as defined by the entirely spontaneous resolution of secondary syphilis. Although interest in naturally acquired immunity and the pathogenesis of infection should lead to questions about the diagnosis of latent syphilis in this situation, it is probably best, from a public health point of view, to treat all such patients as if they actually have latent syphilis.

Tertiary Syphilis

Clinical manifestations of tertiary syphilis develop after a highly variable time period which is dependent, in large measure, upon how carefully an examination is made to detect them (52); usually more than 1 year of latency elapses before late syphilis is detectable. Similarly, the incidence of late or tertiary syphilis varies greatly with how the diagnosis is established. Of a large group of patients who were observed with untreated syphilis for many years, late benign syphilis became clinically apparent in 15%, and cardiovascular syphilis in 10 to 25% (50-52). However, a substantially higher percentage of patients may develop cardiovascular syphilis, and some cardiovascular abnormalities attributable to syphilis have been said to be present at autopsy in up to 80% of affected subjects (53).

"Benign late syphilis" is a term used when nonvital structures such as skin, soft tissue, bones, and cartilage or certain parenchymal organs such as the liver or testes are involved. Lesions are characterized by prominent endothelial proliferation and infiltration of the involved tissues by plasma cells, lymphocytes, histiocytes, and fibroblasts. True granulomas are present with epithelioid and giant cells, and central necrosis is frequently seen; these lesions are called gummas.

Benign late syphilis most commonly involves the skin and subcutaneous tissues; lesions usually occur singly, although asymmetric involvement of a few areas may occur simultaneously. The face, neck, and extremities are most commonly affected. Indurated, noduloulcerated lesions which describe an arc of an irregular full circle are characteristic. Peripheral hyperpigmentation is seen and there is often central scarring. These lesions may be indolent or aggressive; frequently tissue destruction with ulceration results, producing small nodular ulcers which may progress to large confluent ulcerated areas (54,55). If untreated, these may persist for several years. Late syphilis of the bone affects the tibia, fibula, clavicle, and skull, although any bone or multiple areas of bone may be involved. The symptoms of pain and swelling, which are nearly always present, are consistent with the periosteal location of the granulomatous reaction. Destruction of cartilage also plays an important part in determining the clinical appearance of lesions. Large granulomas or gummas of the viscera may be asymptomatic or cause symptoms referable to the organ involved; the liver and testes are most commonly affected. In this form of disease the VDRL reaction is usually positive.

Syphilitic involvement of the vasa vasorum of the aorta with resulting medial necrosis of the aorta produces a spectrum of diseases under the general category of syphilitic aortitis. The majority of patients are asymptomatic. Clinical syndromes that used to be observed relatively frequently and that still occur occasionally include aortic insufficiency, left ventricular hypertrophy, congestive heart failure, and aneurysm of the ascending aorta, sometimes with erosion into the bones of the thorax (56-58). Involvement of the coronary artery ostia occasionally causes symptoms of the ischemic heart disease. Syphilis of the aorta is recognized radiographically by calcifications in the ascending aorta or by an aneurysm of the ascending aorta with or without erosion of adjacent bones. At autopsy, the proximal aorta has a shaggy appearance and the aortic valve is dilated (59). Microscopic examination shows the presence of patchy destruction of the media and obliterating endarteritis of the vasa vasorum with plasma cell infiltration (60). Syphilitic aneurysm may occur years after active disease of the aorta has subsided, probably resulting from continued mechanical stress in an already damaged vital area. This observation is consistent with the finding that the VDRL reaction is negative in one-third of patients at the time that syphilitic disease of the aorta is diagnosed (61). An interesting but unexplained observation is the syphilitic disease of the aorta does not appear in patients who contracted their infection before adolescence.

The pathogenesis of these lesions of late syphilis is obscure. Reports that claimed to identify treponemes in tertiary lesions were based on the silver staining of tissue sections, which tended to produce false positive results (Thomas B. Turner, personal communication, 1979); this is not to say that organisms are definitely not present. Rather than reflecting a response to the presence of large numbers of treponemes, some other kind of poorly defined immunologic reaction is thought to be responsible. The antigenic stimulus is particulary difficult to understand because of the lack of apparent relation between the location of primary or disseminated lesions and the eventual location of gummas. Tertiary skin involvement tends to occur in areas that are frequently traumatized such as the elbows, but the way in which trauma contributes to the development of lesions remains obscure.

A discussion of late syphilis of the nervous system is beyond the scope of this chapter. Suffice it to say that neurosyphilis may cause one of a number of syndromes, including tabes dorsalis, paresis, dementia, or meningitis, or a mixed picture including features of more than one of these syndromes, depending upon which part(s) of the nervous system is/(are) involved. Proving a diagnosis of neurosyphilis or, for that matter, being certain that existing literature includes only proven cases may be exceedingly difficult. The clinical picture is nonspecific; the VDRL reaction in the cerbrospinal fluid may be negative in a substantial percentage of cases and the cerebrospinal fluid is entirely normal in 10-15% of patients who are thought to have the disease (62-65). The FTA-ABS test gives false positive results in the cerebrospinal fluid of an appreciable percentage of syphilitic patients who are not thought to have neurosyphilis (66-68). The pathogenesis of infection is even less well understood than that of other lesions of late syphilis; a further complicating factor is that the central nervous system is, to some extent, immunologically privileged.

Congenital Syphilis

Congenital syphilis is the major exception to the general rule that syphilis usually develops as a result of venereal contact with an infected person. This infection is acquired by transplacental passage of *T. pallidum* from an infected pregnant woman to her fetus. Infection is said not to occur until after the fourth month, and not to be common until after the sixth month of pregnancy (69), when atrophy of the Langhans cell layer permits passage of the treponeme. A recent study has shown light-microscopic structures resembling *T. pallidum* to be present in aborted fetuses in the 9th to 10th week (70). Hager (71) has hypothesized that treponemes may regularly be present in the fetus early in pregnancy but that the search for characteristic syphilitic lesions has been unsuccessful because of the immunologic immaturity of the fetus. Since the fetus acquires infection directly by the hematogenous route, it is not surprising that widespread disseminated disease occurs. Stillbirth may occur, or the newborn may be born with a variety of signs of disseminated disease. An enlarged liver and spleen and hematologic abnormalities are present in nearly all affected infants, and the lymph nodes are enlarged in more than one-half of the cases. Radiologic and histologic findings of periostitis and osteochondritis can be found in nearly all patients. Generally the disease appears in the second to sixth week of life. The first symptom is usually sniffles resulting from involvement of the mucous membranes; skin lesions and mucous patches then appear. The infant may also be febrile. Ultimately, in the absence of treatment, wasting develops, culminating in marasmus and death. This set of symptoms is rapidly reversed by treatment (72).

Late manifestations of congenital syphilis are those which appearance after two years of age. They are divided into two kinds: (1) "stigmata", which become apparent with the development of structures such as the teeth and long bones but actually result from early damage to these tissues by the congenital infection (these changes are prevented completely by treatment before the third month of life); and (2) other late manifestations which resemble, by analogy, the lesions of late (tertiary) syphilis in the adult in that their pathogenesis is obscure and continued signs of inflammation are present in involved tissues. These manifestations include lesions of the eye (keratitis and uveitis) and skin, gummas of the nasal and facial bones, periostitis, and central nervous system disease.

Congenital syphilis used to be extremely common, and two interesting sets of observations, well-documented many years ago, provided early lessons on immunity in syphilis. In 1837 Colles observed that wet nurses who suckled infants with congenital syphilis developed lesions of the nipple, but that their natural mothers did not. A second observation, also made in the 19th century, by Kassowitz noted that as a woman's syphilis progressed without treatment from active disease into late latency, she became progressively less infectious to subsequent progeny, an indication that spirochetemia was prevented by evolving immunity (72).

Yaws

Infection caused by *Treponema pertenue*, yaws or frambesia, has nearly been eradicated, due in large measure to the intensive campaign waged against it by the World Health Organization beginning in the early 1950s. Nevertheless, this disease remains of great interest to those who study the immunology of treponemal infection because of at least three major reasons: (1) The causative organism is indistinguishable from *T. pallidum* morphologically (Chap. 1), serologically, or by analysis of DNA homology (Chap. 3); (2) the disease state, both in terms of clinical manifestations and its prolonged course with early and late manifestations, closely resembles that of syphilis, although there are a few notable exceptions (73,74); and (3) an experimental model of yaws in the hamster is currently being used to study the immunology of treponemal infection (Chap. 7).

Transmission of yaws is nonvenereal, generally occurring among children in hot and humid climates, where open lesions on the skin are common, little clothing is worn, and personal hygiene is poor (75,76). The incubation period is about 3 weeks (range 10-45 days), at the end of which time a solitary primary lesion 2 to 5 cm in diameter appears. These primary lesions are usually proliferative or papillomatous, and they exude serous fluid containing large numbers of treponemes. Ulcerative lesions are sometimes seen. The pathology is similar to that seen in primary syphilis, with edema and cellular infiltration by polymorphonuclear leukocytes, plasma cells, and lymphocytes (73).

Secondary yaws is a systemic disease resulting from the widespread dissemination of treponemes. Patients have fever, systemic symptoms, headache, and widespread skin lesions which resemble those of secondary syphilis, although they are often larger and more exuberant (73, 77). The tendency toward exuberant lesions on the body and disabling hyperkeratosis of the soles of the feet may reflect conditions of the climate, hygiene, and/or undetermined host factors. Secondary bacterial infection and, in the case of plantar lesions, walking barefoot also modify the clinical presentation (73). Just as in the case of primary infection, histologic examination of secondary lesions shows changes that are indistinguishable from those of secondary syphilis. Condylomata occur in the groin and around the anus. Lymphadenopathy is usually absent. Bones of the hands, feet, and wrists and particularly the tibia have painful lesions due to periostitis, and cortical rarefaction may be detected radiographically. A recent study in Surinam (78), a hot but dry country, demonstrated the prevalence of "attenuated" lesions of yaws (79) perhaps due to differences in climate; these lesions more closely resemble the typical skin lesions of secondary syphilis.

Many patients appear to undergo spontaneous cure of secondary yaws, with disappearance of lesions 6-8 months after their onset. For unknown reasons, in some subjects the disease progresses into tertiary stages characterized by gummatous lesions of the skin and soft tissues, bones, and cartilage of the nasal septum and palate. These lesions may be indistinguishable from those of tertiary syphilis (73). Strikingly different from tertiary syphilis is the absence of cardiovascular involvement or disease of the central nervous system. With regard to the former it should be noted that the age of onset of yaws is often quite young and that cardiovascular syphilis does not occur when the infection is contracted in childhood; nevertheless, acquisition of yaws later in life also is not associated with disease of the aorta. One final difference which is potentially of great interest pathogenetically is that, for unknown reasons, congenital yaws has not been documented.

References

1. J. V. Klauder and T. Butterworth. Accidental transmission of syphilis by blood transfusion. *Am. J. Syph. Gonorrhea Vener. Dis.* 21:652-666 (1937).
2. T. J. Fitzgerald, R. C. Johnson, and M. Smith. Accidental laboratory infection with *Treponema pallidum*, Nichols strain. *J. Am. Vener. Dis. Assoc.* 3:76-78 (1976).

3. H. J. Magnuson, H. Eagle, and R. Fleischman. The minimal infectious inoculum of spirochaeta pallida (Nichols strain), and a consideration of its rate of multiplication in vivo. *Am. J. Syph. Gonorrhea Vener. Dis.* 32:1-18 (1948).
4. H. J. Magnuson, E. W. Thomas, S. Olansky, B. I. Kaplan, L. de Mello, and J. C. Cutler. Inoculation syphilis in human volunteers. *Medicine* 35:33-82 (1956).
5. T. A. Chapel. The variability of syphilitic chancres. *Sex. Trans. Dis.* 5:68-70 (1978).
6. A. Notowicz and H. E. Menke. Atypical primary syphilitic lesions on the penis. *Dermatologica* 147:328-333 (1973).
7. M. M. Nazemi, D. M. Musher, R. F. Schell, and S. Milo. Syphilitic proctitis in a homosexual. *J. Am. Med. Assoc.* 231:389 (1975).
8. L. M. Drusin, C. Singer, A. J. Valenti, and D. Armstrong. Infectious syphilis mimicking neoplastic disease. *Arch. Inter. Med.* 137:156-160 (1977).
9. M. B. Moore, Jr., and J. M. Knox. Sensitivity and specificity in syphilis serology: Clinical implications. *South. Med. J.* 48:963-968 (1965).
10. M. F. Garner, J. L. Backhouse, G. Daskalopoulos, and J. L. Walsh. *Treponema pallidum* haemagglutination test for syphilis. Comparison with the TPI and FTA-Abs tests. *Br. J. Vener. Dis.* 48:470-473 (1972).
11. P. O'Neill, R. W. Warner, and C. S. Nicol. *Treponema pallidum* haemagglutination assay in the routine serodiagnosis of treponemal disease. *Br. J. Vener. Dis.* 49:427-431 (1973).
12. J. Lesinski, J. Krauch, and E. Kadziewicz. Specificity, sensitivity, and diagnostic value of the TPHA test. *Br. J. Vener. Dis.* 50:334-340 (1974).
13. A. H. Rudolph. The microhemagglutination assay for *Treponema pallidum* antibodies (MHA-TP), a new treponemal test for syphilis: Where does it fit? *J. Am. Vener. Dis. Assoc.* 3:3-8 (1976).
14. D. M. Musher and R. E. Baughn. Syphilis. In *Immunological Diseases*. 3rd ed., Vol. 1 (M. Samter, ed.). Little Brown, and Co. Boston, Massachusetts, 1978, pp. 639-650.
15. N. J. Fiumara. The treatment of seropositive primary syphilis: An evaluation of 196 patients. *Sex. Transmit. Dis.* 4:92-95 (1977).
15a. T. Putkonen, O. P. Salo, and K. K. Mustakallio. Febrile Herxheimer reaction in different phases of primary and secondary syphilis. *Br. J. Vener. Dis.* 42:181-184 (1966).
16. J. A. Gelfand, R. J. Elin, F. W. Berry, and M. M. Frank. Endotoxemia associated with the Jarisch-Herxheimer reaction. *N. Eng. J. Med.* 295:211-213 (1976).

17. Butler, T. P. Hazen, C. K. Wallace, S. Awoke, and A. Habte-Michael. Infection with *Borrelia recurrentis*: Pathogenesis of fever and petechiae. *J. Infect. Dis. 140*:665-675 (1979).
18. K. W. M. Fulford, N. Johnson, C. Loveday, J. Storre, and R. S. Tedder. Changes in intra-vascular complement and anti-treponemal antibody titres preceding the Jarisch-Herxheimer reaction in secondary syphilis. *Clin. Exp. Immunol. 24*:483-491 (1976).
19. S. A. Lukehart, S. A. Baker-Zander, R. M. C. Lloyd, and S. Sell. Characterization of lymphocyte responsiveness in early experimental syphilis. II. Nature of cellular infiltration and *Treponema pallidum* distribution in testicular lesions. *J. Immunol. 124*:461-467 (1980).
20. R. E. Baughn, D. M. Musher, and J. M. Knox. Effect of sensitization with *Propionibacterium acnes* on the growth of *Listeria monocytogenes* and *Treponema pallidum* in rabbits. *J. Immunol. 118*:109-113 (1977).
21. R. E. Baughn, D. M. Musher, and C. B. Simmons. Inability of spleen cells from chancre-immune rabbits to confer immunity to challenge with *Treponema pallidum*. *Infect. Immun. 17*:535-540 (1977).
22. P. H. Hardy, Jr., D. J. Graham, E. E. Nell, A. M. Dannenberg, Jr. Macrophages in immunity to syphilis: Suppressive effect of concurrent infection with *Mycobacterium bovis* BCG on the development of syphilitic lesions and growth of *Treponema pallidum* in tuberculin-positive rabbits. *Infect. Immun. 26*:751-763 (1979).
23. J. W. Petrozzi, N. A. Lockshin, B. J. Berger. Malignant syphilis. Severe variant of secondary syphilis. *Arch. Dermatol. 109*:387-389 (1974).
24. K. Lejman and Z. Starzycki. Early malignant syphilis observed during infection and reinfection in the same patient. *Br. J. Vener. Dis. 54*:278-282 (1978).
25. R. J. Pariser and K. A. Mehr. Pustules in secondary syphilis. *Sex. Transmit. Dis. 5*:115-118 (1978).
26. P. S. Friedman and D. J. Wright. Observations on syphilis in Addis Ababa. 2. Prevalence and natural history. *Br. J. Vener. Dis. 53*:276-280 (1977).
27. R. K. Pandhi, T. R. Bedi, and L. K. Bhutani. Leucoderma in early syphilis. *Br. J. Vener. Dis. 53*:19-22 (1977).
28. W. C. Butz, J. C. Watts, S. Rosales-Quintana, and M. D. Hicklin. Erosive gastritis as a manifestation of secondary syphilis. *Am. J. Clin. Pathol. 63*:895-900 (1975).
29. P. Jeerapaet and A. B. Ackerman. Histologic patterns of secondary syphilis. *Arch. Dermatol. 107*:373-377 (1973).

30. E. Abell, R. Markes, and E. W. Jones. Secondary syphilis: A clinicopathological review. *Br. J. Dermatol.* 93:53-61 (1975).
31. R. E. I. Cochran, J. Thomson, K. A. Fleming, A. M. M. Strong. Histology simulating reticulosis in secondary syphilis. *Br. J. Dermatol.* 95:251-254 (1976).
32. D. M. Musher. An unusual case of FUO. *Hosp. Pract.* 13(10): 134-135 (1978).
33. J. C. Gerster, A. Weintraub, T. L. Vischer, and G. H. Fallet. Secondary syphilis revealed by rheumatic complaints. *J. Rheumatol.* 4:197-200 (1977).
34. A. J. Reginato, H. R. Schumacher, S. Jimenez, and K. Maurer. Synovitis in secondary syphilis. Clinical, light and electron microscopic studies. *Arthritis Rheum.* 22:170-176 (1979).
35. U. J. Wile and F. E. Senear. A study of the involvement of the bones and joints in early syphilis. *Am. J. Med. Sci.* 151:689-693 (1916).
36. R. G. Thompson and R. H. Preston. Lesions of the skull in secondary syphilis. *Am. J. Syph.* 36:332-341 (1952).
37. I. Ehrlich and M. E. Krican. Radiographic findings in early acquired syphilis: Case report and critical review. *Am. J. Roentgenol.* 127:789-792 (1976).
38. W. E. Dismukes, D. G. Delgado, S. V. Mallernee, and T. C. Myers. Destructive bone disease in early syphilis. *J. Am. Med. Assoc.* 236:2646-2648 (1976).
39. R. R. Tight and J. F. Warner. Skeletal involvement in secondary syphilis detected by bone scanning. *J. Am. Med. Assoc.* 235:2326 (1976).
40. R. N. Shore, H. A. Kiesel, and H. D. Bennett. Osteolytic lesions in secondary syphilis. *Arch. Intern. Med.* 137:1465-1467 (1977).
41. H. J. Sobel, E. H. Wolf, and N. J. Passaic. Liver involvement in early syphilis. *Arch. Pathol.* 93:565-568 (1972).
42. J. Feher, T. Somogyi, M. Timmer, and L. Jozsa. Early syphilitic hepatitis. *Lancet* 2:896-899 (1975).
43. L. Jozsa, M. Timmer, T. Somogyi, and J. Feher. Hepatitis syphilitica. A clinico-pathological study of 25 cases. *Acta Hepatogastroenterol.* 24:344-347 (1977).
44. A. McMillian, J. R. Anderson, and D. H. Robertson. Hepatitis in early syphilis. Report of three cases. *Br. J. Vener. Dis.* 53:295-298 (1977).
45. W. F. Falls, Jr., K. L. Ford, and C. T. Answorth. The nephrotic syndrome in secondary syphilis: Report of a case with renal biopsy findings. *Ann. Intern. Med.* 63:1047-1058 (1965).
46. G. D. Braunstein, E. J. Lewis, E. G. Galvanek, A. Hamilton, and W. R. Bell. The nephrotic syndrome associated with secondary syphilis. *Am. J. Med.* 48:643-648 (1970).

47. M. S. Bhorade, H. B. Carag, H. J. Lee, E. V. Potter, and G. Dunea. Nephropathy of secondary syphilis. A clinical and pathological spectrum. *J. Am. Med. Assoc. 216*:1159-1166 (1971).
48. B. S. Kaplan, F. W. Wiglesworth, M. I. Marks, and K. N. Drummond. The glomerulopathy of congenital syphilis — An immune deposit disease. *J. Pediatr. 81*:1154-1156 (1972).
49. N. J. Fiumara. The treatment of secondary syphilis: An evaluation of 204 patients. *Sex. Transmit. Dis. 4*:96-99 (1977).
50. E. G. Clark and N. Danbolt. The Oslo study of the natural course of untreated syphilis. An epidemiologic investigation based on a re-study of the Boeck-Bruusgaard material. *Med. Clin. North Am. 48*:613-623 (1964).
51. W. R. Gschwandtner and J. Zelger. Latent syphilis. *Z. Hautkr. 41*:735-741 (1976).
52. J. E. Kemp and K. D. Cochems. Studies in cardiovascular syphilis: Influence of treatment of early syphilis upon incidence of cardiovascular syphilis. *Am. J. Syph. Gonorrhea Vener. Dis. 21*:625-633 (1937).
53. R. H. Kampmeier. The late manifestations of syphilis: Skeletal, visceral and cardiovascular. *Med. Clin. North Am. 48*:667-697 (1964).
54. S. Olansky. Late benign syphilis (gumma). *Med. Clin. North Am. 48*:653-665 (1964).
55. S. Olansky and L. C. Norins. Venereal diseases: Syphilis and other treponematoses. In *Dermatology in General Medicine* T. B. Fitzpatrick et al. Eds. McGraw-Hill, New York, 1971, pp. 1955-1989.
56. T. A. Prewitt. Syphilitic aortic insufficiency. Its increased incidence in the elderly. *J. Am. Med. Assoc. 211*:637-639 (1970).
57. R. J. Weiser, Jr., and R. J. Marshall. Syphilitic aneurysms with bone erosion and rupture. *W. V. Med. J. 72*:1-4 (1976).
58. W. Grabau, R. Emanuel, D. Ross, J. Parker, and M. Hedge. Syphilitic aortic regurgitation. An appraisal of surgical treatment. *Br. J. Vener. Dis. 52*:366-373 (1976).
59. K. Hiraoka, S. Okawa, and M. Suguira. Clinico-pathological study of the syphilitic aortic regurgitation in the aged. *Jpn. Heart J. 14*:22-31 (1973).
60. H. A. Heggtveit. Syphilitic aortitis. A clinicopathologic autopsy study of 100 cases, 1950 to 1960. *Circulation 29*:346-355 (1964).
61. S. Olansky and L. C. Norins. Current serodiagnosis and treatment of syphilis. *J. Am. Med. Assoc. 198*:165-168 (1966).
62. H. Hooshmand, M. R. Escobar, and S. W. Kopf. Neurosyphilis, a study of 241 patients. *J. Am. Med. Assoc. 219*:726-729 (1972).
63. R. D. Catterall. Neurosyphilis. *Br. J. Hosp. Med. 17*:585-604 (1977).

64. O. J. Kolar and J. E. Burkhart. Neurosyphilis. *Br. J. Vener. Dis.* 53:221-225 (1977).
65. L. Luxon, R. J. Greenwood, and A. J. Lees. Neurosyphilis today. *Lancet* 1:90-93 (1979).
66. M. R. Escobar, H. P. Dalton, and M. J. Allison. Fluorescent antibody tests for syphilis using cerebrospinal fluid: Clinical correlation in 150 cases. *Am. J. Clin. Pathol.* 53:88-90 (1976).
67. H. W. Jaffe, S. A. Larsen, M. Peters, D. F. Jove, B. Lopez, and A. L. Schroeter. Tests for treponemal antibody in CSF. *Arch. Intern. Med.* 138:252-255 (1978).
68. G. LeClerc, M. Giroux, A. Birry, and S. Kasatiya. Study of fluorescent treponemal antibody test on cerebrospinal fluid using nonspecific anti-immunoglobulin conjugates IgG, IgM and IgA. *Br. J. Vener. Dis.* 54:303-308 (1978).
69. A. L. Dippell. The relationship of congenital syphilis to abortion and miscarriage, and the mechanism of intrauterine protection. *Am. J. Obstet. Gynecol.* 47:369-379 (1944).
70. C. Harter and K. Benirschke. Fetal syphilis in the first trimester. *Am. J. Obstet. Gynecol* 124:705-711 (1976).
71. W. D. Hager. Transplacental transmission of spirochetes in congenital syphilis: A new perspective. *Sex. Transmit. Dis.* 5:122-123 (1978).
72. D. Ingall and D. M. Musher. Syphilis. In *Infectious Diseases of the Fetus and Newborn Infant*, 2nd ed. (J. S. Remington and J. O. Klein, Eds.). W. B. Saunders, Phildelphia, 1983.
73. H. U. Williams. Pathology of yaws, especially the relation of yaws to syphilis. *Arch. Pathol.* 20:596-630 (1935).
74. J. Wilson. Syphilis and yaws: Diagnostic difficulties and case reports. *N. Z. Med. J.* 78:18-21 (1973).
75. C. J. Hackett. The transmission of yaws in nature. *J. Trop. Med. Hyg.* 60:159-168 (1957).
76. T. Guthe. Clinical, serological and epidemiological features of Framboesia tropica (yaws) and its control in rural communities. *Acta Derm. Vener.* 49:343-368 (1969).
77. P. E. C. Manson-Bahr. Treponematoses. In *Manson's Tropical Diseases*, 17th ed. (C. Wilcocks and P. E. C. Manson-Bahr, Eds.). Williams and Wilkins, Baltimore, Maryland, 1972, pp. 559-583.
78. P. L. Niemel, E. A. Brunings, and H. E. Menke. Attenuated yaws in Surinam. *Br. J. Vener. Dis.* 55:99-101 (1979).
79. G. C. Ramsay. The influence of climate and malaria on yaws. *J. Trop. Med. Hyg.* 28:85-86 (1925).

7
Rabbit and Hamster Models of Treponemal Infection

RONALD F. SCHELL
Hahnemann University School of Medicine
Philadelphia, Pennsylvania

The Rabbit Model   122
The Hamster Model   126
Relevance to Human Disease   131
References   132

Despite the wealth of clinical, diagnostic, and therapeutic information available on treponemal disease in humans (Chap. 6), more remains to be learned before the treponematoses can be eradicated from the world. Animal models are becoming increasingly important for elucidating the mechanisms of pathogenesis and immunity. Such models increase our understanding of the basic infectious process by providing data not otherwise obtainable, since the experimentation cannot be done in humans. Transmission of treponemal disease to lower animals enables a detailed exploration of the host-parasite relationship. The host's pathologic, physiologic, and immunologic responses can be monitored and modified at the cellular and molecular level. Findings derived from animal models, however, can become clinically relevant only to the degree that the experimental disease mimics the infectious process and pathogenesis of the disease in humans.

Fortunately treponemal research is endowed with two animal models, the rabbit and the hamster, which respond rapidly to infection with virulent treponemes and develop a clinical syndrome reasonably analogous to treponemal disease in humans. Other animals, such as guinea pigs (1), mice (2-5), rats (6), monkeys, and apes (7), can also be used. In those species, however, clinical manifestations of treponemal disease cannot be regularly induced, or else the labor and expense of handling makes them less suitable for laboratory investigations. Studies dependent upon the production of clinical manifestations are therefore limited to the rabbit and the hamster. Important future investigations may focus on the inherent mechanisms in the other species which prevent the induction of overt treponemal disease.

The Rabbit Model

The rabbit is considered the animal model of choice for investigation of treponemal infection (8). This preference is based partly on the historical development of treponemal research. Rabbits were first successfully inoculated with *Treponema pallidum* in the anterior chamber of the eye by Haensell (9) in 1881. The ability to produce keratitis was confirmed in 1906 by Bertarelli (10), who also successfully transferred the disease between rabbits. Parodi (11) in 1907 demonstrated that rabbits are susceptible to intratesticular infection. Nichols (12), Hoffmann (13), and Noguchi (14) showed that *T. pallidum* could be readily propagated in the testes of rabbits.

In the 1920s Brown and Pearce (15-22) firmly established the rabbit as the animal model of choice with their classic description of the clinical picture of experimental treponemal disease in this species. Turner and associates (23-29) placed further emphasis on the rabbit by making improvements in experimental designs and clarifying the role of environmental, pathologic, and immunologic factors affecting the course of the disease. The failure of other animal models (mice, rats, and guinea pigs) to develop symptomatic disease after infection with *T. pallidum* spurred investigators to concentrate research on the rabbit.

Rabbits can be easily infected with virulent *T. pallidum* by inoculation of the eye, blood, skin, testes, or scrotum. Testicular, cutaneous, or intravenous inoculations are used almost exclusively. The route of inoculation depends upon the design of the experiment. Testicular inoculation is used frequently to infect animals and to transfer the organism between rabbits, thereby maintaining the treponemes' pathogenicity, since virulent treponemes cannot be cultivated in vitro. The host's immunologic status is generally determined by intravenous or intracutaneous inoculation (Chaps. 13-15). The latter routes produce characteristic local or generalized lesions that can be quantitated. Absence or delay of the appearance of these lesions, or the development of atypical lesions, may demonstrate the induction of resistance in vaccinated or infected rabbits.

Development of syphilitic lesions can be observed most readily after intracutaneous inoculation of a rabbit's shaved back. The lesions usually become visible over periods ranging from a few days to several months, although the absence of a lesion does not preclude infection. Temperature greater than 70°F, the quality and number of organisms, and the strains of rabbit and treponeme can influence the appearance of lesions. The minimal infective inoculum varies from one to five virulent treponemes (30,31). Izzat et al. (31) showed that the time required for formation of cutaneous lesions varied inversely with the size of the inoculum. Intracutaneous inoculations of 10^6, 10^5, 10^4, and 10^3 motile *T. pallidum* induced chancres (syphilomata) approximately 6, 10, 13, and 16 days after infection, respectively. In general the incubation period increases by approximately 3 to 4 days with each 10-fold decrease in inoculum.

Lesions induced by cutaneous inoculation are characteristically indurated and surrounded by erythema. During the early stage of development the lesion is well circumscribed and elevated, with a flat surface. Both induration and size increase rapidly for 10 or 12 days before obliterative endoarteritis causes local ischemia with necrosis and ulceration. The lesion may then regress and heal with minimal scarring. Complete resolution may require 10 days to 8 weeks. Cutaneous infection with *Treponema pertenue* elicits less of a reaction. The lesion is raised and erythemic, seldom ulcerates, and heals within 2 to 3 weeks after appearance.

After intravenous infection with 10^7 *T. pallidum* generalized lesions develop within approximately 17 to 21 days and involve all external areas (Fig. 1) Orchitis with extreme scrotal edema develops in about 28 days. The cutaneous lesions may coalesce and begin to regress 35 to 40 days after infection.

Intratesticular inoculation usually results in orchitis. After a quiescent period of 7 to 10 days the entire testicle becomes swollen and enlarged, followed by marked scrotal edema. The scrotum and scrotal sac contain gelatinous material or clear serous fluid which coagulates quickly. Fitzgerald and assoociates (32-34) have shown this material to be a mucopolysaccharide with immunosuppressive activity. Within a few days the congestion and edema subside. The syphilitic testicle is nodular and often becomes ulcerated; some nodular epididymitis may remain after the testicular lesion has healed. Testicular infection with *T. pertenue* produces tiny miliary nodules on the tunic of the testis. This granular periorchitis occurs about 21 to 28 days after infection and is one of the most characteristic features distinguishing frambesial from syphilitic rabbits.

Local multiplication and dissemination of treponemes to regional lymph nodes and blood occur soon after treponemal infection, regardless of the route of inoculation (8). Raiziss and Severac (35) recovered *T. pallidum* from blood within minutes after intratesticular inoculation. Treponemes were recovered within 2 hr from the dermis after inoculation of the intact mucous membrane. Hematogenous and lymphatic spread carry treponemes to the liver, spleen, bone marrow, testes,

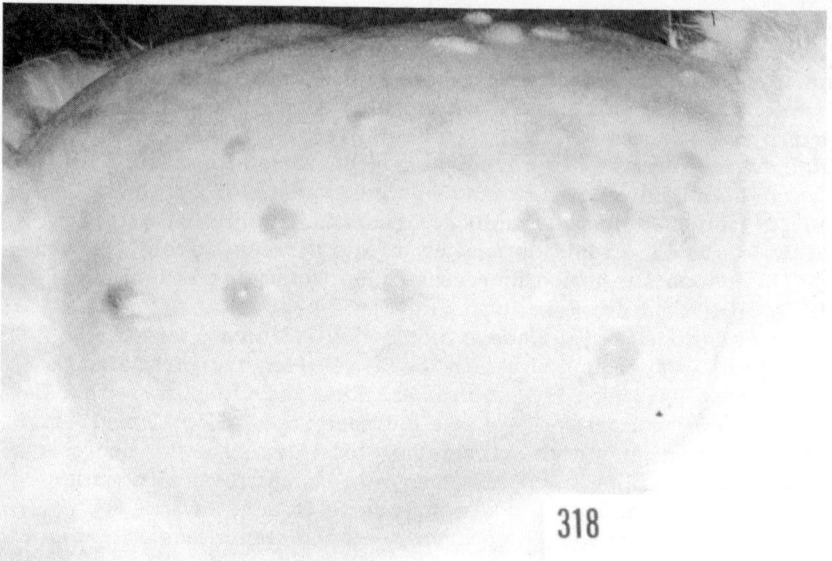

Figure 1 Syphilitic lesions 28 days after intravenous infection with 10^7 Treponema pallidum.

and other organs. Metastatic lesions involving the bones of the foreleg, metatarsals, nose, base of the ears, and tail have been reported (18,36-38). Visceral lesions occur only rarely. In contrast, generalized lesions in rabbits infected with T. pertenue are limited to bone (39).

During the early stage of infection treponemal multiplication is not appreciably influenced by immune factors. Since treponemes multiply every 24 to 33 hr, considerable numbers can be obtained by extracting the testis with tissue culture medium 7 to 12 days after infection. Turner and Hollander (8) calculated that there were 2×10^8 treponemes in a rabbit's testicle 22 days after infection with 10^5 T. pallidum. The number of treponemes isolated depends upon the quality of the inoculum and the duration of syphilitic infection. If the testicles are harvested after peak orchitis, the number of treponemes recovered is reduced precipitously. A 10-fold or greater increase in the spirochetal content of the rabbit testicle can be achieved by administration of adrenocorticosteroid. Brause et al. (40) have shown that treatment with methylprednisolone reduces testicular mononuclear cell infiltration while increasing the treponemal content of the testes 660%.

Serologic reactivity is one of the most consistent findings in treponemally infected rabbits. Their sera are reactive in three serologic tests—the Venereal Disease Research Laboratory (VDRL), fluorescent treponemal antibody absorption (FTA-ABS), and *Treponema pallidum* immobilization tests (TPI)—by the time their testicular or cutaneous syphilomas have fully developed. Both VDRL and FTA-ABS antibodies can be detected within 2 weeks of infection. VDRL antibody titers increase to an early peak (64 to 256) 3 to 5 weeks after infection and thereafter rapidly decline. TPI and FTA-ABS antibodies peak approximately 2 to 4 months after infection, but only FTA-ABS antibodies are regularly detected 8 to 12 months after infection.

Although several kinds of antibodies can be demonstrated, the exact nature of their contribution to immunity is not yet clear (Chap. 13). The results of in vitro serologic assays do not correlate with the state of immunity in experimental treponemal disease. Repeated injections of killed treponemes into rabbits, for example, leads to development of antibodies but usually does not confer protection against challenge with virulent treponemes.

It is generally accepted that rabbits begin to develop resistance within 3 weeks of infection. In untreated rabbits resistance gradually increases during subsequent weeks. Between 3 and 6 months after infection they develop complete resistance to cutaneous reinfection with treponemes; however, if infection is terminated by treatment with penicillin in less than 3 months, the rabbits can be consistently reinfected (8).

Paradoxically rabbits cannot eradicate treponemes after primary infection, even though they develop resistance. During a prolonged course of primary treponemal disease rabbits acquire complete resistance to exogenous reinfection; yet they are incapable of eradicating the primary infectious agent from regional lymph nodes, cerebral spinal fluid, or aqueous humor. Lymph nodes are regularly found to be infectious (8) by inoculating this tissue into normal animals. Frazier et al. (41,42) also demonstrated that after an infection had been asymptomatic for 1 or 2 years, blood remained intermittently infectious for at least another 3 years.

An area that merits further investigation is cross-resistance in the rabbit to infection with *T. pallidum*, *T. pertenue*, and other virulent treponemes. These organisms have not been distinguished by morphologic or immunologic criteria or by hybridization studies and antibodies produced in response to these infections. Some investigators believe that the treponemes are identical and that differences in expression result from varying host responses, perhaps mediated in part by climatic conditions; others propose that although the virulent treponemes evolved from a common precursor, they now have biologic differences.

Human patients with frambesia are protected against syphilis (43-45), and rabbits infected with frambesia or syphilis show some resistance to challenge with heterologous treponemes (46,47). There is also evidence that infection of rabbits with *T. pallidum* Nichols induces cross-immunity to *T. pallidum* Bosnia A, the causative agent of endemic syphilis. Turner and Hollander (48) inoculated rabbits intratesticularly with the Nichols strain. Between 3 and 4 months after infection the rabbits were challenged intradermally with Bosnia A. No lesions developed, although control rabbits developed characteristic lesions. Similar results were obtained when rabbits were infected with the Nichols strain and challenged with another strain of endemic *T. pallidum*, Bosnia B. Turner and Hollander concluded that both Bosnia strains are closely related immunologically to the Nichols strain.

Demonstration of cross-immunity suggests that similar or identical mechanisms of resistance are induced by the virulent treponemes (Chap. 17). This relationship must be clarified before a general or specific vaccine can be developed.

The Hamster Model

The nature of the immune response to treponemal infection is still poorly understood (Chaps. 13-18). A major obstacle has been the unavailability of a suitable inbred animal model for elucidating the roles of humoral and cell-mediated immunity. With outbred animals the efficacy of the treponemal immune cells or serum in recipients cannot be guaranteed due to allogeneic differences. Although the rabbit is considered the animal model of choice, inbred rabbit strains are not readily available.

We have shown that the inbred LSH/Ss LAK strain of hamster is especially suitable for studies of passive transfer of resistance to infection with the agent of endemic syphilis (49,50). Use of the hamster for studies of treponemal disease had been virtually ignored during the last two decades because clinical manifestations of syphilis cannot be regularly induced (8). Inbred LSH hamsters, however, develop extensive chronic skin lesions after infection with *T. pallidum* Bosnia A. Two additional responses are elicited which are amenable to quantitation; changes in lymph node weights and growth of treponemes in the lymph nodes (51). By these parameters it has been possible to compare treponemal infections in normal animals and in animals that have been transfused with immune serum and cells (Chap. 17). In addition, LSH hamsters infected with *T. pallidum* Bosnia A are resistant to reinfection with homologous or heterologous virulent treponemes (51).

In one of these studies a large group of hamsters was infected with 4×10^5 *T. pallidum* and examined daily for inflammation. Each week for 12 weeks three of these syphilitic hamsters were killed, along with three age-matched noninfected hamsters that served as controls. Each site of inoculation became erythematous 3 weeks after infection in all hamsters. The intensity of erythema increased until day 26 after infection, at which time the skin appeared roughened and scaly. Within

Table 1 Approximate Number of Treponemes in Inguinal Lymph Nodes of LSH Hamsters Infected with *T. pallidum* Bosnia A

Week after infection	Treponemes $(\times 10^3)$[a]
1	9
2	2
3	90
4	330
5	2000
6	3000
7	2500
8	2000
9	1000
10	700
11	400
12	200

[a] Three hamsters per week.

Source: Reference 51.

24 to 48 hours thereafter the skin ulcerated and became either a larger, crusted lesion or an open lesion, while the periphery of the lesion continued to expand. Central healing of the lesions began 4 months after infection (Fig. 2).

The inguinal nodes of syphilitic hamsters gradually increased in weight, reaching a peak 10 weeks after infection (Fig. 3). The number of treponemes detected in the lymph nodes increased concomitantly for 6 weeks (Table 1). After 10 weeks both the node weights and the number of treponemes were decreasing. The specific treponemal antibody rose slowly during the first 4 weeks after infection and then increased rapidly (Fig. 3). A peak titer was reached 8 to 9 weeks after infection and was maintained until 9 months after infection.

When infected with *T. pallidum* Bosnia A, LSH hamsters are resistant to reinfection with homologous or heterologous virulent treponemes. Infection with 4×10^5 *T. pallidum* Bosnia A was timed so that 12 groups of experimental hamsters could be studied stimultaneously after 6, 8, 10, and 16 weeks of infection. For each time period there were three groups of six hamsters each. Three groups of six normal hamsters were included as controls. Each animal in the 15 groups (12 infected, 3 control) was given 4000 units of penicillin. After 10 days each was challenged with 10^6 *T. pallidum* Bosnia A, *T. pallidum* Nichols, or *T. pertenue*.

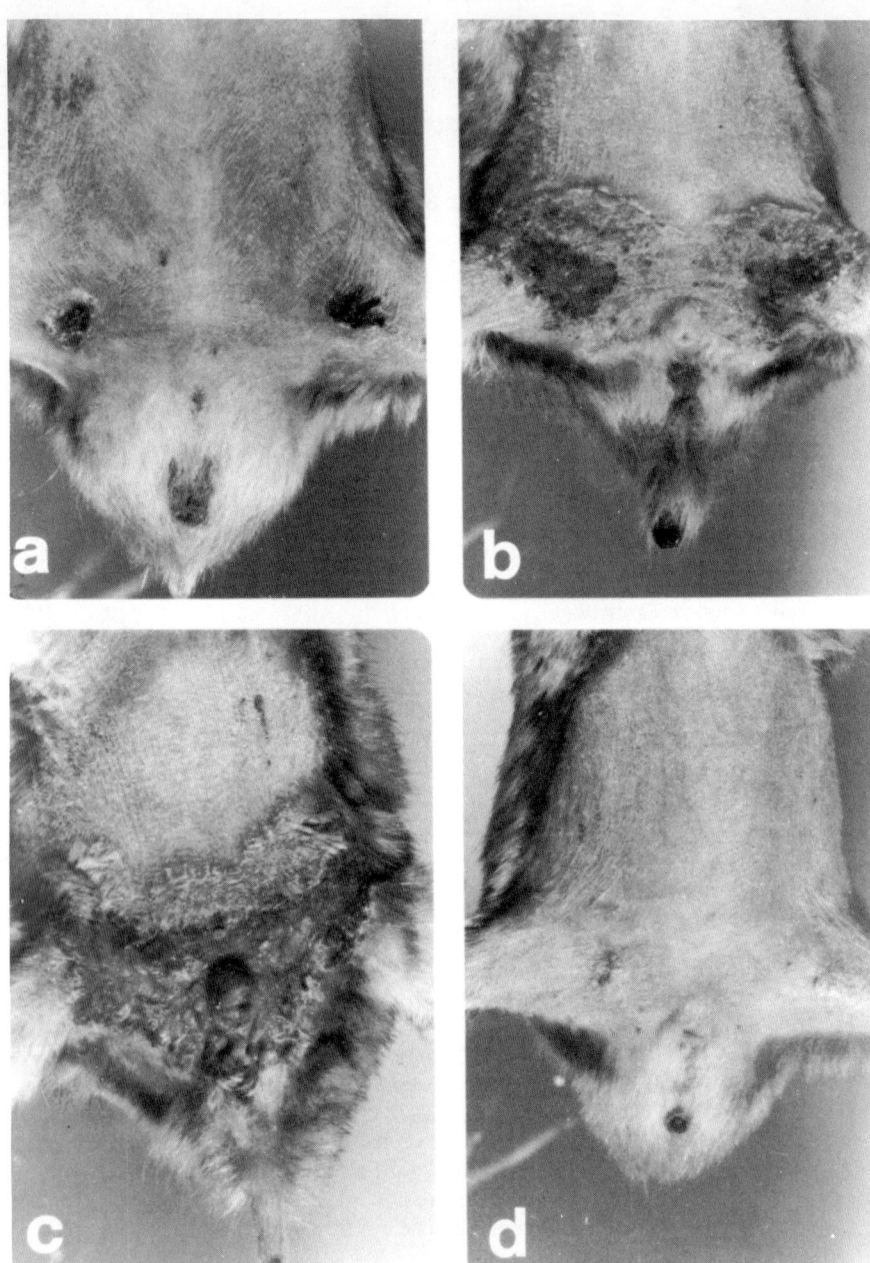

Figure 2 Development and regression of cutaneous lesions in representative LSH hamsters at (a) 4, (b) 8, (c) 16, and (d) 36 weeks after infection with *T. pallidum* Bosnia A. (*Source*: Reference 51.)

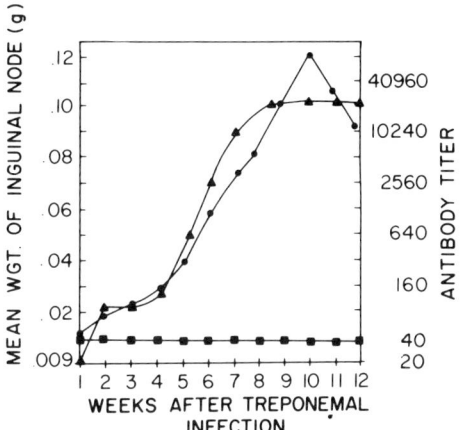

Figure 3 Mean weights of inguinal lymph nodes in normal LSH hamsters (■) and in hamsters infected with 4×10^5 T. pallidum Bosnia A (●). Standard error for each mean = 0.005. Antitreponemal antibody response is also shown (▲).

Reinfection with T. pallidum Bosnia A produced lesions after 21 ± 4 days (mean ± standard deviation) in the controls and after 31 days in most animals which had been previously infected with this strain for 8 weeks or less (Table 2). In contrast, hamsters previously infected with this strain for 10 to 16 weeks developed no lesions during a prolonged observation period of 20 weeks after reinfection.

Twenty-eight days after reinfection three hamsters from each experimental group and three control hamsters were sacrificed. Very few treponemes were detected in lymph nodes of hamsters previously infected for 6, 8, or 10 weeks, compared to the controls (Table 2). No treponemes were detected in hamsters previously infected for 16 weeks.

Thus after 10 weeks of infection with T. pallidum Bosnia A, the hamsters had mounted an effective immune response to this strain.

Hamsters infected with T. pallidum Bosnia A also developed a substantial resistance to heterologous reinfection. The number of T. pallidum Nichols or T. pertenue treponemes detected 28 days after reinfection was lower in all the experimental groups than in the controls (Table 2). Hamsters previously infected for 16 weeks with T. pallidum Bosnia A developed no lesions and had no treponemes after reinfection with T. pallidum Nichols or T. pertenue. Infection of control hamsters with T. pallidum Nichols produced no lesions but an abundance of treponemes. These results demonstrated that hamsters exposed to T. pallidum Bosnia A are protected against challenge with other virulent treponemes.

It has also been found that the CB/Ss LAK strain of hamsters responds rapidly to infection with T. pertenue, the causative agent of frambesia (52). When infected, this strain developed cutaneous lesions which lasted for 6 or 7 months, even in the presence of peak titers of antitreponemal antibody. The rates of appearance and resolution of these lesions varied with the size of the inoculum. The infected

Table 2 Development of Resistance in Hamsters Infected with *T. pallidum* Bosnia A to Reinfection with the Same or Other Treponemes

Week after initial infection	*Treponema pallidum* Bosnia A		*Treponema pallidum* Nichols[a]		*Treponema pertenue*	
	Lesions/sites[b]	Treponemes ($\times 10^3$) per node	Lesions/sites	Treponemes ($\times 10^3$) per node	Lesions/sites	Treponemes ($\times 10^3$) per node
6	12/12	5.6	0/12	67	12/12	100
8	8/12	2.2	0/12	49	12/12	78
10	0/12	1	0/12	2	4/12	4
16	0/12	0	0/12	0	0/12	0
Controls	12/12	310	0/12	150	12/12	1750

[a]Lesions rarely develop in hamsters infected with *T. pallidum* Nichols, but the lymph nodes teem with treponemes.
[b]Six animals per group; each animal was inoculated at two sites.
Source: Reference 51.

hamsters' inguinal lymph nodes increased significantly in weight and teemed with treponemes for several weeks. Animals infected for 8 or 10 weeks obtained quick resolution of their lesions by treatment with penicillin and were thereafter resistant to reinfection.

The ultimate goal of treponemal research is to develop an effective vaccine. For this purpose it is especially important that treponemal infections of vaccinated and nonvaccinated inbred hamsters can be compared in three parameters: lymph node weight, the number of treponemes per inguinal lymph node, and the development of cutaneous lesions. In the rabbit model only the cutaneous lesions can be readily measured.

For experimental studies of the immune mechanism of syphilitic and frambesial infection, inbred LSH and CB hamsters have several distinct advantages: (1) They are readily available. (2) Infection with *T. pallidum* Bosnia A or *T. pertenue* produces extensive chronic skin lesions that can be measured easily. (3) Syphilitic or frambesial lymph nodes can be easily detected, and their increased weight is a useful measure of pathogenicity and infectivity. (4) The lymph nodes of infected animals teem with treponemes, whose numbers can be readily estimated by dark-field microscopy. (5) Infection with *T. pallidum* Bosnia A or *T. pertenue* induces cross-resistance to homologous and heterologous virulent treponemes. Because of this ability to acquire resistance to reinfection, they are appropriate models for studies of passive transfer of resistance to normal recipients with sera or cells from immune animals (Chap. 17) (6). They have no known treponemal disease that might influence an experimental infection. (7) They are relatively inexpensive and do not require elaborate animal facilities.

Relevance to Human Disease

Experimental animal models should faithfully duplicate most aspects of human disease. To what extent are the rabbit and hamster models relevant to human treponemal disease?

Syphilis of the rabbit and hamster does not present the diverse clinical syndromes of human syphilis. The disease in rabbits is short-lived, and relapses rarely occur, even though treponemes are harbored for years in the lymph nodes. This latency is usually permanent. Hamsters are easily infected; they develop extensive chronic skin lesions that persist for 6 to 9 months and their lymph nodes remain infected for the rest of their lives. However, clinical manifestations of syphilis are restricted to a few strains of *T. pallidum*, such as *T. pallidum* Bosnia A. Therefore the classical sequence of primary, secondary, and tertiary syphilis with periods of latency—the disease as it occurs in man (Chap. 6)—is only partially mimicked in syphilitic rabbits and hamsters. Moreover, the offspring of syphilitic rabbits and hamsters do not develop congenital syphilis.

Nevertheless, most clinical aspects of primary syphilis, as well as its pathology (Chap. 15) and serology, have been duplicated in these models. Experimental syphilis in the rabbit has contributed significantly to our knowledge during the past 80 years; from it we have learned a great deal about the humoral response (Chap. 13), cross-protection among treponemal strains, histopathology (Chap. 15), immunity (Chaps. 15-17), therapeutic techniques, and the spread and dissemination of the disease. The hamster has provided direct evidence that immune cells, particularly T cells, can confer resistance to syphilitic and frambesial infection (Chap. 17). Hamsters have also demonstrated the similarity of cell-mediated immune reactions to various treponemes. Further exploration of these animal models should elucidate many other important aspects of human treponemal disease.

References

1. K. Wicher and A. Jakubowski. Effect of cortisone on the course of experimental syphilis in the guinea pig. I. Effect of previously administered cortisone on guinea pigs infected with *Treponema pallidum* intradermally, intratesticularly, and intravenously. *Br. J. Vener. Dis. 40*:213-216 (1964).
2. A. Bessemans and A. DeMoor. Rèceptivité des petits animaux de laboratoire à la syphilis et à la pallidoidose. *Ann. Inst. Pasteur Paris 63*:569-591 (1939).
3. B. Gueft and P. D. Rosahn. Experimental mouse syphilis, a critical review of the literature. *Am. J. Syph. Gonorrhea Vener. Dis. 32*:59-88 (1948).
4. Y. Ohta. *Treponema pallidum* antibodies in syphilitic mice as determined by immunofluorescence and passive hemagglutination techniques. *J. Immunol. 108*:921-926 (1972).
5. A. Vaisman. *La Syphilis Inapparente Expérimentale chez la Souris*. Imprimerie Tancrede, Paris, 1936, p. 67.
6. J. Schereschewsky. Culture de spirochètes pâles provenant de la rate de la souris blanche. *Bibl. Soc. Fr. Dermatol. Syph. 43*:1063-1064 (1936).
7. G. S. Wilson and A. A. Miles. The spirochaetes. In *Topley and Wilson's Principles of Bacteriology and Immunity*, 4th ed. Williams & Wilkins, Baltimore, 1955, pp. 2027-2044.
8. T. B. Turner and D. H. Hollander. Biology of the Treponematoses. *WHO Monogr. Ser. 35*:193-197 (1957).

9. P. Haensell. Vorläufige Mittheilung über Versuche von Impfsyphilis der Iris und Cornea des Kanichenauges. *Arch. Ophthal. Berlin* 27:93-100 (1881).
10. E. Bertarelli. Sulla transmissione della sifilide al coniglio. *Riv. Ig. San. Pubbl.* 17:646-660 (1906).
11. U. Parodi. Sulla transmissione della sifilide al testicole del coniglio. *G. Accad. Med. Torino* 13:288 (1907).
12. H. J. Nichols. Experimental yaws in the monkey and rabbit. *J. Exp. Med.* 12:616-622 (1910).
13. E. Hoffmann. Die Übertragung der Syphilis auf Kaninchen mittels reingezuchteter Spirochäten von Menschen. *Dtsch. Med. Wochenschr.* 37:1546-1547 (1911).
14. H. Noguchi. A method for the pure cultivation of pathogenic *T. pallidum* (Spirochaeta pallida). *J. Exp. Med.* 14:99-108 (1911).
15. W. H. Brown and L. P. Pearce. Experimental syphilis in the rabbit. I. Primary infection in the testicle. *J. Exp. Med.* 31:475-498 (1920).
16. W. H. Brown and L. P. Pearce. Experimental syphilis in the rabbit. II. Primary infection in the scrotum. Part I. Reaction to infection. *J. Exp. Med.* 31:709-727 (1920).
17. W. H. Brown and L. P. Pearce. Experimental syphilis in the rabbit. II. Primary infection in the scrotum. Part 2. Scrotal lesions and the character of the scrotal infection. *J. Exp. Med.* 31:729-748 (1920).
18. W. H. Brown and L. P. Pearce. Experimental syphilis in the rabbit. III. Local dissemination, local recurrence, and involvement of regional lymphatics. *J. Exp. Med.* 31:749-764 (1920).
19. W. H. Brown and L. P. Pearce. Experimental syphilis in the rabbit. IV. Cutaneous syphilis. Part I. Affections of the skin and appendages. *J. Exp. Med.* 32:445-471 (1920).
20. W. H. Brown and L. P. Pearce. Experimental syphilis in the rabbit. IV. Cutaneous syphilis. Part 2. Clinical aspects of cutaneous syphilis. *J. Exp. Med.* 32:473-495 (1920).
21. W. H. Brown and L. P. Pearce. Experimental syphilis in the rabbit. VII. Affections of the eye. *J. Exp. Med.* 34:167-181 (1921).
22. W. H. Brown and L. P. Pearce. Note on the preservation of stock strains of *Treponema pallida* and on the demonstration of infection in rabbits. *J. Exp. Med.* 34:185-188 (1921).
23. T. B. Turner. Studies on the relationship between yaws and syphilis. *Am. J. Hyg.* 25:477-506 (1937).
24. T. B. Turner. Some features of the biology of syphilitic infection. *P. Med. J.* 41:777-782 (1938).
25. T. B. Turner. Protective antibodies in the serum of syphilitic rabbits. *J. Exp. Med.* 69:867-890 (1939).

26. T. B. Turner and C. McLeod. Cross immunity in experimental syphilis, yaws and venereal spirochetosis of rabbits. *Trans. Assoc. Am. Physicians* 57:265-266 (1942).
27. T. B. Turner, C. McLeod, and E. L. Updyke. Cross immunity in experimental syphilis, yaws and venereal spirochetosis of rabbits. *Am. J. Hyg.* 46:287-295 (1947).
28. T. B. Turner and D. H. Hollander. Cortisone in experimental syphilis—A preliminary note. *Bull. Johns Hopkins Hosp.* 87: 505-509 (1950).
29. T. B. Turner and D. H. Hollander. Studies on the mechanism of action of cortisone in experimental syphilis. *Am. J. Syph.* 38: 371-387 (1954).
30. H. J. Magnuson, H. Eagle, and R. Fleischman. The minimal infectious inoculum of *Spirochaeta pallida* (Nichols strain) and a consideration of its rate of multiplication *in vivo*. *Am. J. Syph.* 32:1-18 (1948).
31. N. N. Izzat, J. M. Knox, J. A. Werth, and W. G. Dacres. Evolution of syphilitic chancres with virulent *Treponema pallidum* in the rabbit. *Br. J. Vener. Dis.* 47:67-72 (1970).
32. R. F. Bey, R. C. Johnson, and T. J. Fitzgerald. Suppression of lymphocyte response to concanavalin A by mycopolysaccharide material from *Treponema pallidum* infected rabbits. *Infect. Immun.* 26:64-69 (1979).
33. T. J. Fitzgerald and R. C. Johnson. Surface mucopolysaccharides of *Treponema pallidum*. *Infect. Immun.* 24:244-251 (1979).
34. T. J. Fitzgerald and R. C. Johnson. Influence of testicular fluid infected with *Treponema pallidum* on intradermal lesions. *Br. J. Vener. Dis.* 56:125-128 (1980).
35. G. W. Raiziss and M. Severac. Rapidity with which Spirochaeta pallida invades the blood stream. *Arch. Dermatol. Syphilol.* 35:1101-1119 (1937).
36. W. H. Brown, L. P. Pearce, and W. D. Witherbee. Experimental syphilis in the rabbit. VI. Affections of bone, cartilage, tendons and synovial membranes. Part I. Lesions of the skeletal system. *J. Exp. Med.* 33:495-514 (1921).
37. W. H. Brown, L. P. Pearce, and W. D. Witherbee. Experimental syphilis in the rabbit. VI. Affections of bone, cartilage, tendons and synovial membranes. Part 2. Clinical aspects of the skeletal system. Affections of the facial and cranial bones and the bones of the forearm. *J. Exp. Med.* 33:515-523 (1921).
38. W. H. Brown, L. P. Pearce, and W. D. Witherbee. Experimental syphilis in the rabbit. VI. Affections of bone, cartilage, tendons and synovial membranes. Part 3. Syphilis of the posterior extremities with other affections of a miscellaneous type. *J. Exp. Med.* 33:525-538 (1921).

39. H. U. Williams. Pathology of yaws, especially the relation of yaws to syphilis. *Arch. Pathol.* 20:596-630 (1935).
40. B. D. Brause, S. Qualls, and R. B. Roberts. Testicular cultivation of *Treponema pallidum* (Nichols strain) facilitated by sustained-release steroid administration. *J. Clin. Microbiol.* 10:937-939 (1979).
41. C. N. Frazier, A. Bensel, and C. S. Keuper. Phenomena of disease in rabbits fed cholesterol and inoculated with *Treponema pallidum*. II. Infectivity of blood. *Am. J. Syph.* 34:453-459 (1950).
42. C. N. Frazier, A. Bensel, and C. S. Keuper. Further observations on the duration of spirochetemia in rabbits with asymptomatic syphilis. *Am. J. Syph.* 36:167-173 (1952).
43. K. R. Hill. Non-specific factors in the epidemiology of yaws. *Bull. WHO* 8:17-47 (1953).
44. O. Schobl and I. Miyao. Immunologic relation between yaws and syphilis. *Philipp. J. Sci.* 40:91-109 (1929).
45. T. B. Turner. The resistance of yaws and syphilis patients to reinoculation with yaws spirochetes. *Am. J. Hyg.* 23:431-448 (1936).
46. C. P. McLeod and H. J. Magnuson. Study of cross immunity between syphilis and yaws in treated rabbits. *J. Vener. Dis. Inf.* 32:305-309 (1951).
47. T. B. Turner, C. P. McLeod, and E. L. Updyke. Cross immunity in experimental syphilis, yaws, and venereal spirochetosis of rabbits. *Am. J. Hyg.* 46:287-295 (1947).
48. T. B. Turner and D. H. Hollander. Studies on treponemes from cases of endemic syphilis. *Bull. WHO* 7:75-81 (1952).
49. R. F. Schell, J. K. Chan, and J. L. LeFrock. Endemic syphilis: Passive transfer of resistance with serum and cells in hamsters. *J. Infect. Dis.* 140:378-383 (1979).
50. R. F. Schell, J. K. Chan, J. L. LeFrock, and O. Bagasra. Endemic syphilis: Transfer of resistance to *Treponema pallidum* strain Bosnia A in hamsters with a cell suspension enriched in thymus-derived cells. *J. Infect. Dis.* 141:752-758 (1980).
51. R. F. Schell, J. L. LeFrock, J. K. Chan, and O. Bagasra. LSH hamster model of syphilitic infection. *Infect. Immun.* 28:909-913 (1980).
52. R. F. Schell, J. L. LeFrock, J. P. Babu, and J. K. Chan. Use of CB hamster in the study of *Treponema pertenue*. *Br. J. Vener. Dis.* 55:316-319 (1979).

Part III
The Immune Response

8
Immunopathology of Syphilis

KONRAD WICHER
New York State
Department of Health
Albany, and
The State University
of New York at Buffalo
Buffalo, New York

VICTORIA WICHER
New York State
Department of Health
Albany, New York

Histopathology 140
Cellular Location of *Treponema pallidum* 140
Immune Response 141
Persistence of *Treponema pallidum* 144
Reactivation of Syphilis 145
Immunopathologic Mechanism: An Overview 145
Other Pathogenic Treponemes 148
References 153

In the past two decades the study of immunopathology has progressed rapidly from a phenomenologic description of the immune reaction in a number of diseases to the more fundamental molecular and cellular analysis of the underlying mechanisms. Current recognition of the variety of cells participating in the immunologic reactions has contributed significantly to a better understanding of the immunopathologic mechanisms of some diseases; however, syphilology has not advanced as rapidly as might have been anticipated.

In the immunopathology of syphilis each element contributing to the host-parasite interaction is important: the morphophysiologic characteristics of *Treponema pallidum*, its mode of infection, the host's humoral and cellular responses, the pathologic changes induced, the persistence of the organism in the infected host, and the reactivation of the disease. All these topics are described in earlier chapters, and the discussion in this review will be limited to a hypothetical scheme of the immunopathologic mechanisms of *T. pallidum* infection; hypothetical, because very little of the complex host-*T. pallidum* interaction is known with certainty.

Histopathology

The histopathological changes in *T. pallidum*-infected tissue consists of a perivascular accumulation of plasma cells, lymphocytes, and endothelial cells. The number of cells varies, depending on the stage and severity of infection. In chancres and secondary lesions the tissue is infiltrated predominantly with lymphocytes and plasma cells, and the number and proportion of cells depend on the age of the lesions; macrophages and rarely giant cells may be present. The enlarged lymph nodes in primary and secondary syphilis show marked follicular lymphoid hyperplasia of the cortical area, with concomitant histiocytic infiltration of the otherwise atrophic paracortical area (1-4). The presence of immature and mature plasma cells in the germinal centers has been stressed by some investigators (3,4); others disagree (Chap. 15).

In late active syphilis the granulomatous lesion (gumma), characteristic of this stage, is a focal nonsuppurative, inflammatory lesion with the consistency of rubber and an opaque appearance. The gumma shows a massive infiltration of lymphocytes, plasma cells, macrophages, and occasionally giant cells. A similar cell makeup is seen in late active syphilis involving the cardiovascular and central nervous systems. The histopathology of congenital syphilis resembles that of early or late syphilis in adults.

Cellular Location of *Treponema pallidum*

A number of studies have demonstrated the presence of *T. pallidum* in a variety of cell types. Electron microscopy of ultrathin sections of material from human syphilitic lesions has shown *T. pallidum* within the cytoplasm of neutrophils, plasma cells, macrophages, endothelial perivascular connective tissue cells, and even in the nucleus of epithelial cells (5-8). In *T. pallidum*-infected rabbit testes the organisms have been found in Leydig's cells, fibroblasts, interstitial cells, spermatocytes (9), macrophages, plasma cells, and lymphocytes (10). The mechanism whereby treponemes penetrate such a variety of strict and facultative phagocytic cells is unknown, and the possibility remains that artifact may be responsible. If true penetration occurs, this intracellular residence may have some relevance to the persistence of treponemes in the infected host.

Immune Response

The phagocytosis of *T. pallidum*, at least during the early stage of infection, is questionable. Several lines of evidence seem to indicate a selective failure of the afferent limb of the immune response. This failure seems to reside in the biological properties of the virulent treponemes, rather than in the phagocytic cells (11-14). The microorganism's ability to evade host defense mechanisms may be attributed to the ease with which it coats itself with mucoid material and host proteins (15-17); however Harris and Thoen [*Abst. Annu. Meet. Am. Soc. Microbiol.* E32:86 (1977)] and more recently Hardy et al. (18) have demonstrated in more elaborate experiments that *T. pallidum* can be phagocytized when injected adjacent to areas of intradermal bacille Calmette Guérin (BCG) challenge in BCG-presensitized rabbits. Hardy and colleagues admit that virulent *T. pallidum* must be "processed" in order to be phagocytized. Even when the *T. pallidum* is "processed," the number of phagocytic cells exhibiting the organism intracellularly is suspiciously low. The complexity of the phenomenon may explain the discrepancies in results and interpretations (11-14, 18,19).

Although phagocytosis in the early stage of syphilis is questionable, treponemal antigens are ingested and processed by the phagocytic cells, as demonstrated by the production of antibodies. It is possible that during the early stage only nonvirulent or dead treponemes are phagocytized and processed by the immunologically competent cells. The various humoral and cellular responses thus invoked do not provide effective resistance to reinfection. Resistance in syphilis appears, unlike that in a number of other diseases, only after many months of infection, when, it may be assumed, the phagocytes are equipped with the degree of reactivity needed to cope with virulent treponemes.

In the naturally infected host, antibodies to *T. pallidum* are detected first by the fluorescent treponemal antibody absorption (FTA-ABS) test, followed by the cardiolipin (Wassermann) antibodies. The host responds first with the production of IgM and then IgG and IgA antibodies (20). Very recently (21) IgE antibodies to *T. pallidum* were demonstrated by the FTA-ABS test using monospecific antiserum to IgE. The antitreponemal IgE appeared simultaneously with the IgG and IgA antibodies and was found in early as well as latent and late active syphilis. The latter finding may explain the increased level of serum IgE observed in syphilitic patients (22). It may be anticipated that the IgE antibody may also be present on the basophil granulocytes and mast cells of infected patients and may play an important role in cell degranulation during the treatment of syphilis, especially during secondary syphilis. The treponemal antigen released during the antibiotic action on the organisms may react with the cell-bound IgE antibodies, causing the release of histamine and other pharmacologically active mediators, contributing to the Jarisch-Herxheimer reaction. Another clinical aspect of treponemal IgE antibody is its possible role in the development of immune complexes, which may be of importance in the etiology of some lesions in secondary syphilis (23). Immune complexes in secondary syphilis, regretfully, have not been studied extensively enough. They may play an important role in the development of lesions.

The IgE synthesis is under T suppressor-cell control and has been found to be increased in the sera of patients with disorders of the thymus-dependent functions, as the Wiskott-Aldrich syndrome, thymic alymphoplasia, etc. The decreased number of circulating T cells observed in syphilitic patients (21) would fit well in the picture of the increased synthesis of IgE antibodies.

It has not yet been established whether the order of detection of treponemal and cardiolipin antibodies is due to the sensitivity of the tests or represents the true order of host responses. The source of the immunogenic component inducing cardiolipin antibodies is not known for certain, although it may originate from both host and treponemes. Indirect evidence of host origin has been provided by Kumar et al. (24), who found a transient but significant increase of cardiolipin at the third day of infection in the spleen of rabbits injected intratesticularly with 2×10^7 T. pallidum. This increase could not be attributed to the inoculum, since 10^{12} washed microorganisms could not provide a detectable amount of cardiolipin with the procedure used. Matthews et al. (25) demonstrated cardiolipin in a suspension of 5×10^9 unwashed T. pallidum. However, Magnuson et al. (26) could not observe any increase in cardiolipin antibody titers in syphilitic patients who received 5×10^7 heat-killed T. pallidum Nichols strain; an anamnestic rise in Treponema pallidum immobilization (TPI) antibodies was observed. Moreover, the finding by Wright et al. (27) of antibodies against mitochondrial cardiolipin in syphilitic patients suggests that T. pallidum interacts not only with the mammalian cell membrane but also with intracellular organelles. The mitochondrial cardiolipin antibody differs from the Wasserman antibody.

During the course of infection a number of treponemal antibodies demonstrated by various methods are produced. These antibodies might be directed to various components of the treponeme. The carbohydrate fraction has been suggested to give rise to species-specific antibodies (28), and the protein component to group-specific antibodies, which have a wide range of cross-reactivities (29). Lipid fractions have been isolated from both cultivable and pathogenic treponemes, but since lipids are abundant in a variety of host cells, antibodies to the lipid fraction do not warrant high specificity.

In spite of the assumed autoimmune mechanism prevailing in syphilis, patients do not show an increase of tissue-specific autoantibodies, such as occurs in a variety of autoimmune disorders (30). In experimental

8. Immunopathology of Syphilis

syphilis, however, transient tissue autoantibodies (31) and cellular response to homologous tissues have been demonstrated (32), suggesting that the process of syphilitic infection may render host tissue components into self-antigens. Other diseases also exist in which immunologic tolerance is broken, but not always with irreversible and damaging consequences (33,34). This does not preclude the possibility that later contact with treponemes, either endogenous or exogenous, might trigger a specific response in the primed host. Although the clinical implications of these observations can hardly be evaluated in rabbits, where symptoms of late active syphilis are not known, they might have some relevance for man. Moreover, in the experimental rabbit model, where the infection is carried out with treponemes obtained from rabbit testes, the presence of host proteins on the surface, especially immunoglobulins (17,35) has been considered responsible for inducing antiglobulin in the recipient host (35). Although these antibodies cannot confer immunity to the host, the opposite may prove to be the case. These antibodies, acting alone or together with other serum factors (36,37), may protect the infectious treponemes against the host immune response, allowing them to occupy a niche in various organs (38) for a long period of time.

Attempts to demonstrate a humoral mechanism of resistance by the passive transfer of immune serum have been encouraging, though for unknown reasons not totally successful (39-42). Moreover, no correlation has been found between the presence of known treponemal antibodies and host resistance to treponemal challenge (43-45). If there is a protective antibody, it is not detectable by the available laboratory tests for syphilis (see Chap. 13).

The fact that the humoral response does not seem to be effective in abolishing syphilitic infection has led investigators to examine the cellular response (46,47; Chaps. 16 and 17). The results of such investigations in natural infection are controversial. The limited number of studies on human subjects and, most of all, the wide variations in the reagents and techniques employed may in part explain the difficulty of drawing definite conclusions.

More general agreement has been reached in the experimental model, i.e., the rabbit. A state of anergy, which may be attributed not only to humoral factors (36,37) but also to intrinsic cellular impairment (36), has been observed during the early stage of syphilitic infection. This conclusion has been recently challenged by Lukehart et al. (48), who, using lymph node and spleen lymphocytes from *T. pallidum*-infected animals, found no impairment of the in vitro cellular response to treponemal antigen or mitogen. Furthermore the authors (49) observed a rapid clearance of *T. pallidum* (after the 13th day) from the orchitic testes which they attributed to the simultaneous increase in the T-cell infiltration. This assumption requires further confirmation; while the functional capability of the infiltrating cells remains to be proven, the prolonged presence of large numbers of T. pallidum in the testes has been repeatedly observed by us [Yeagle et al., Abstr. Annu. Meet. Am. Soc. Microbiol. B20:17 (1978)], using wet imprints of fresh testes and dark-field microscopy. Difficulties encountered in the histological localization of T. pallidum as indicated by the same investigators (49) may be explained by the different techniques used and also by the difference in the localization of treponemes in the tissue. The number of organisms decreases significantly from the center to the distal part, and their location depends on the technique of the intratesticular inoculation.

Persistence of Treponema pallidum

The mechanism by which the spirochetes are eliminated from the body of the host is not known. Several investigators have shown in natural (50-52) and experimental infections (53) that even after a prolonged and intensive penicillin therapy viable organisms can still be found in certain body tissues and fluids. Some of these results, however, should be taken with reservation. Negative in vitro results are not an absolute criterion that the host is free of T. pallidum, and positive in vitro results where only T. pallidum-like organisms are observed do not indicate the presence of pathogenic T. pallidum in the tissue or fluid examined. In this regard, it must be recognized that the available methods for examination of the persistence of T. pallidum, especially in patients, are not the most reliable, and that neither an absolute test of the persistent infection nor a criterion of cure is available.

Assuming that the T. pallidum persist in the host, the following possible mechanisms of surviving may be suggested:

1. *Treponema pallidum* coats itself easily with mucoid material (16) and a variety of host proteins, including immunoglobulins (17, 35). This property not only enables the treponemes to escape recognition as a foreign substance but may also enhance its survival by abrogating the cellular immune response.
2. *Treponema pallidum* may establish residence in immunologically privileged sites, such as the brain and eyes. The physiology of these organs renders them relatively impervious to circulating antibodies and to the antibiotics used for treatment (54,55).
3. *Treponema pallidum* may be affected by antibiotics only when they are actively proliferating. Organisms which are not multiplying may survive even in the presence of high concentrations of penicillin (56).

Reactivation of Syphilis

The experiments on inoculation syphilis in human volunteers by Magnuson and associates (26) provided complex but unique information. Patients with untreated latent syphilis did not respond clinically or serologically to experimental challenge with 10^5 *T. pallidum* Nichols strain and could be considered resistant to reinfection. In contrast, those who had previously been treated for early syphilis developed lesions with increased antibody production after experimental challenge. Volunteers who had been previously treated for latent syphilis responded to challenge in variable fashions: one-half did not respond clinically or immunologically, as was the case in the patients with untreated latent syphilis; others (40%) developed lesions that were usually dark-field negative with an increase in cardiolipin antibody response. One subject developed a gumma.

These results suggest that at a certain point in the evolution of syphilis the host becomes refractory to exogenous reinfection with *T. pallidum*. The relation of these observations to clearance of endogenous *T. pallidum* remains obscure. These studies also do not provide clues to the mechanism involved and events leading to this state of relative immunity to syphilis. The results of Magnuson and associates suggest that the formation of gummas may require the presence of *T. pallidum*. It is possible that late syphilis occurs only in those who are not completely immune to endogenous reinfection as a result of the interaction between surviving *T. pallidum* and lymphocytes sensitized to various treponemal and/or host tissue antigens. Consistent with observations that *T. pallidum* persists in the host for a long period of time is the concept of a prolonged, continuous lymphocyte sensitization, and the persistence of treponemal antibodies may also suggest continuous sensitization to treponemal antigens.

What triggers the reactivation in tertiary syphilis is a matter of pure speculation. Unfavorable conditions may tilt the host's immunoregulatory balance toward tolerating the multiplication of *T. pallidum* in the skin, blood vessels, or elsewhere. This growth would attract or trap lymphocytes and other cells. Lymphocytes sensitized to various antigens, including host tissue, would then initiate a process of autoaggression. The ensuing tissue destruction may include "amputation" of part of an organ, as in cavitary tuberculosis. The role of local trauma in inducing skin lesions of tertiary syphilis is also not understood.

Immunopathologic Mechanism: An Overview

Attachment of *T. pallidum* to the host cells may be an important precursor of infection. The eagerness of the organism to adhere to cells has long been known (57), but only recently has this characteristic been definitely associated with virulence and infectivity (58,59).

During the incubation period an accumulation of mucoid material parallels the multiplication of *T. pallidum* at the site of entry (60, Chap. 11). It has been assumed for many years that this material provides a physical barrier against host defense mechanisms; only recently has the material been shown to have immunosuppressive activity (61,62), which delays the appearance of the inflammatory process at the site of entry. It is difficult to assess whether virulent *T. pallidum* itself exerts chemotactic activity in vivo, since it may trigger very complex reactions when coated with mucoid material and host proteins, including immunoglobulins and complement components (17,35). In preliminary in vitro studies on chemotaxis we have observed that treponemal extract, as prepared for inoculation, and washed *T. pallidum* did not exert any significant chemotactic activity on normal rabbit peritoneal leukocytes [Kalinka et al. *Abstr. Annu. Meet. Am. Soc. Microbiol.* B41:24 (1980)]. An alternative explanation—that the chemotactic substance locally produced at the site of the inoculation is of cellular origin—is difficult to accept in view of the immunosuppressive activity of the mucoid material at the site of infection. We are therefore inclined to believe that the inoculation site behaves as a trapping place for cells sensitized elsewhere by a less virulent *T. pallidum*. This may explain why such a long time is needed to mount an infiltrate of mononuclear cells, in particular T and B cells, sensitive enough to curb the local infection yet unable to prevent the systemic infection.

Thus in early syphilis, while the invading *T. pallidum* multiplies, favored by the production of mucoid material, and spreads freely throughout the body, a depletion of lymphocytes in thymus-dependent areas of lymphoid tissues has been observed in man (2,3) and animals (1,4). Cell-mediated reasponses (T dependent) are held in restraint, as indicated by negative skin reaction to treponemal antigen and by in vitro tests (for a review, Refs. 46 and 47). Some aspects of the humoral response (B dependent) progress undisturbed, whereas suppression can be demonstrated in yet others. (Chaps. 13 and 14). The mechanism by which the suppression of cell-mediated responses occurs remains to be established. Substances exhibiting immunosuppressive activity have been found in the serum of infected subjects (36,37,63). In addition, an intrinsic impairment of the lymphocytes, independent of the serum factor(s), has been observed in early stages of infection (36). Conceivably the suppressed responsiveness could be effected directly by treponemal substances released into circulation, but syphilitic infection may also act indirectly and may affect differently the various subpopulations of lymphocytes. The latter case may entail some imbalance in favor of cells with immunosuppressive or

8. Immunopathology of Syphilis

immunoregulatory function, which may express themselves by direct cell-to-cell interaction or indirectly through factors released into their microenvironment. Substances with inhibitory activity have been found in serum-free supernatants of *T. pallidum*-infected rabbit lymph node lymphocytes cultured with treponemal antigen. Those substances were capable of inhibiting both DNA synthesis in purified protein derivative-sensitized lymphocytes and allogeneic stimulation of normal rabbit lymphocytes (64).

Thus in early syphilis an apparently paradoxical situation occurs: While the humoral response, represented by treponemal and non-treponemal antibodies, increases parallel to the development of the disease, the cell-mediated response seems to be suppressed or not actively involved in protecting the host. How can one explain this phenomenon? The concept of a two-organism disease is attractive, particularly in view of the morphophysiologic heterogeneity within virulent strains of *T. pallidum* observed by several investigators (56, 65,66).

Treponema pallidum with little or no protective extracellular mucopolysaccharide would be an easy prey for the host phagocytic cells and could be used for immune processing, leading to antibody prodduction and cell sensitization. *Treponema pallidum* with the protective cover might evade defense mechanisms and multiply unaffected by the rising antibody titers. This population would be responsible for the clinical course of the disease. Even some early-stage manifestations of delayed hypersensitivity, such as leukocyte migration inhibition (67) and macrophage activation (68), do not seem to affect the clinical course of the disease. This is consistent with the observation that delayed hypersensitivity alone does not produce antimicrobial resistance (69), which is a late manifestation of sustained antigenic stimulation. In a natural infection with *T. pallidum* the protective delayed hypersensitivity appears in the latent period. The difference between the non-immunity-conferring delayed hypersensitivity of the early stage and the resistance-conferring delayed hypersensitivity of the late stage may depend not only on the length of exposure to the antigen, but also on the availability of relevant sensitizing antigens during the course of infection.

As the disease progresses, sensitization of the host becomes more evident. The treponemes are either eliminated (spontaneous cure) or forced to retreat to various organs in order to evade the host immune response and the action of therapeutic drugs (54,55). The disease enters a noninfective latent stage. The duration of the latent stage cannot be predicted, and there can be no firm prognosis as to whether the disease may cease, whether secondary infection recur, or whether the tertiary stage will begin. The outcome is most likely determined by the balance between the host's immune stage, expressed by sensitization, and the virulence of the invading strain. Needless to say, host sensitization must vary widely, since it may, in some instances, be overcome by the treponemes.

Prolonged coexistence between *T. pallidum* and the host may depend on the degree of interaction in the early stage. As *T. pallidum*, invades selected organs, it may cause the release of organ-specific substances, which then coat the treponemes, helping the organisms evade the host's immune reaction. This intimate relationship between the host and the parasite may exist for years. At some point, however, the check of the host immune response may wane, and the disease may be reactivated. The intensity of the host reaction will then depend less on the number of treponemes than on the degree of host sensitization. The biologic properties of the virulent treponemes and the requirement for its survival (35,58,59,17) in the host are highly suggestive that tissue damage and, most likely, modification of host proteins play a role in eliciting an autoaggressive reaction. This could explain why in most, if not all, patients with tertiary lesions the reaction is out of proportion to the number of treponemes found; it could also account for the irreversible damage, including interstitial keratitis, sensorineural deafness, and Clutton's joints, which is observed during the late stage of congenital syphilis and that does not respond to antisyphilitic treatment.

Other Pathogenic Treponemes

The nonsyphilitic treponemes and the diseases they cause (Table 1) have several features which are similar to syphilis and some which are dissimilar. The morphology of these treponemes is undistinguishable under dark-field microscopy from that of *T. pallidum*. Some of the clinical symptoms may mimic early or late active syphilis, and the cardiolipin and treponemal antibodies produced during the infection can be detected by the same antigens and techniques as in syphilis. However, as indicated by the variations in host susceptibility, cross-immunity, and the time of appearance of antibodies, the mechanisms of pathogenicity of the nonsyphilitic treponemes differ in some aspects from that of syphilis.

Infection

In natural infections *T. pertenue*, *T. carateum*, and *T. pallidum endemicum* invade the host through injured skin or mucous membrane and spread via the lymphatics to the regional lymph nodes. The mechanism of attachment of these organisms to cells has not been extensively studied. Fieldsteel et al. (70) observed that *T. pertenue* attaches to tissue culture cells of human, rabbit, or mouse origin, but in smaller numbers than *T. pallidum*. In elegantly executed experiments Baseman

Table 1 Nonsyphilitic Treponematoses

Disease	Organism	Production of antibodies[a]	Cross immunity	Susceptible animals
Yaws	Treponema pertenue	Within weeks of infection	Protection against T. pallidum	Philippine monkey Rabbit[b] Hamster
Pinta	Treponema carateum	Very slow seroconversion 3 months after primary lesions	No protection against T. pallidum	Chimpanzee only
Bejel	Treponema pallidum (T. pallidum endemicum)	Within weeks of infection	Protection against T. pallidum	Rabbit[b] Hamster

[a]Cardiolipin and treponemal.
[b]Rabbits respond differently to experimental infection with these treponemes than with T. pallidum.

and Hayes (71) identified three fractions of proteins from *T. pallidum* Nichols strain which were responsible for attachment to tissue culture cells and reacted with treponemal antibodies from *T. pallidum-* or *T. pertenue-*infected individuals. The authors inferred that some of the antigenic molecules were homologous among the pathogenic treponemes, and they postulated that the three protein fractions may also be responsible for attachment of *T. pertenue* to tissue culture cells. However, they also found protein fractions in *T. pallidum* which differ from *T. pertenue*. The similarities of antibody production in individuals infected by *T. pertenue, T. carateum,* and *T. pallidum endemicum* indicate that the organisms must have some common antigens. Species-specific antigens may be expected, but the latter have not been identified.

The mode of infection in the nonsyphilitic treponematoses has not been well established. It may resemble that of syphilis, but because of the late seroconversion observed in pinta, some deviations would be expected. Yaws appears to attack only skin and bone, and pinta attacks only skin. The pathologic changes in bejel are similar to those of venereal syphilis, except that primary lesions are very rarely seen. In all three diseases the lesions undergo progressive changes, and the course of the untreated disease may be categorized in primary, secondary, and tertiary stages, or at least in early and late stages. Children are more frequently affected by nonsyphilitic treponemes than by *T. pallidum*.

Clinical Manifestations

The clinical manifestations of yaws have been discussed in Chap. 6. Pinta is characterized by a large variety of dyschromic skin lesions affecting, as does yaws, adolescents and young adults. The early stage is characterized by erythematous papules; secondary lesions are associated with the dissemination of treponemes; and the late stage is characterized by depigmented areas of the skin. In some instances, however, depigmentation may develop in the early stage of the disease.

Yaws and pinta are restricted to tropical countries, but endemic syphilis (bejel) has also been reported in Europe and North America. Bejel is usually acquired in childhood, but primary lesions are rarely, if ever, observed. In the secondary stage patches appear on the mucous membrane of the oropharynx. The late manifestations are similar to those of syphilis: Gummatous lesions may involve the skin and nasopharyngeal area and the bones may become involved. In bejel (unlike in yaws and pinta) the cardiovascular and neural systems may be affected, but this happens very infrequently and the symptoms are mild.

Pathology

Yaws

The primary skin lesions of yaws and syphilis show a similar cell infiltration. Depending on the depth at which the skin is involved, the lesions contain polymorphonuclear leukocytes, numerous plasma cells, fewer lymphocytes, and occasionally eosinophils. The lymphatics and capillary vessels are dilated, and the endothelial cells are swollen. Treponemes are present. The secondary lesions in yaws are the consequence of *T. pertenue* dissemination and are infiltrated much like the primary lesions, except that macrophages and giant cells may also be found and treponemes are usually absent. The late, destructive manifestations of yaws are indistinguishable from those of syphilis: The long bones are quite frequently involved, with localized gummatous nodes on the tibia, radius, and ulna.

Ferris and Turner (72) observed that the histologic criteria for differentiating lesions of yaws and syphilis in man are unreliable. The authors (73) also compared the cutaneous lesions produced in rabbits infected intracutaneously with various strains of *T. pertenue* and *T. pallidum*. They concluded that *T. pertenue* causes less severe skin lesions which appear more slowly than the syphilitic lesions, but that qualitatively the cell infiltration of the lesion and the histology are very similar.

Pinta

The early and late lesions of pinta are infiltrated by plasma cells, lymphocytes, histiocytes, and occasionally eosinophils. The most characteristic feature of this disease is the unique changes in the pigmentation of the skin affected: bluish discoloration in the early stage, followed by total depigmentation in the later stages. The pathophysiologic mechanism of these changes is not known.

Bejel

The lesions in bejel resemble clinically and pathologically the secondary eruptions of syphilis but may be complicated by superimposed infection. Lymphadenopathy is common. As in syphilis, the lesions are infiltrated predominantly by plasma cells and lymphocytes.

Immune Responses

As in syphilis, patients with yaws, pinta, and bejel produce both treponemal and cardiolipin antibodies, which are detected by a variety of treponemal-antibody (*Treponema pallidum* immobilization, FTA-ABS, treponemal hemagglutination) and cardiolipin-antibody (Venereal Disease Research Laboratories, rapid plasma reagin) tests. The treponemal antibodies can be detected earlier than the cardiolipin antibodies. In pinta, however, the antibodies appear later than in syphilis. In experimentally controlled conditions, when chimpanzees were infected with *T. carateum*, dark-field positive lesions were observed between 35 and 70 days later (74), treponemal antibodies (FTA-ABS test) appeared at day 121, and cardiolipin antibodies (VDRL) appeared at day 155 (75). However, this pattern does not necessarily apply to humans, since the material used to infect the chimpanzees was of human origin, which might influence the incubation time. There is very little information on experimental infection in man. Varela and Olarte (76), studying humans who had received, experimentally, an intradermal inoculation of *T. carateum*, found positive serology 3 months after inoculation.

In the *T. carateum*-infected host treponemal antibodies persist for about as long as in syphilis, but cardiolipin antibodies sometimes persist for longer than in syphilis (77).

Immunologic differences and cross-immunity have been demonstrated among experimental syphilis, yaws, and venereal spirochetosis in rabbits (78,79). There is definite cross-reactivity and immunity between *T. pallidum*, *T. pertenue*, and *Treponema cuniculi*.

The immunologic relationship between syphilis and yaws has also been studied in the monkey (80) and man (81,82). Reciprocal immunity between these two diseases was established convincingly. Furthermore, the monkey experiments showed that infection with *T. pallidum* confers a greater degree of immunity to infection with *T. pertenue* than vice versa.

In recent years interest in the immunology of nonsyphilitic treponematosis has been reactivated. Guerraz et al. (83) used *Treponema Freibourg-Blanc*, a variant strain of *T. pertenue* isolated from a lymph node of a cynocephalus baboon (84), for experiments in hamsters. Schell and associates (85) studied the mechanism of passive transfer of resistance to *T. pertenue* in hamsters and (86,87) also examined resistance to bejel in the hamster using *T. pallidum* strain Bosnia A.

Immunopathologic Mechanism

The gross morphology and immunogenic properties of *T. pertenue*, *T. carateum*, and *T. pallidum endemicum* are similar to those of *T. pallidum*. However, the treponemes appear to have different properties when injected into laboratory animals; moreover, the infections they cause are differentiated by the portal of entry (sexual versus nonsexual infection and venereal versus endemic syphilis), the age of the affected host (nonsyphilis treponemes more frequently infect children), the incubation and seroconversion times, and clinical and geographic

8. Immunopathology of Syphilis

features. Differences in the sensitivity of various laboratory animals and in the degree of cross-immunity suggest that there might also be a difference in the immunopathologic course.

Evidence for attachment of *T. pertenue* to tissue culture cells has been reported (71). Partial resistance to infection in hamsters with *T. pertenue* has been demonstrated to be antibody related, but suggestive evidence lets us assume that total resistance may be T-cell-mediated (85). Recent studies (87) have similarly demonstrated that total resistance to infection with *T. pallidum endemicum* Bosnia A is T-cell-mediated.

References

1. H. Festenstein, C. Abrahams, and V. Bokkenheuser. Runting syndrome in neonatal rabbits infected with *Treponema pallidum*. *Clin. Exp. Immunol.* 2:311-320 (1967).
2. G. M. Levene, D. J. M. Wright, and J. L. Turk. Cell mediated immunity and lymphocyte transformation in syphilis. *Proc. R. Soc. Med.* 64:14-16 (1971).
3. D. R. Turner and D. J. M. Wright. Lymphadenopathy in early syphilis. *J. Pathol.* 110:305-308 (1973).
4. R. W. Lapushin, R. E. Baughn, D. M. Musher, and P. Gyorkey. Ultrastructural study of satellite lymph nodes in syphilitic rabbits. *Br. J. Vener. Dis.* 55:168-172 (1979).
5. L. M. Drusin, G. C. Rouiller, and G. B. Chapman. Electron microscopy of *Treponema pallidum* occurring in a human primary lesion. *J. Bacteriol.* 97:951-955 (1969).
6. T. Hasegawa. Electron microscopic observations on the lesions of condyloma latum. *Br. J. Dermatol.* 81:367-374 (1969).
7. H. A. Azar, T. D. Pham, and A. K. Kurban. An electron microscopic study of a syphilitic chancre: Engulfment of *T. pallidum* by plasma cells. *Arch. Pathol.* 90:143-150 (1970).
8. J. A. Sykes, J. N. Miller, and A. J. Kalan. *Treponema pallidum* within cells of a primary chancre from a human female. *Br. J. Vener. Dis.* 50:40-44 (1974).
9. J. A. Sykes and J. N. Miller. Intracellular location of *Treponema pallidum* (Nichols strain) in the rabbit testis. *Infect. Immun.* 4:307-314 (1971).
10. N. M. Ovcinnikov and V. V. Delektorskij. Electron microscopy of phagocytosis in syphilis and yaws. *Br. J. Vener. Dis.* 48:227-248 (1972).
11. R. F. Schell, D. M. Musher, K. Jacobson, P. Schwethelm, and C. Simmons. Effect of macrophage activation on infection with *T. pallidum*. *Infect. Immun.* 12:505-511 (1975).

12. S. R. Graves and R. C. Johnson. Effect of pretreatment with *Mycobacterium bovis* (strain BCG) and immune syphilitic serum on rabbit resistance to *T. pallidum*. Infect. Immun. *12*: 1029-1036 (1975).
13. R. E. Baughn, D. M. Musher, and J. M. Knox. Effect of sensitization with *Propionibacterium acnes* on the growth of *Listeria monocytogenes* and *T. pallidum* in rabbits. J. Immunol. *118*: 109-113 (1977).
14. V. Wicher, S. Blakowski, and K. Wicher. Nitroblue tetrazolium test in experimental syphilis. Br. J. Vener. Dis. *53*: 292-294 (1977).
15. T. B. Turner and D. H. Hollander. Cortisone in experimental syphilis. Johns Hopkins Hosp. Bull. *87*:505-509 (1950).
16. J. A. Zeigler, A. M. Jones, R. H. Jones, and K. M. Kubica. Demonstration of extracellular material at the surface of pathogenic *T. pallidum* cells. Br. J. Vener. Dis. *52*:1-8 (1976).
17. J. F. Alderete and J. B. Baseman. Surface-associated host proteins on virulent *T. pallidum*. Infect. Immun. *26*:1048-1056 (1979).
18. P. H. Hardy, Jr., D. J. Graham, E. E. Nell, and A. M. Danneberg, Jr. Macrophages in immunity to syphilis: Suppressive effect of concurrent infection with *Mycobacterium bovis* BCG on the development of syphilitic lesions and growth of *Treponema pallidum* in tuberculin-positive rabbits. Infect. Immun. *26*:751-763 (1979).
19. S. A. Lukehart and J. N. Miller. Demonstration of the in vitro phagocytosis of *Treponema pallidum* by rabbit peritoneal macrophages. J. Immunol. *121*:2014-2024 (1978).
20. W. Manikowska-Lesinska and A. Jakubowski. Relationship of antibodies detected by the immunofluorescence method with the various classes of immunoglobulins in cases of untreated syphilis. Br. J. Vener. Dis. *46*:380-382 (1970).
21. J. D. Bos, F. Hamerlinck, and R. H. Cormane. Antitreponemal IgE in early syphilis. Br. J. Vener. Dis. *56*:20-25 (1980).
22. R. L. Green, R. W. Scales, and S. J. Kraus. Increased serum immunoglobulin E concentrations in venereal diseases. Br. J. Vener. Dis. *52*:257-260 (1976).
23. J. Sølling, K. Sølling, K. U. Jacobsen, S. Olsen, and E. From. Circulating immune complexes in syphilitic nephropathy. Br. J. Verner. Dis. *54*:53-56 (1978).
24. V. Kumar, J. D. Klingman, and K. Wicher. Host response to *T. pallidum*. I. Quantitative changes of lipids in rabbits organs. Int. Arch. Allergy Appl. Immunol. *55*:476-480 (1979).

25. H. M. Matthews, T. K. Yang, and H. M. Jenkin. Unique lipid composition of Treponema pallidum (Nichols virulent strain). Infect. Immun. 24:713-719 (1979).
26. H. J. Magnuson, E. V. Thomas, S. Olansky, B. I. Kaplan, L. DeMello, and J. C. Cutler. Inoculation syphilis in human volunteers. Medicine 35:33-82 (1953).
27. D. J. M. Wright, M. G. Lessof, A. S. Grimble, D. Doniach, J. L. Turk, and R. D. Catterall. New antibody in early syphilis. Lancet 1:740-743 (1970).
28. E. E. Nell and P. H. Hardy. Studies on the chemical composition and immunologic properties of a polysaccharide from the Reiter treponeme. Immunochemistry 3:233-245 (1966).
29. G. D'Alessandro, P. Zaffiro, G. Fichera, and G. DiChiara. Rapporti tra antigene polisaccaridico e reazione d'immobilizzazione del Treponema di Reiter. Riv. Ist. Sieroter. Ital. 37: 521-531 (1962).
30. D. Doniach. Autoantibodies in syphilis and in chronic biological false positive reactors. In Sexually Transmitted Diseases (R. D. Catteral and C. S. Nichol, Eds.). Academic, New York, 1976, pp. 210-218.
31. C. H. Casavant, V. Wicher, and K. Wicher. Host response to T. pallidum infection. III. Demonstration of autoantibodies to heart in sera from infected rabbit. Int. Arch. Allergy Appl. Immunol. 56:171-178 (1978).
32. V. Wicher and K. Wicher. Host response to T. pallidum infection. II. Rabbit leukocyte migration inhibition in the presence of homologous organ extract. Int. Arch. Allergy Appl. Immun. 55:481-486 (1977).
33. M. H. Kaplan. The concept of autoantibodies in rheumatic fever and in the postcommisurotomy state. Ann. N.Y. Acad. Sci. 86:774-791 (1960).
34. M. H. Kaplan. Autoimmunity to heart and its relation to heart disease. Prog. Allergy 13:408-429 (1969).
35. L. C. Logan. Rabbit globulin and antiglobulin factors associated with Treponema pallidum grown in rabbits. Br. J. Vener. Dis. 50:421-427 (1974).
36. V. Wicher and K. Wicher. In vitro cell response of Treponema pallidum infected rabbits. II. Inhibition of lymphocyte response to phytohemaglutinin by serum of T. pallidum-infected rabbits. Clin. Exp. Immunol. 29:487-495 (1977).
37. C. S. Pavia, J. D. Folds, and J. B. Baseman. Selective in vitro response of thymus-derived lymphocytes from Treponema pallidum-infected rabbits. Infect. Immun. 18:603-611 (1977).

38. M. A. Medici. The immunoprotective niche. A new pathogenic mechanism for syphilis, the systemic mycoses and other infectious diseases. *J. Theor. Biol.* 36:617-625 (1972).
39. T. B. Turner, P. H. Hardy, B. Newman, and E. E. Nell. Effects of passive immunization on experimental syphilis in the rabbit. *Johns Hopkins Med. J.* 133:241-251 (1973).
40. P. L. Perine, R. S. Weiser, and S. J. Klebanoff. Immunity to syphilis. Passive transfer in rabbits with hyperimmune serum. *Infect. Immun.* 8:787-790 (1973).
41. M. Sepetjian, D. Salussola, and J. Thivolet. Attempt to protect rabbits against experimental syphilis by passive immunization. *Br. J. Vener. Dis.* 49:335-337 (1973).
42. R. S. Weiser, D. Erickson, P. L. Perine, and N. N. Pearsall. Immunity to syphilis: Passive transfer in rabbits using serial doses of immune serum. *Infect. Immun.* 13:1402-1407 (1976).
43. C. P. McLeod and H. J. Magnuson. Production of immobilizing antibodies unaccompanied by active immunity to *Treponema pallidum* as shown by injecting rabbits and mice with killed organisms. *Am. J. Syph.* 37:9-22 (1953).
44. M. Metzger and W. Smogor. Artificial immunization of rabbits against syphilis. I. Effect of increasing intramuscular doses of treponemes. *Br. J. Vener. Dis.* 45:308-312 (1969).
45. J. N. Miller. Immunity in experimental syphilis. VI. Successful vaccination of rabbits with *Treponema pallidum*, Nichols strain, attenuated by irradiation. *J. Immunol.* 110:1206-1215 (1973).
46. D. M. Musher, R. F. Schell, and J. M. Knox. The immunology of syphilis. *Int. J. Dermatol.* 15:566-576 (1976).
47. C. S. Pavia, J. D. Folds, and J. B. Baseman. Cell-mediated immunity during syphilis. A review. *Br. J. Vener. Dis.* 54:144-150 (1978).
48. S. A. Lukehart, S. A. Baker-Zander, and S. Sell. Characterization of lymphocyte responsiveness in early experimental syphilis. I. In vitro response to mitogens and *Treponema pallidum* antigens. *J. Immunol.* 124:454-460 (1980).
49. S. A. Lukehart, S. A. Baker-Zander, R. M. C. Lloyd, and S. Sell. Characterization of lymphocyte responsiveness in early experimental syphilis. II. Nature of cellular infiltration and *Treponema pallidum* distribution in testicular lesions. *J. Immunol.* 124:461-467 (1980).
50. P. Collart, L. J. Borel, and P. Durel. Etude de l'action de la pénicilline dans la syphilis tardive. Persistance du tréponème pâle aprés traitement. II. La syphilis tardive humaine. *Ann. Inst. Pasteur Paris* 102:693-704 (1962).

51. J. L. Smith, C. W. Israel, J. A. McCrory, and R. E. Harner. Recovery of *Treponema pallidum* from aqueous humor removed at cataract surgery in man by passive transfer to rabbit testis. *Am. J. Ophthalmol.* 65:242-247 (1969).
52. L. Yogeswari and C. W. Chacko. Persistence of *T. pallidum* and its significance in penicillin-treated seropositive late syphilis. *Br. J. Vener. Dis.* 47:339-347 (1971).
53. P. Collart, L. J. Borel, and P. Durel. Etude de l'action de la pénicilline dans la syphilis tardive. Persistance du tréponème pâle après traitement. I. La syphilis tardive expérimentale. *Ann. Inst. Pasteur Paris* 102:596-615 (1962).
54. E. E. Goldman, J. H. McLain, and J. L. Smith. Penicillin and aqueous humor. *Am. J. Ophthalmol.* 65:717-721 (1968).
55. W. E. Gager, C. W. Israel, and J. L. Smith. Presence of spirochetes in paresis despite penicillin therapy. *Br. J. Vener. Dis.* 44:177-282 (1968).
56. P. Collart, J. C. Pechere, P. Franceschini, and P. Dunoyer. Persisting virulence of *T. pallidum* after incubation with penicillin in Nelson-Mayer medium. *Br. J. Vener. Dis.* 48:29-31 (1972).
57. M. I. Wright. Exploratory studies in tissue culture of *T. pallidum*. *Proc. XII Int. Congr. Dermatol.* 2:884-887 (1962).
58. T. J. Fitzgerald, J. N. Miller, and J. A. Sykes. *Treponema pallidum* (Nichols strain) in tissue culture: Cellular attachment, entry survival. *Infect. Immun.* 11:1133-1140 (1975).
59. T. J. Fitzgerald, R. C. Johnson, J. N. Miller, and J. A. Sykes. Characterization of the attachment of *Treponema pallidum* (Nichols strain) to cultured mammalian cells and the potential relationship of attachment to pathogenicity. *Infect. Immun.* 18:467-478 (1977).
60. T. B. Turner and D. H. Hollander. Biology of the treponematoses. *WHO Monogr. Ser.* 35:35-37 (1957).
61. T. J. Fitzgerald and R. C. Johnson. Influence of testicular fluid infected with *Treponema pallidum* on intradermal lesions. *Br. J. Vener. Dis.* 56:125-128 (1980).
62. K. Wicher, V. Wicher, and D. Kaminski. Effect of *T. pallidum*-infected testis supernatants on the cellular response of normal rabbit lymphocytes. *Infect. Immun.* 27:846-850 (1980).
63. G. M. Levene, J. L. Turk, D. J. M. Wright, and A. G. S. Grimble. Reduced lymphocyte transformation due to plasma factors in patients with active syphilis. *Lancet* 2:246-247 (1969).
64. V. Wicher and K. Wicher. *In vitro* cell response of *Treponema pallidum*-infected rabbits. III. Impairment in production of lymphocyte mitogenic factor. *Clin. Exp. Immunol.* 29:496-500 (1977).

65. T. J. Fitzgerald, P. Cleveland, R. C. Johnson, J. D. Miller, and J. A. Sykes. Scanning electron microscopy of *Treponema pallidum* (Nichols strain) attached to cultured mammalian cells. *J. Bacteriol.* 130:1333-1344 (1977).
66. J. B. Baseman, J. C. Nichols, J. W. Rumpp, and N. S. Hayes. Purification of *Treponema pallidum* from infected rabbit tissue: Resolution into two treponemal populations. *Infect. Immun.* 24: 1062-1067 (1974).
67. V. Wicher and K. Wicher. Cell response in rabbits infected with *T. pallidum* as measured by the leukocyte migration inhibition test. *Br. J. Vener. Dis.* 51:240-245 (1975).
68. R. F. Schell and D. M. Musher. Detection of non-specific resistance to *Listeria monocytogenes* in rabbits infected with *T. pallidum*. *Infect. Immun.* 9:658-662 (1974).
69. G. B. Mackaness and R. V. Blanden. Cellular Immunity. *Progr. Allergy* 11:89-140 (1967).
70. H. A. Fieldsteel, J. G. Stout, and F. A. Becker. Comparative behavior of virulent strains of *Treponema pallidum* and *Treponema pertenue* in gradient culture of various mammalian cells. *Infect. Immun.* 24:337-345 (1979).
71. J. B. Baseman and E. C. Hayes. Molecular characterization of receptor binding proteins and immunogens in virulent *Treponema pallidum*. *J. Exp. Med.* 151:573-586 (1980).
72. H. W. Ferris and T. B. Turner. Comparative histology of yaws and syphilis in Jamaica. *Arch. Pathol.* 24:703-737 (1937).
73. H. W. Ferris and T. B. Turner. Comparison of cutaneous lesions produced in rabbits by intracutaneous inoculation of spirochetes from yaws and syphilis. *Arch. Pathol.* 26:491-500 (1941).
74. U. S. G. Kuhn III, G. Varela, F. W. Chandler, Jr., and G. G. Osuna. Experimental pinta in the chimpanzee. *J. Am. Med. Assoc.* 206:829 (1968).
75. U. S. G. Kuhn III, R. Medina, P. G. Cohen, and M. Vegas. Inoculation pinta in chimpanzees. *Br. J. Vener. Dis.* 46: 311-312 (1970).
76. G. Varela and J. Olarte. Unpublished data quoted in Ref. 74.
77. J. Mesa, A. Restrepo, and A. Cortes. A study of fluorescent treponemal antibody absorption (FTA-ABS) and VDRL test in pinta. *Int. J. Dermatol.* 12:135-138 (1973).
78. A. S. Khan, R. A. Nelson, Jr., and T. B. Turner. Immunological relationships among species and strains of virulent treponemes as determined with the treponemal immobilization test. *Am. J. Hyg.* 53:296-316 (1951).
79. T. B. Turner, C. McLeod, and E. L. Updyke. Cross immunity in experimental syphilis, yaws, and venereal spirochetosis in rabbits. *Am. J. Hyg.* 46:287-295 (1947).

80. O. Schobl and I. Miyao. Immunologic relation between yaws and syphilis. *Philipp. J. Sci. 40*:91-109 (1929).
81. T. B. Turner. The resistance of yaws and syphilis patients to reinoculation with yaws spirochetes. *Am. J. Hyg. 23*: 431-448 (1936).
82. T. B. Turner. Studies on the relationship between yaws and syphilis. *Am. J. Hyg. 25*:477-506 (1937).
83. F. T. Guerraz, M. Sepetjian, J. C. Monier, and D. Salussola. Changes in the susceptibility of the golden hamster to cutaneous treponemal infection after transfer of lymphoid cells from infected donors. *Br. J. Vener. Dis. 53*:146-147 (1977).
84. A. Fribourg-Blanc, G. Niel, and H. H. Mollaret. Confirmation sérologique et microscopique de la tréponèmose du cynocéphale de guinée. *Bull. Soc. Pathol. Exot. 59*:54-59 (1966).
85. R. F. Schell, J. L. LeFrock, and J. P. Babu. Passive transfer of resistance to frambesial infection in hamsters. *Infect. Immun. 21*:430-435 (1978).
86. Schell, R. F., J. K. Chan, and J. L. LeFrock. Endemic syphilis: Passive transfer of resistance with serum and cells in hamsters. *J. Infect. Dis. 140*:378-383 (1979).
87. R. F. Schell, J. K. Chan, J. L. LeFrock, and O. Bagasra. Endemic syphilis: Transfer of resistance to *Treponema pallidum* strain Bosnia A in hamsters with a cell suspension enriched in thymus-derived cells. *J. Infect. Dis. 141*:752-758 (1980).

9
The Jarisch–Herxheimer Reaction

EDWARD J. YOUNG
Baylor College of Medicine and
Veterans Administration Medical Center
Houston, Texas

Clinical Characteristics of the Jarisch-Herxheimer Reaction   161
Herxheimer-Like Reactions in Other Diseases   163
Theories of the Etiology of the Jarisch-Herxheimer Reaction   164
Experimental Models of the Jarisch-Herxheimer Reaction   166
Summary   167
References   168

Jarisch in 1895 (1) and Herxheimer and Krause in 1902 (2) described a transient exacerbation in the appearance of the mucocutaneous lesions of early syphilis after treatment with mercury. This phenomenon, now known as the Jarisch-Herxheimer reaction (JHR), had apparently been recognized by syphilologists since the 16th century, when the mercury ointment was used to treat the "great pox" (3). The JHR was subsequently reported to occur during the treatment of syphilis with other heavy metals (bismuth and arsenic), immune serum, and antibiotics (penicillin and erythromycin). Because of the transient nature and the infrequency of serious sequelae of the JHR, interest has waxed and waned; however, the etiology of the reaction remains speculative to this day (4-7).

Clinical Characteristics of the Jarisch-Herxheimer Reaction

The JHR occurs in seropositive and seronegative phases of primary syphilis but is more common when the serologic reaction is positive (8,

9). In early secondary syphilis the incidence is as high as it is in late primary disease, occurring in 75 to 100% of cases, depending upon the care with which symptoms are sought. The incidence decreases in late secondary infection, and the reaction does not usually occur in latent disease. More than 75% of patients with neurosyphilis are said to experience a JHR and it is reported to be especially common in general paresis or in patients with abnormal cerebrospinal fluid (CSF) (10).

Occasional deaths have been attributed to the JHR in patients with neurosyphilis (11). The occurrence of the JHR in cardiovascular syphilis is difficult to ascertain from the literature. Autopsy reports have shown acute inflammation in blood vessels of patients dying with cardiovascular involvement which has been attributed to the JHR (5, 12), but how this differs from vascular lues without a JHR is not clear. A review of patients treated for congenital syphilis failed to document any with a JHR, regardless of the mode of therapy (4).

The JHR is characterized by the triad of fever, exacerbation of skin lesions, and a variety of physiologic disturbances such as hyperventilation, vasoconstriction, and hypertension. Additional nonspecific complaints which may also accompany the JHR include rigors, sore throat, headache, tachycardia, malaise, anorexia, myalgias, arthrlagias, nausea, and vomiting (13). All of these manifestations are transient and resolve within 24 to 48 hr. The temperature characteristically begins to rise approximately 3 to 4 hr after the initiation of treatment, peaks at 6 to 10 hr, and returns to normal within 24 to 48 hr. In neurosyphilis the fever is reported to occur later, an observation which has been attributed to the delayed penetration of penicillin into the CSF. A double fever curve has been reported in both children and adults who have received an initial low dose of penicillin followed by larger amounts of the drug. In patients who become reinfected, a second course of treatment can result in a recurrence of the JHR.

Skin biopsies of human and rabbit syphilitic lesions during the JHR were made by Sheldon and Heyman (14). They reported a transient inflammation consisting of vascular dilation, endothelial swelling, and an influx of polymorphonuclear leukocytes (PMN). The inflammation was reported to subside within 18 hr without producing vascular damage or thrombosis. These investigators felt that the skin changes were a more sensitive measure of the JHR than any other symptoms, including fever. They also emphasized the resemblance of this tissue response to that seen when large amounts of tuberculoprotein are injected into the skin of tuberculin-sensitive individuals, suggesting that the JHR might represent an allergic reaction. Other investigators were unable to verify these observations in a group of patients with early syphilis during the JHR (15), instead, they observed a perivascular mononuclear cell infiltrate and PMN leukocytes were found in only 2 of 13 patients. Unfortunately these data do not allow one to differentiate an allergic reaction from a toxic response to a microbial product such as endotoxin. Greisman and Hornick (16) reported that the injection of gram-negative bacterial endotoxin into the skin of normal volunteers resulted in an early mononuclear cell reaction similar to the response observed following the injection of purified protein derivative (PPD) into the skin of tuberculin-sensitive individuals. In contrast, large doses of either of these substances produced a granulocytic infiltrate, as did smaller doses of gram-positive bacteria or nonbacterial inflammants. To assess the possibility that the exacerbation of skin lesions might be due to an immunologic reaction involving immune complexes, we performed skin biopsies in patients with secondary syphilis during the JHR and found no evidence of immunoglobulin or complement deposition by immunofluorescent techniques (17). Aronson et al. (18) were also unable to detect immunoglobulin in the skin of syphilitic rabbits during the JHR.

Examination of the peripheral blood smear during the JHR revealed lymphopenia and granulocytosis (19). This is distinct from the reaction in louse-borne relapsing fever, where a Herxheimer-like reaction (HLR) during treatment with tetracycline is associated with profound granulocytosis which is preceeded by lymphopenia and granulocytopenia. Since some animal species exhibit granulocytopenia followed by granulocytosis after treatment with endotoxin (20), this reaction in louse-borne relapsing fever has been used as evidence that the HLR and presumably also the JHR are due to endotoxin (21). Once again, the peripheral white blood cell responses do not permit one to define the etiology of the JHR, since some humans do not experience a granulocytopenia when injected with endotoxin (22).

A variety of drugs have been used to treat the symptoms of the JHR. Antihistamines are reported to have no effect (5), whereas corticosteroids were shown to reduce the fever but not to alter the white cell response (23, 24).

Herxheimer-Like Reactions in Other Diseases

Transient exacerbations of fever and other symptoms during treatment of a variety of infections have been considered analogous to the JHR. These HLRs have been reported in both spirochetal and nonspirochetal infections; these include louse-borne relapsing fever (borreliosis) (20), yaws (*Treponema pertenue*), Vincent's angina (fusospirochetal infection), leptospirosis, brucellosis, tularemia, anthrax, and glanders (5). A severe HLR has also been reported in both Gambian and Rhodesian African trypanosomiasis (25). While these reactions each resembles the JHR in some ways, it seems unwise to assume that they have the same pathogenesis as long as the etiology remains unknown.

Theories of the Etiology of the Jarisch-Herxheimer Reaction

Several theories have been advanced to explain the pathogenesis of the JHR. When mercury and arsenic were the primary treatments for syphilis, a direct vasotoxic action of these heavy metals was suspected. This theory was abandoned when the JHR was produced by penicillin and immune serum.

Bryceson and his colleagues performed detailed studies of patients with louse-borne relapsing fever (borreliosis) in which a severe and occasionally lethal HLR occurs following treatment with tetracycline (7,13,21,26). These investigators concluded that HLR was caused by the release of endotoxin from spirochetes dying in the blood stream. By analogy they suggested that the JHR in syphilis was due to a similar mechanism and that the differences in clinical findings were due either to differences in endotoxins from different organisms or the location of dying spirochetes (Table 1). In support of the endotoxin hypothesis for the JHR was the observation that some patients with the HLR of borreliosis had evidence of endotoxemia by the limulus amoebocyte lysate (LAL) test (7,21,22). Butler et al. (28) challenged these findings when they isolated a heat-stable, particulate pyrogen distinct from endotoxin in the serum of patients with borreliosis. In

Table 1 Comparison between the JHR in Syphilis and the Herxheimer-Like Reaction in Borreliosis

Characteristic	Syphilis	Borreliosis
System effects	Variable severity	Always severe
Latent period before onset of fever	3-4 hr	1 hr
Peak fever after treatment	6-10 hr	2 hr
Fever curve	Slow onset, prolonged	Rapid onset, rapid defervescence
Effect on white blood cell count	Granulocytosis	Leukopenia (PMN + lymphs) followed by leukocytosis
Site of spirochetes	Tissues	Blood
Effect of steroid of fever	Prevents fever	No effect

Source: After Ref. 13

addition, they found that most patients with louse-borne relapsing fever did not have positive LAL tests. When a positive LAL test was observed, the patients were either more severely ill or had concomitant bacterial infection to explain the endotoxemia.

As seen in Table 1, there are distinct differences between the JHR and the HLR in borreliosis. It has been suggested that these differences could be explained on the basis of differences in endotoxins from different organisms or by the fact that organisms are in the tissues in syphilis, whereas they are intravascular in borreliosis. An alternative explanation is that the mechanisms underlying these reactions are not identical.

A fundamental objection to the endotoxin theory of the JHR is the conflicting evidence for endotoxin in the cell wall of *Treponema pallidum* (29). Heyman et al. (5) were unable to demonstrate a treponemal toxin by injecting young mice with living or dead spirochetes. In 1961 Mergenhagen et al. (30) detected endotoxin-like activity in *Borelia buccalis* and *Borrelia vincenti*, both oral cavity spirochetes. Others found chemical and morphologic evidence of an endotoxic lipopolysaccharide in phenol-water extracts of *T. pallidum* (31,32). On the other hand, Hardy was unable to detect endotoxin in *T. pallidum* (33) and Johnson (34) found no pyrogenic activity in extracts of *Treponema phagedenis* or *Leptospiria interrogens*. Gelfand et al. (35) presented evidence for endotoxemia during the JHR when they reported that two patients with secondary syphilis had a positive LAL test at the height of the JHR. We were unable to confirm this observation in 19 consecutive patients with secondary syphilis, 15 of whom developed a JHR during treatment with penicillin. In addition, we found no evidence of endotoxemia by the LAL test in syphilitic rabbits undergoing an experimental JHR during treatment with penicillin (17).

A second major hypothesis to explain the JHR is an allergic reaction possibly mediated by immune complexes (5,36). Herxheimer originally postulated that the JHR was caused by the release of treponemal breakdown products reacting with "sensitized" syphilitic tissues (2). Most investigators agree that the direct effect of an "endotoxin" on the tissues is by itself insufficient to cause the JHR, otherwise the incidence and severity of the reaction would always depend on the number of treponemes in a given individual at the time of treatment and the quantity of organisms destroyed by treatment (4). This is clearly not the case, since the JHR occurs with the same frequency in primary syphilis, where there are presumably small numbers of spirochetes, as in secondary syphilis, where there are large numbers of spirochetes. An immunologic reaction is also the most likely explanation for the JHR produced by the administration of specific immune serum (37,38). In African trypanosomiasis as in syphilis (39-41) there is evidence for antigen-antibody complexes in the circulation. Immune complexes have also been reported in brucellosis (42), another infection which is occasionally associated with a HLR. Immune complexes appear to be involved in a rare form of glomerulonephritis which occurs in syphilis (43-45). Fulford et al. (46) were unable to detect circulating immune complexes in secondary syphilis by the C1q-solid phase assay (C1q-SPA); however their negative results could have been due to the low sensitivity of this assay. These investigators were able to show a decrease in total hemolytic complement and in complement components C4, C3, C6, C7, and C1 INH preceding the JHR. Solling et al. (39) found normal levels of C1q, C3PA, C3, and C4, but did detect circulating immune complexes by the C1q-SPA and an anticomplement test in patients with secondary syphilis. This is in contrast to patients with early syphilis, where several investigators (47,48) found no depression of total hemolytic complement. These assays vary in the sensitivity with which they detect circulating immune complexes, and the failure to detect immune complexes in the serum does not mitigate against an immune reaction taking place in the tissues. We have detected immune complexes in the serum of patients with secondary syphilis, but found no correlation between the absolute level of immune complexes and the JHR (17). In addition, we detected immune complexes in the serum of rabbits infected intravenously with *T. pallidum*, but again could find no correlation with the JHR (17).

Further studies are needed to determine the role of delayed hypersensitivity (type IV allergy) in the manifestations of the JHR. Similarities in the histologic picture in the JHR and cell-mediated immune reactions have been noted by several investigators (4). Recent studies indicate that depending upon the techniques of sensitization, febrile responses to various microbial antigens may be due to cell-mediated immunity or humoral (antibody-mediated) immunity (49). With the development of an animal model of the JHR the role of humoral and cellular factors can now be tested.

Experimental Models of the Jarisch-Herxheimer Reaction

Until 1949 data regarding the JHR came exclusively from clinical observations of patients treated for syphilis. Sheldon and Heyman (14) first performed experimental animal studies of the JHR. These investigators described morphologic and histologic changes in primary and secondary skin lesions of syphilitic rabbits treated with penicillin or immune serum (37,38). These skin changes were reported to be a more sensitive measurement of the JHR than other objective parameters, but Skog and Gudjonsson (15) were unable to confirm these observations in human syphilitic lesions. Putkonen and Hull (50) were the first to attempt to demonstrate fever in syphilitic rabbits during treatment with penicillin, but they were unsuccessful.

Gudjonsson and co-workers (51-53) also attempted unsuccessfully to develop a fever model of the JHR in syphilitic rabbits. These investigators showed that rabbits infected with the Stockholm substrain of *T. pallidum* became febrile, but they could not develop a reproducible model of the JHR, because more than half of their animals died spontaneously from a contaminating agent which was felt to be a virus (52). In a subsequent report, they were unable to induce fever in rabbits infected with *T. pallidum* by the intratesticular route during treatment with penicillin or erythromycin (53).

We have developed a reproducible animal model of the JHR, using rabbits infected intravenously with virulent *T. pallidum* (17). Following the intravenous injection of 4×10^7 treponemes the rabbits were housed in a cold room (ambient temperature 18°C) and the fur on the back was shaved three to four times a week. Untreated, these animals regularly developed disseminated cutaneous lesions of the shaved skin 17 to 21 days later, which mimicked the secondary stage of syphilis in man. At various times after infection groups of rabbits were treated with penicillin and monitored for the development of fever. Rabbits were lightly restrained in Plexiglas stalls with a thermistor probe inserted 15 cm into the rectum and connected to a central recording telethermometer. Penicillin G was administered intravenously and rectal temperatures were recorded at $\frac{1}{2}$-hr intervals for 18 to 24 hr. When syphilitic rabbits were treated with penicillin between 1 and 18 days after infection, only 2 of 12 (17%) developed a febrile JHR. In contrast, 14 of 19 (74%) rabbits treated between 19 and 28 days after infection developed a JHR. The character of the fever was similar to the JHR in man, with a temperature beginning to rise approximately 4 hr after penicillin was given and remaining elevated for 10-18 hr. Rabbits which developed a fever also had other manifestations of JHR, including an exacerbation of skin lesions, agitation, and hyperventilation. A serologic test for syphilis (VDRL) became positive on or about the 18th day of infection, but did not correlate with the JHR, since some animals with a positive VDRL reaction did not develop a fever during treatment with penicillin. Serum samples drawn before, during, and after the experimental JHR were negative for endotoxemia by the LAL test. Immune complexes were detected in the serum of syphilitic rabbits by several assay methods after the second week of infection, but these too did not correlate with the JHR. Further studies with this experimental animal model may help to define the pathogenesis of the JHR in man.

Summary

The JHR is a constellation of events occurring in patients with syphilis following treatment with treponemicidal agents, including heavy metals, immune serum, and antibiotics. The reaction is characterized by the exacerbation of skin lesions, fever, and transient physiologic reactions, including hyperventilation and hypertension. The etiology of the JHR remains unknown, but it is believed to be due to the release of toxic products of dying treponemes reacting with "sensitized" tissues. In experimental animals fever can be induced to heterologous proteins or microbial products by several mechanisms, including direct toxicity, immune complexes, and cell-mediated immunity (54-58). The final mediator of such reactions is believed to be endogenous pyrogen, a small-molecular-weight protein released from granulocytes, monocytes, eosinophils, and fixed phagocytic cells of the reticuloendothelial system. The mechanism by which this reaction occurs in the JHR remains to be elucidated.

References

1. A. Jarisch. Therapeutische Versuche bei Syphilis. *Wein Med. Wochenschr.* 45:721-724 (1895).
2. K. Herxheimer and N. Krause. Uber eine Bei Syphilitischen vorkomende Quecksilberreaktion. *Dtsch. Med. Wochenschr.* 28:895-897 (1902).
3. C. C. Dennie. *A History of Syphilis.* Charles C Thomas, Springfield, Illinois, 1962, pp. 3-19.
4. I. K. Aronson and K. Soltani. The enigma of the pathogenesis of the Jarisch-Herxheimer reaction. *Br. J. Vener. Dis.* 52: 313-315 (1976).
5. A. Heyman, W. H. Sheldon, and L. D. Evans. Pathogenesis of the Jarisch-Herxheimer reaction: A review of clinical and experimental observations. *Br. J. Vener. Dis.* 28:50-60 (1952).
6. Editorial: The Jarisch-Herxheimer reaction. *Lancet* 1:340-341 (1977).
7. A. D. M. Bryceson. Clinical pathology of the Jarisch-Herxheimer reaction. *J. Infect. Dis.* 133:696-704 (1976).
8. T. Putkonen, O. P. Salo, and K. K. Mustakallio. Febrile Herxheimer reaction in different phases of primary and secondary syphilis. *Br. J. Vener. Dis.* 42:181-184 (1966).
9. T. Putkonen and K. Rehtijarvik. The febrile Herxheimer reaction in early infectious and latent syphilis treated with penicillin. *Acta Derm. Venereol* 30:503-506 (1950).
10. M. T. Hoekenga and T. W. Farmer. Jarisch-Herxheimer reaction in neurosyphilis treated with penicillin. *Arch. Intern. Med.* 82:611-622 (1948).
11. B. Shaffer and H. A. Shenkin. Fatal Herxheimer reaction following penicillin therapy. *Am. J. Syph.* 34:78-82 (1950).
12. C. M. Wharton and S. W. Denham. The occurrence of the Jarisch-Herxheimer reaction in a patient with gummatous syphilitic aortitis. *Am. J. Syph.* 35:255-262 (1951).

13. D. A. Warrell, P. L. Perine, A. D. M. Bryceson, E. H. O. Parry, and H. M. Pope. Physiologic changes during the Jarisch-Herxheimer reaction in early syphilis: A comparison with louse-borne relapsing fever. *Am. J. Med.* 51:176-185 (1971).
14. W. H. Sheldon and A. Heyman. Morphologic changes in syphilitic lesions during the Jarisch-Herxheimer reaction. *Am. J. Syph.* 33:213-224 (1949).
15. E. Skog and H. Gudjonsson. On the allergic origin of the Jarisch-Herxheimer reaction. *Acta Derm. Venereol.* 46:136-143 (1966).
16. S. E. Greisman and R. B. Hornick. Cellular inflammatory responses of man to bacterial endotoxin: A comparison with PPD and other bacterial antigens. *J. Immunol.* 109:1210-1222 (1972).
17. E. J. Young, N. Weingarten, R. E. Baughn, and W. C. Duncan. Studies on the pathogenesis of the Jarisch-Herxheimer reaction: Development of an animal model and evidence against a role for classical endotoxin. *J. Infect. Dis.* (in press).
18. I. K. Aronson, K. Soltani, and F. Brickman. Jarisch-Herxheimer reaction in complement-depleted rabbits. Histologic and immunofluorescent studies of early cutaneous lesions. *Br. J. Vener. Dis.* 57:226-231 (1981).
19. F. McDowell. Occurrence of a transient leukocytosis during the Jarisch-Herxheimer reaction. *Proc. Soc. Exp. Biol. Med.* 71:568-569 (1949).
20. L. Olitzki, S. H. Avinery, and J. Bendersky. The leukopenic action of different microorganisms and the antileukopenic immunity. *J. Immunol.* 41:361-373 (1941).
21. A. D. M. Bryceson, K. E. Cooper, D. A. Warrell, P. L. Perine, and E. H. O. Parry. Studies of the mechanism of the Jarisch-Herxheimer reaction in louse-borne relapsing fever: Evidence for the presence of circulating borrelia endotoxin. *Clin. Sci.* 43:343-354 (1972).
22. S. M. Wolff. Biological effects of bacterial endotoxins in man. *J. Infect. Dis.* 128:S259-S264 (1973).
23. P. de Graciansky and C. Grupper. Cortisone in the prevention of the Herxheimer reaction in early syphilis. *Br. J. Vener. Dis.* 37:247-251 (1961).
24. H. Zachariae and E. Nielson. Plasma kinins and the Jarisch-Herxheimer reaction. *Acta Derm. Venereol* 54:401-402 (1974).
25. H. C. Whittle and H. M. Pope. The febrile response to treatment in Gambian sleeping sickness. *Ann. Trop. Med. Parisitol.* 66:7-14 (1972).
26. D. A. Warrell, H. M. Pope, E. H. Parry, P. L. Perine, and A. D. M. Bryceson. Cardiorespiratory disturbances associated with infective fever in man: Studies of Ethiopian louse borne relapsing fever. *Clin. Sci.* 39:123-145 (1970).

27. R. E. Galloway, J. Levin, T. Butler, G. B. Naff, G. H. Goldsmith, H. Saito, S. Awoke, and C. K. Wallace. Activation of protein mediators of inflammation and evidence for endotoxemia in Borrelia recurrentis infection. *Am. J. Med.* 63: 933-938 (1977).
28. T. Butler, P. Hazen, C. K. Wallace, S. Awoke, and A. Habte-Michael. Infection with Borrelia recurrentis: Pathogenesis of fever and petechiae. *J. Infect. Dis.* 140:665-675 (1979).
29. *Lancet* (editorial): The Jarisch-Herxheimer reaction. *Lancet* 1:340-341 (1977).
30. S. E. Mergenhagen, E. G. Hampp, and H. W. Scherp. Preparation and biological activities of endotoxins from oral bacteria. *J. Infect. Dis.* 108:304-310 (1961).
31. A. H. Christiansen. Studies on the antigenic structure of *Treponema pallidum. Acta Pathol. Microbiol. Scand.* 56:166-176 (1962).
32. S. W. Jackson and P. N. Zey. Ultrastructure of lipopolysaccharide isolated from *Treponema pallidum. J. Bacteriol.* 113:838-844 (1973).
33. P. Hardy. Personal communication to D. M. Musher (1980).
34. R. C. Johnson. Comparative spirochete physiology and cellular composition. In *The Biology of Parasitic Spirochetes* (R. C. Johnson, Ed.). Academic, New York, 1976, pp. 39-48.
35. J. A. Gelfand, R. J. Elin, F. W. Berry, and M. M. Frank. Endotoxemia associated with the Jarisch-Herxheimer reaction. *N. Engl. J. Med.* 295:211-213 (1976).
36. A. D. M. Bryceson. Immune complexes and the Jarisch-Herxheimer reaction. In *International Symposium on Immune Complexes* (L. Bonemo and J. L. Turk, Eds.). Carlo Erba Foundation, Milan, 1970, pp. 110-121.
37. W. H. Sheldon, A. Heyman, and L. D. Evans. The pathogenesis of the Jarisch-Herxheimer reaction in rabbit syphilis: Its production by the injection of syphilitic serum. *Am. J. Syph.* 35:405 (1951).
38. W. H. Sheldon, A. Heyman, and L. D. Evans. Production of Herxheimer like reactions in rabbits with *Spirilium minus* infections by administration of penicillin or immune serum. *Am. J. Syph.* 35:441 (1951).
39. J. Solling, K. Solling, K. Jacobsen, and E. From. Circulating immune complexes in syphilis. *Acta Derm. Venereol.* 58:263-267 (1978).
40. S. Engel and W. Diezel. Persistent serum immune complexes in syphilis. *Br. J. Vener. Dis.* 56:221-222 (1980).
41. R. E. Baughn, K. S. K. Tung, and D. M. Musher. Detection of circulating immune complexes in the sera of rabbits with

experimental syphilis: Possible role in immunoregulation. *Infect. Immun.* 29:575-582 (1980).
42. T. Bocanegra, E. Gotuzzo, G. Alarcon, F. B. Vasey, B. F. Germain, and L. R. Espinoza. Circulating immune complexes in acute typhoid fever and brucellosis: Correlation with disease severity. *Clin. Res.* 29:381A (1981).
43. V. Scott and E. G. Clark. Syphilitic nephrosis as a manifestation of a renal Herxheimer reaction following penicillin therapy for early syphilis. *Am. J. Syph.* 30:463-467 (1946).
44. G. D. Braunstein, E. J. Lewis, E. G. Galvenek, A. Hamilton, and W. R. Bell. The nephrotic syndrome associated with secondary syphilis: An immune deposit disease. *Am. J. Med.* 48:643-648 (1970).
45. C. N. Gamble and J. B. Reardon. Immunopathogenesis of syphilis glomerulonephritis: Elution of antitreponemal antibody from glomerular immune-complex deposits. *N. Engl. J. Med.* 292:449-454 (1975).
46. K. W. M. Fulford, N. Johnson, C. Loveday, J. Storey, and R. S. Tedder. Changes in intravascular complement and antitreponemal antibody titers preceeding the Jarisch-Herxheimer reaction in secondary syphilis. *Clin. Exp. Immunol.* 24: 483-491 (1976).
47. D. J. M. Wright and A. S. Grimble. Why is the infectious stage of syphilis prolonged? *Br. J. Vener. Dis.* 50:45-49 (1974).
48. C. O. Kindmark, H. Moller, and K. Persson. C-reactive protein, C3, C4 and properdin during the Jarisch-Herxheimer reaction in early syphilis. *Acta Med. Scand.* 204:287-290 (1978).
49. H. A. Bernheim, L. Francis, and E. Atkins. Hypersensitivity fever: Cell-mediated and antibody-mediated mechanisms. In *Fever* (J. M. Lipton, Ed.). Raven Press, New York, 1980, pp. 11-21.
50. T. Putkonen and J. Hull. Rabbit syphilis and the Herxheimer reaction. *Ann. Med. Exp. Biol. Fenn.* 29:137-140 (1951).
51. H. Gudjonsson and E. Skog. Fever after inoculation of rabbits with *Treponema pallidum*. *Br. J. Vener. Dis.* 46:318-322 (1970).
52. H. Gudjonsson, B. Newman, and T. B. Turner. Demonstration of a virus-like agent contaminating material containing the Stockholm substrain of the Nichols pathogenic *Treponema pallidum*. *Br. J. Vener. Dis.* 46:435-440 (1970).
53. H. Gudjonsson. Experiments to induce febrile Jarisch-Herxheimer reaction in syphilitic rabbits with penicillin or erythromycin. *Acta Derm. Venereol.* 52:493-496 (1972).

54. H. M. Grey, W. Briggs, and R. S. Farr. The passive transfer of sensitivity to antigen induced fever. *J. Clin. Invest.* 40:703-706 (1961).
55. R. K. Root and S. M. Wolff. Pathogenetic mechanisms in experimental immune fever. *J. Exp. Med.* 128:309-323 (1968).
56. I. D. Mickenberg, R. Snyderman, R. K. Root, S. E. Mergenhagen, and S. M. Wolff. Immune fever in the rabbit: Responses of the hematologic and complement systems. *J. Immunol.* 107:1457-1465 (1971).
57. E. Atkins and L. Francis. Pathogenesis of fever, in delayed hypersensitivity: Factors influencing release of pyrogen-inducing lymphokines. *Infect. Immun.* 21:806-812 (1978).
58. E. Atkins and P. Bodel. Clinical fever: Its history, manifestations and pathogenesis. *Fed. Proc. Fed. Am. Soc. Exp. Biol.* 38:57-63 (1979).

10

Toxic Activities of *Treponema pallidum*

T. J. FITZGERALD and L. A. REPESH
University of Minnesota
School of Medicine
Duluth, Minnesota

Tissue pathology in syphilis 173
In vitro toxic effects 174
Applications to clinical manifestations 187
References 191

Tissue Pathology in Syphilis

Treponema pallidum infects most tissues of the body, localizing predominantly in perivascular areas. Characteristic histopathology involves endarteritis, periarteritis, inhibited blood supply, necrosis, and ulceration. As discussed in Chaps. 6 and 8, some of the clinical manifestations of syphilis are of host rather than treponemal origin. Tissue pathology in syphilis may also be attributed to toxic action of the organisms. Summary findings of four recent papers (3-6) will be presented in this chapter. These findings demonstrate specific toxic activities of *T. pallidum* that result in the morphologic destruction of numerous types of tissue culture cells. In addition, treponemes inhibit electrophysiologic responses of cultured nerve cells, interfere with the beating of cultured cardiac muscle cells, and penetrate into skeletal muscle and capillaries.

In Vitro Toxic Effects

Cultured mammalian cells have provided a model system for studying certain aspects of the pathogenesis of T. pallidum (Chap. 11). Treponemal attachment to cultured cells usually does not harm the cells. As many as 50 treponemes may be attached per cell, and active motility may be retained for 5 to 7 days. The cultured cell surface, however, is not morphologically altered and cell viability remains high (7,8).

The cultivation and maintenance of normal rabbit testicular cells, Hep-2 cells, human foreskin cells, rat cardiac muscle cells, rat skeletal muscle cells, and rat nerve cells have been described (3-5). Four different preparations were added to each of these cell types: viable treponemes that were pelleted via high-speed centrifugation and resuspended in fresh medium, heat-inactivated treponemes, the high-speed supernatant from the infected testicular extract which contains soluble treponemal, inflammatory, and testicular materials; and culture medium alone. Treponemal preparations were adjusted to 7×10^7 to 3×10^8 organisms per milliliter. Incubation was performed at $37°C$ in an atmosphere of 2.5% O_2 oxygen/5% CO_2/92.5% N_2.

Normal rabbit testis cells were incubated in Sykes-Moore chambers (9) with viable treponemes, heated treponemes, the high-speed supernatant, and culture medium. One additional chamber contained viable treponemes; this chamber was incubated inverted, with the cultured cells topside. After 24 to 48 hr, the morphology of the cells exposed to the three control preparations appeared normal (Fig. 1A). In contrast, cells exposed to viable treponemes exhibited altered morphology (Fig. 1B). The cells were highly vacuolated or rounded and detached from the glass substratum. Some cells appeared more condensed with an absence of nuclear detail. In the inverted chamber, most of the organisms settled to the bottom. The morphology of the cultured cells on top of the chamber appeared identical to the morphology of the three control preparations (Fig. 1C). Similar findings were observed using Hep-2 and human foreskin cells.

In the next series of experiments, cultured cardiac muscle cells were used. These cells retain the ability to beat in vitro for 2 to 3 weeks. Numerous groups of 5 to 10 cells beat synchronously. Preliminary experiments indicated that T. pallidum interfered with the beating process; cells beat spasmodically with loss of synchrony, then stopped beating altogether. In further experiments different concentrations of treponemes were added to the cardiac cells, and subsequent effects on beating were assessed (Table 1). Beating stopped within 14 hr in the presence of 2×10^8 treponemes per militer, and within 39 hr in the presence of 4×10^7 treponemes per milliliter. Beating was still detected in the control preparation and in the presence of treponemes at 2×10^7 and 1×10^7 organisms per milliliter after 70 hr.

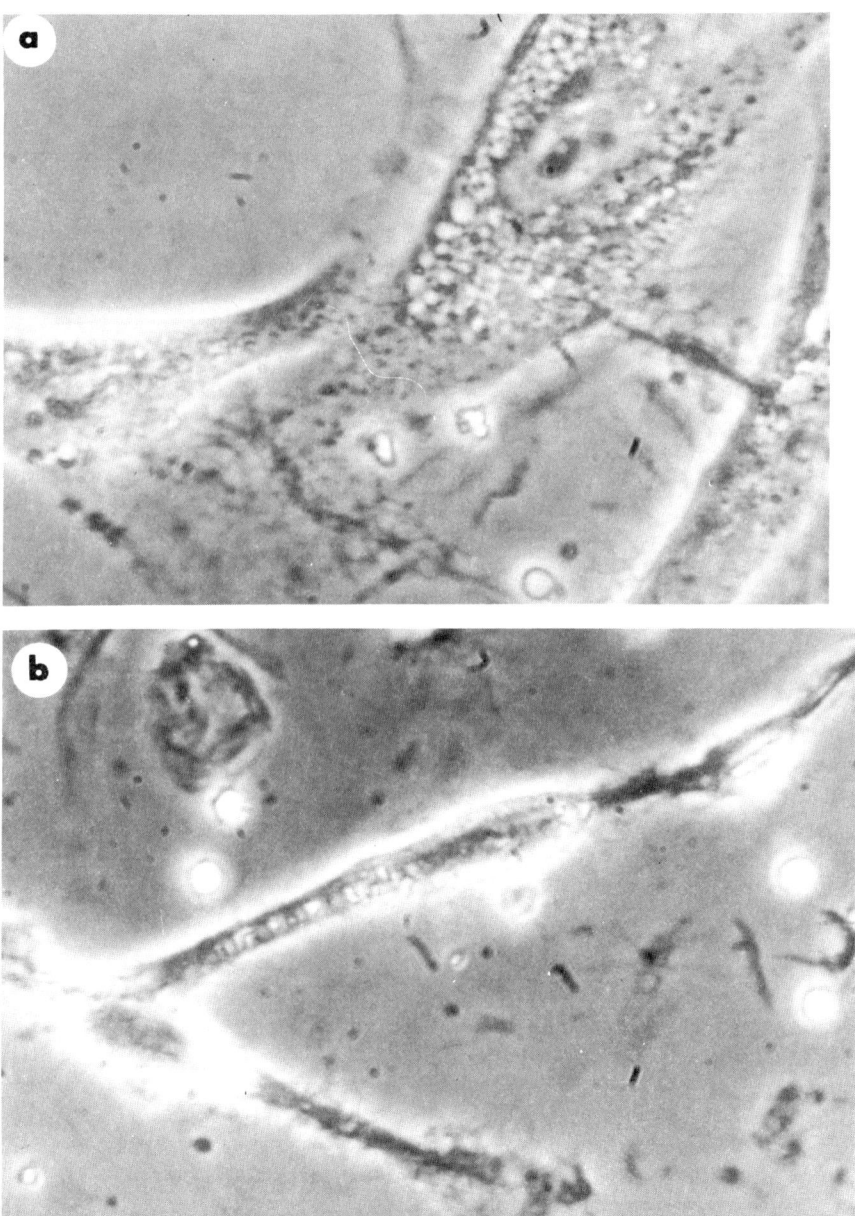

Figure 1 Cultured cells derived from normal rabbit testicular tissue: (a) control preparation of heat-inactivated treponemes, (b) preparation of viable treponemes, and (c) preparation of viable treponemes incubated with cultured cells topside (×400). (From Ref. 5.)

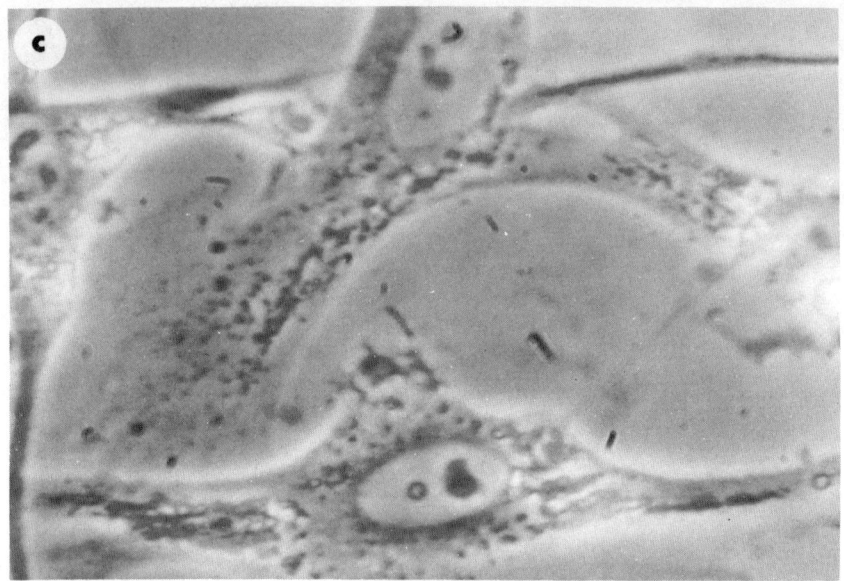

Figure 1 (Continued)

Cardiac muscle cells were then incubated with viable treponemes, heat-inactivated treponemes, the high-speed supernatant, and culture medium to determine potential morphologic damage. After 24 to 48 hr, the morphology of the three control preparations appeared normal (Fig. 2A); the preparation containing viable treponemes was severely damaged (Fig. 2B). In these experiments, beating of the cells stopped

Table 1 Treponeme-Mediated Dysfunction of the Beating of Cultured Heart Cells

Time (hr)	Control	Beats per min			
		2×10^8	4×10^7	2×10^7	1×10^7
0	19	27	18	21	19
14	33	0	50	38	32
23	50	0	31	50	35
30	83	0	31	77	66
39	51	0	0	35	22
70	34	0	0	30	28

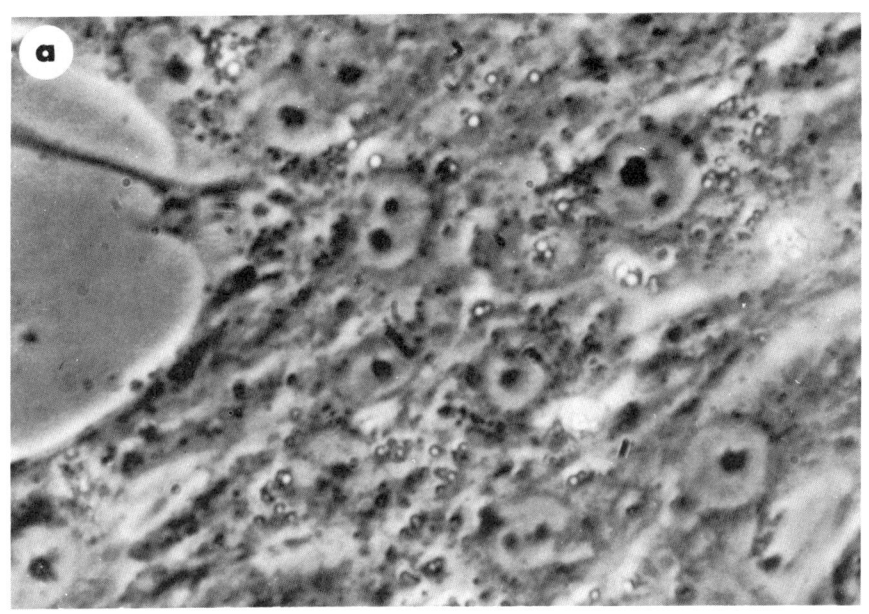

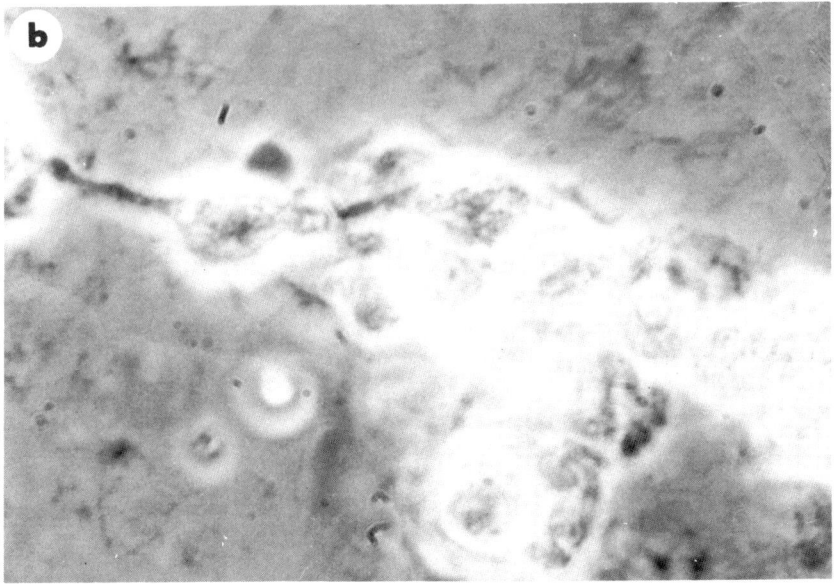

Figure 2 Cultured cells derived from rat cardiac muscle: (a) Control preparation of heat-inactivated treponemes and (b) preparation of viable treponemes (×400). (From Ref. 5.)

after 19 hr in the presence of viable organisms. At this time, morphologic damage was not yet apparent. In contrast, beating of the cells was detected after 280 hr in the presence of heat-inactivated treponemes and their morphology was normal.

Cultured skeletal muscle cells were incubated with viable treponemes, heat-inactivated treponemes, the high-speed supernatant, and culture medium. These muscle cells are readily differentiated from the background fibroblasts by their excessive length. Individual myoblasts coalesced to form characteristic long myotubes containing multiple nuclei (Fig. 3A). After 24 to 48 hr morphologic damage occurred in preparations exposed to viable organisms (Fig. 3B). The long myotubes were attenuated and the processes retracted to form round cells. The three control preparations retained normal morphology (Fig. 3A).

Scanning electron microscopy provided a three-dimensional visualization of the treponeme-mediated morphologic alterations to the skeletal muscle cells. Cultured cells exposed to the three control preparations exhibit normal morphology (Fig. 4A). The myotubes are elongated and characteristically grow on top of the background fibroblasts.

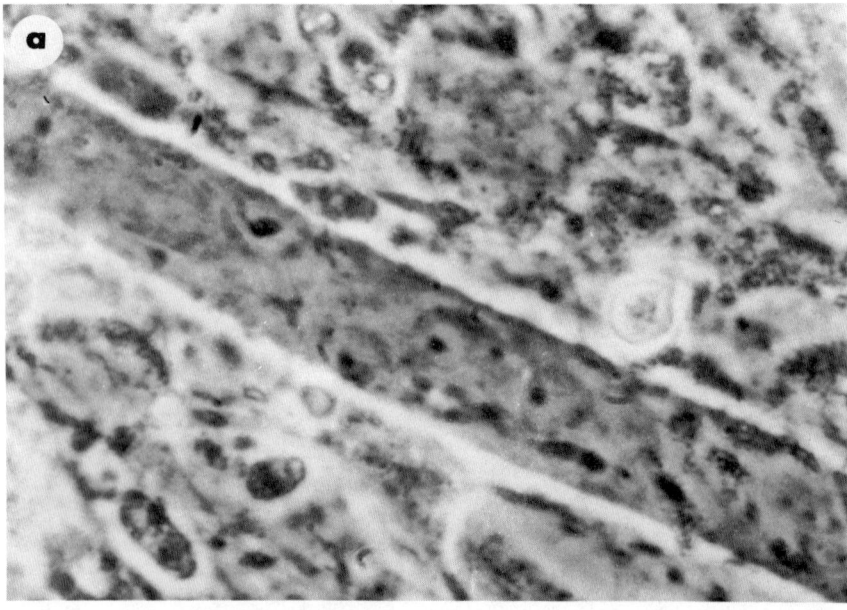

Figure 3 Cultured cells derived from rat skeletal muscle: (a) control preparation incubated with heat-inactivated treponemes and (b) preparation incubated with viable treponemes (×400). (From Ref. 5.)

10. Toxic Activities of Treponema pallidum

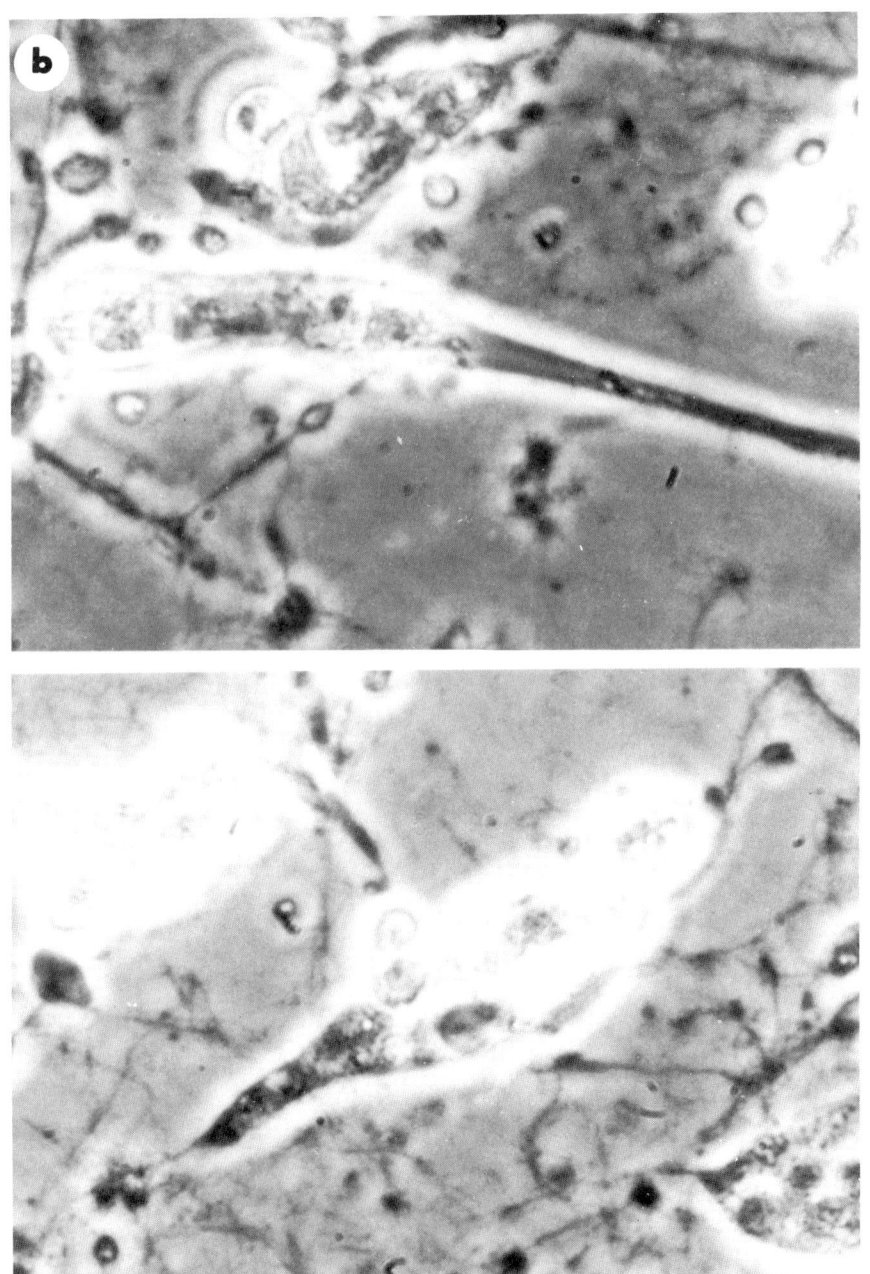

Figure 3 (Continued)

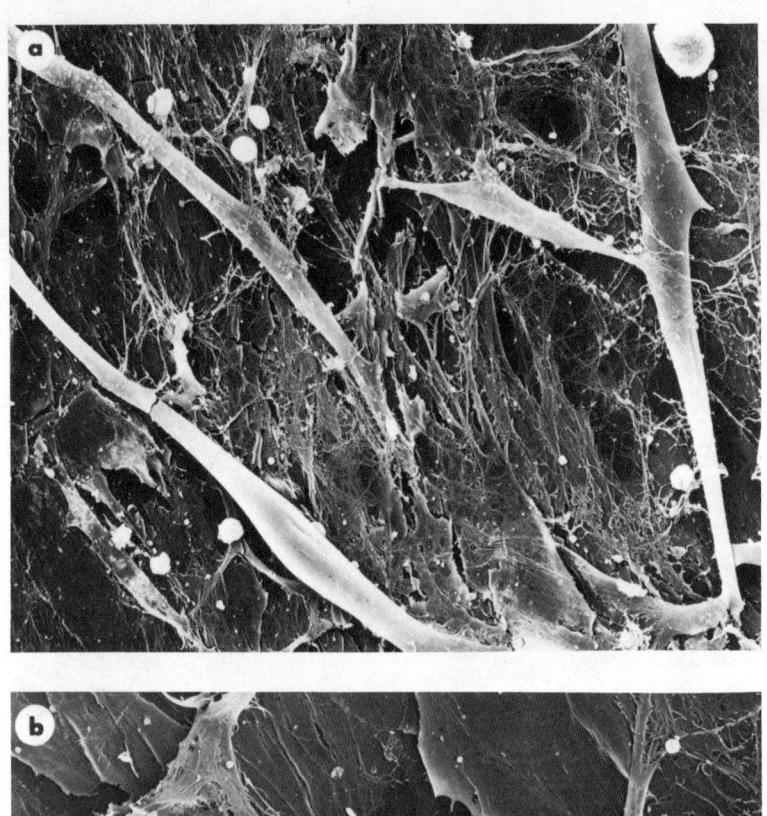
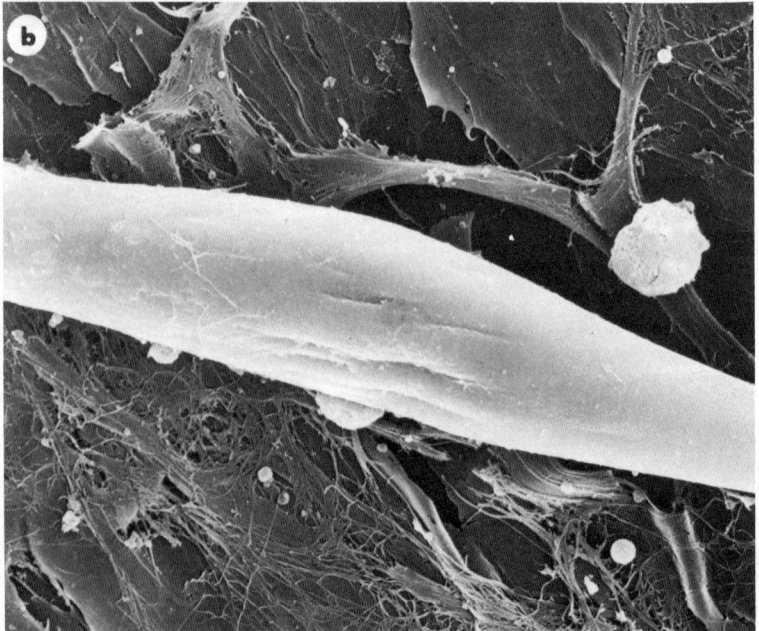

Figure 4 Cultured cells derived from rat skeletal muscle after incubation with: (a) high-speed supernatant control (×500), (b) high-speed supernatant control (×2000), and (c) viable treponemes (×2200). (From Ref. 5.)

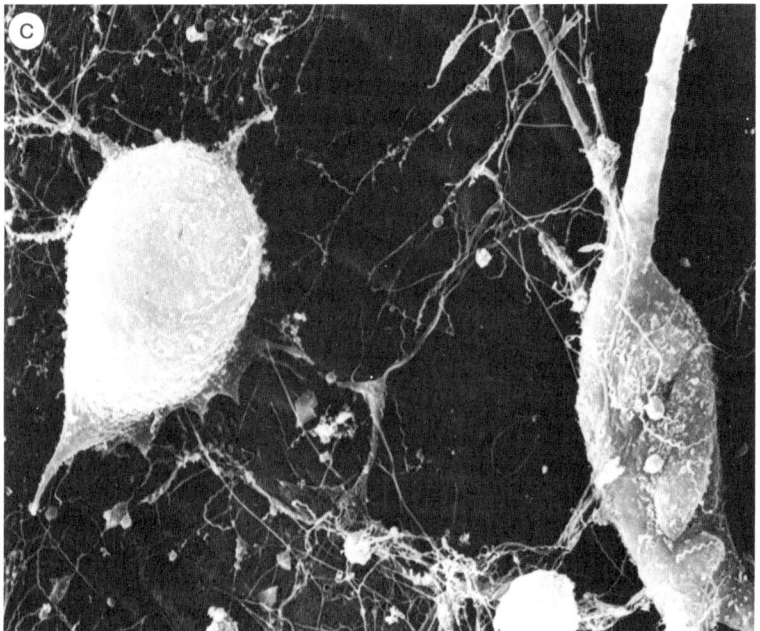

Figure 4 (Continued)

A higher magnification of this control preparation (Fig. 4B) shows that the myotube surface is smooth with gently rounded contours. The background fibroblasts are apparent beneath this portion of the myotube. Following incubation with viable treponemes for 24 hr, the myotubes exhibited various stages of degradation resulting in pleomorphism. Some were beginning to retract and others to have a round morphology. Figure 4C shows a higher magnification of treponeme-damaged muscle cells. The cell at the right of the micrograph is apparently retracting; the cell at the left is almost completely rounded and contains numerous surface projections not present on cells in control preparations. At this magnification, treponemes can be observed. Initially, large numbers of actively motile organisms attach along the full length of the myotubes. Morphologic damage to the muscle cells results in detachment of treponemes.

The treponemes also damaged the background fibroblasts, as shown in Fig. 5. Irregular holes and numerous attached treponemes are apparent at the surface of a group of fibroblasts. The underlying substratum is visualized through these damaged cellular areas. In the three control preparations, the morphology of the fibroblasts is unaltered.

One other significant observation was made. A few treponemes were observed attached to the cultured muscle cells that were exposed to the high-speed supernatant. These treponemes were apparently not

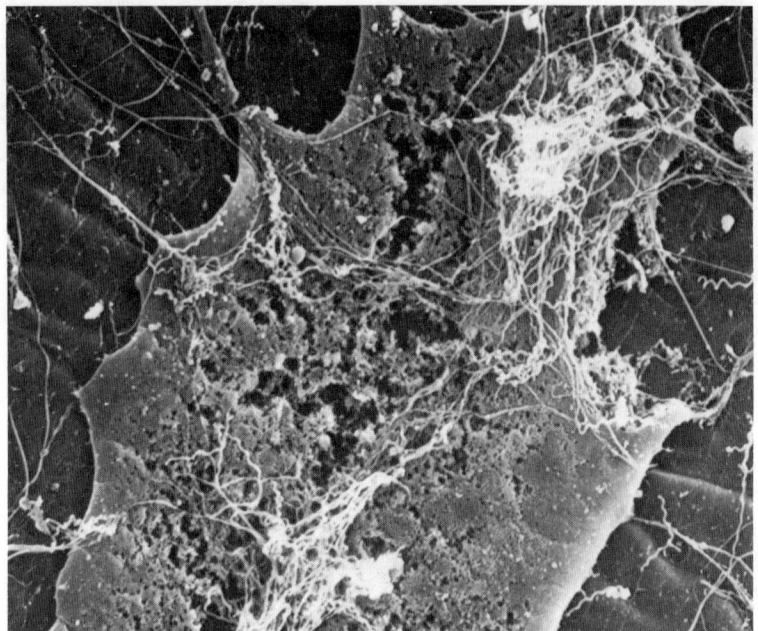

Figure 5 Destruction of background fibroblasts in a preparation of cultured cells from skeletal muscle (×3000). (From Ref. 5.)

pelleted during the high-speed centrifugation, or were inadvertantly resuspended during the removal of the supernatant. Figure 6 shows a portion of a myotube with an attached "half-treponeme". Note the short length and few coils relative to the other attached treponemes. This organism appears to be penetrating into the myotube.

Experiments were then performed with cultured cells derived from different nerve tissues. Treponemes were found to attach to cells from dorsal root ganglia, superior cervical ganglia (Fig. 7), and from spinal cord. *Treponema pallidum* attached to the neuronal cell body as well as to the neuritic extensions.

Neuronal cells were presumptively identified by their characteristic morphology. Definitive identification is based on the ability of these cells to respond to electrical stimulation with an action potential. Attempts were made to evaluate the influence of *T. pallidum* on the genesis and character of the action potential of cultured nerve cells. Figure 8 shows representative action potentials of control cells (Fig. 8A) and test cells (Figs. 8B and 8C) incubated with viable treponemes for 13 hr. Normal action potentials are readily distinguished from abnormal action potentials.

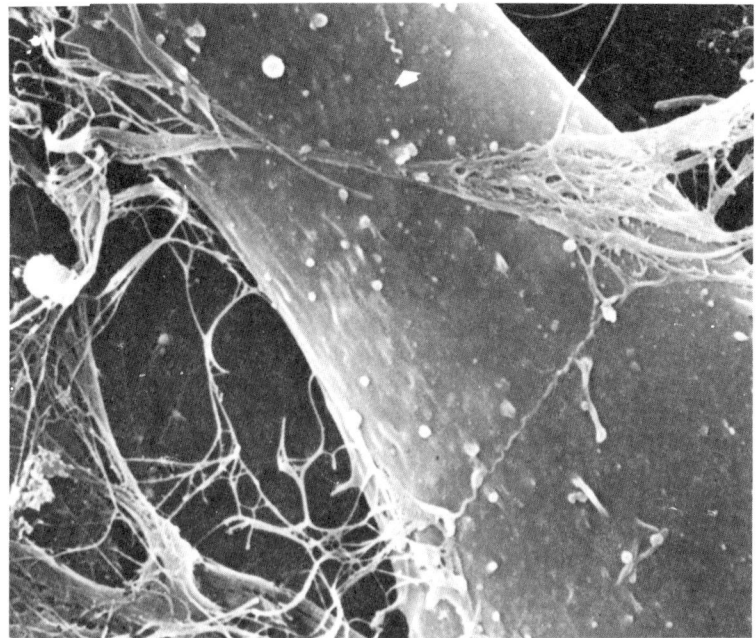

Figure 6 Portion of a half-treponeme at the surface of a myotube (×5400). (From Ref. 5.)

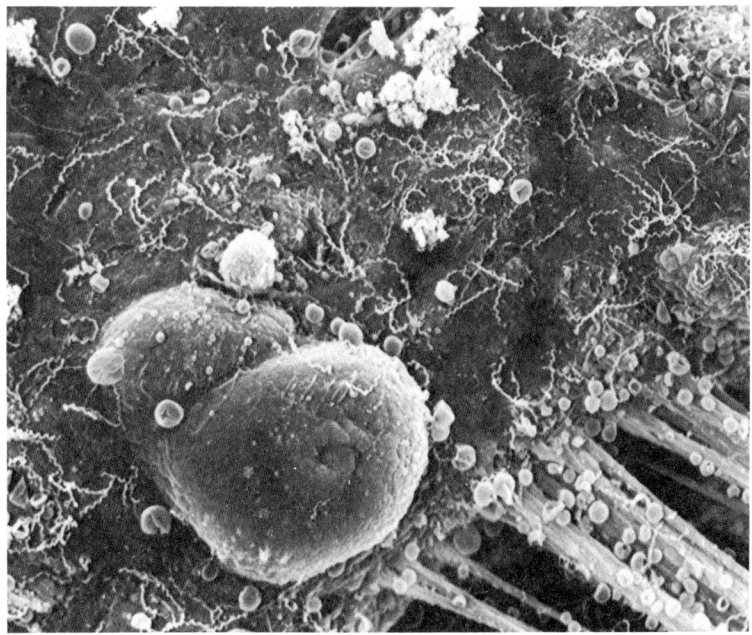

Figure 7 Treponemes attached to cultured cells derived from superior cervical ganglia (×1500). (From Ref. 5.)

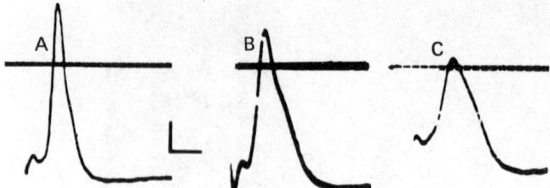

Figure 8 Action potentials elicited from cultured dorsal root ganglia: (A) action potentials of nerve cells exposed to control medium and (B and C) viable treponemes. (From Ref. 3.)

The results of a typical experiment are shown in Table 2. Normal responses were defined as those that fell within one standard deviation of the resting membrane potential, the maximum rate of rise, the afterhyperpolarization maximum, and the spike amplitude for the controls not containing treponemes. At 0 hr the nerve cells exposed to control medium and to the two different concentrations of *T. pallidum* exhibited normal functioning. After incubation for 26 hr, 10 of 10 cells in the control preparation responded normally. With 2×10^8 treponemes per milliliter, abnormal responses were detected after 13 hr; only 3 of 11 cells responded normally. After 18 hr action potentials could no

Table 2 Treponemal Interference with Electrophysiologic Responses of Cultured Dorsal Root Ganglia

	Normal[a] response/total tested		
Time (hr)	Without treponemes	2×10^8 treponemes per milliliter	1×10^8 treponemes per milliliter
0	5/5	5/5	
5		5/5	
7		5/5	
10		5/5	
13		3/11	5/5
18		0/5	6/6
26	10/10	0/5	10/12

[a]Normal responses are defined as those that fall within one standard deviation of the resting membrane potential, the maximum rate of rise, the afterhyperpolarization maximum, and the spike amplitude for the controls not containing treponemes.
Source: Reference 4.

longer be elicited. With 1×10^8 treponemes per milliliter, normal responses were detected in 5 of 5 cells after 18 hr and in 10 or 12 cells after 26 hr.

In further experiments, cultures of nerve cells were inoculated with viable treponemes or controls of culture medium, heated treponemes, and high-speed supernatant. Cultures were examined with phase-contrast microscopy. After incubation for 24 hr, pronounced damage to both neuronal and fibroblastic cells was apparent in cultures exposed to viable treponemes. Neuronal morphology was not altered in the three control preparations.

Treponemal degradation of neuronal cells was visualized with scanning electron microscopy. Figure 9A shows the atypical morphology of a nerve cell after 16 hr of incubation with viable treponemes. In contrast to the round, elevated appearance of normal neurons, the cells assumed a flattened morphology and their surfaces were marked with irregular holes. Various stages of treponeme-mediated nerve cell degradation were observed. Figure 9B shows the ghost-like remnant of an apparent dorsal root ganglion cell. The nuclear profile in the center of the cell has deteriorated to a coagulated matrix. Remnants of cellular substratum attachment processes are visualized peripherally. The edge of the cell is demarcated by fibrous extensions which are associated with small bleblike particles. These may represent the cytoskeletal cores of radially extending retraction fibers. Other preparations showed further degradation, with loss of differentiation between cytoplasm and nucleus and degradation of fibrous extensions of the cellular margin.

Preparations of capillaries were obtained from rabbit brain cortex. *Treponema pallidum* was incubated with capillaries and visualized using dark-field and phase-contrast microscopy. The attachment of treponemes was identical to that previously described for numerous types of cultured cells derived from different mammalian tissues. Within minutes after inoculation treponemes attached in random fashion along the length of the capillary vessels. With increasing times of incubation, higher numbers of organisms attached. Attachment was mediated through the tip of the treponemes, usually at one end but occasionally at both ends, and attached treponemes retained motility longer than unattached organisms.

The addition of *T. pallidum* to capillary preparations results in the immediate precipitation of an insoluble fibrinlike network. The capillaries strongly adhere to the glass cover slips. Initially, this was advantageous, in that specimen fixation, dehydration, and critical-point drying were facilitated. Visualization of treponemal attachment to capillaries, however, is obscured by this network of fibrillar strands.

If the treponemal preparations were centrifuged at high speed and resuspended in fresh medium, this precipitation did not occur. In order to attain adherence of the capillaries for subsequent fixation and processing, cover slips were coated with poly-L-lysine. Figure 10 shows capillaries incubated with *T. pallidum* for 20 hr. Numerous

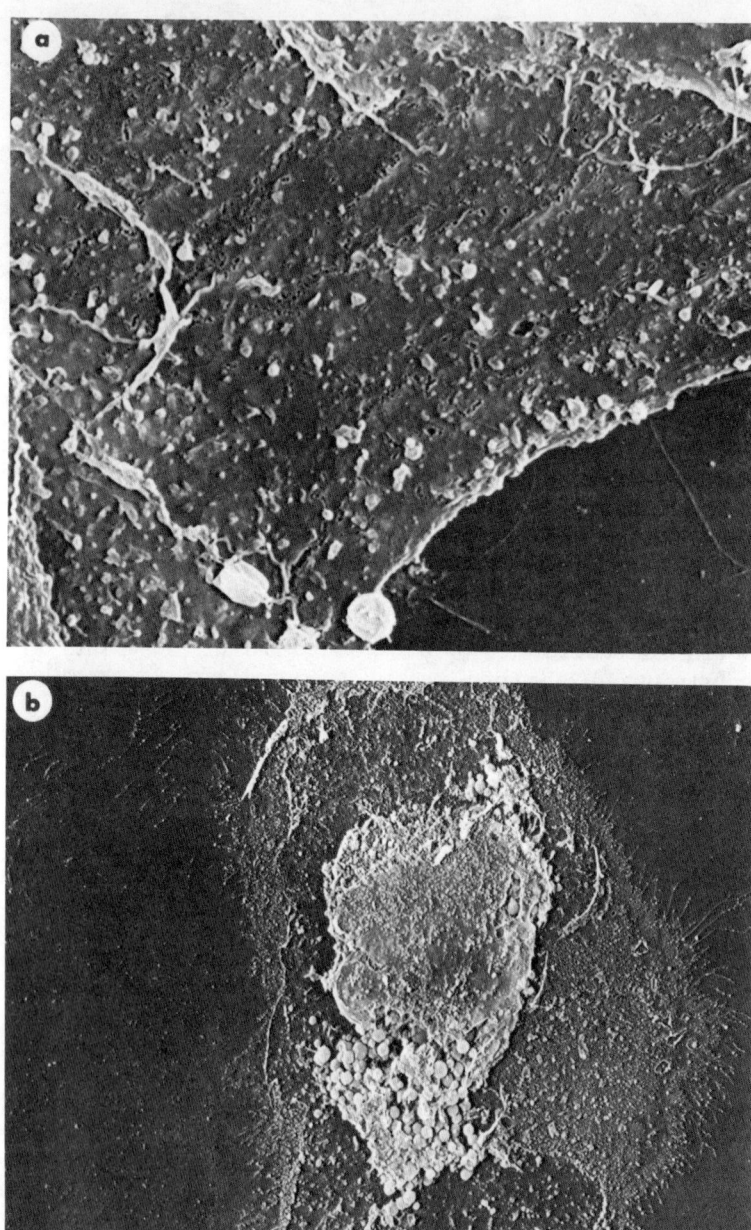

Figure 9 Treponeme-mediated destruction of dorsal root ganglia: (a) flattened cellular morphology with irregular holes in the membrane (×3900) and (b) ghostlike remnant with coagulated nuclear matrix and peripheral cellular substratum attachment processes (×2000). (From Ref. 4.)

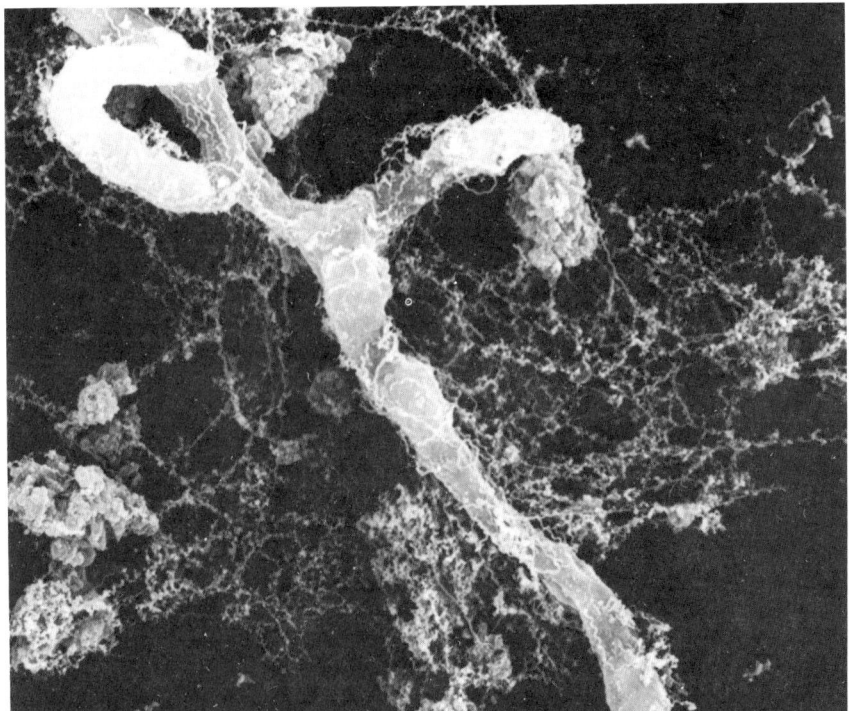

Figure 10 Capillaries isolated from rabbit brain cortex after incubation with viable treponemes for 20 hr (×1600). (From Ref. 4.)

organisms are attached to the outer surface. An extracellular patchy meshwork was associated with areas of treponemal aggregation. In the two control preparations this material was not detected or was observed in minimal amounts. A few half-treponemes were observed attached to outer capillary surface (Fig. 11). These organisms were approximately 5 µm in length (instead of 10 to 20 µm) and contained only 3 to 5 coils (instead of 10 to 12).

Applications to Clinical Manifestations

Numerous other studies using lower inocula of treponemes have indicated that *T. pallidum* interacts with cultured cells without damaging them (10). The findings presented in this chapter demonstrate the disruptive influences of *T. pallidum* at higher inocula. Three observations indicate that disruption of the various cultured cells was mediated through the specific attachment of treponemes to the cells: First, heat-inactivated organisms that failed to attach did not damage the cells; second, the high-speed supernatant which contains soluble

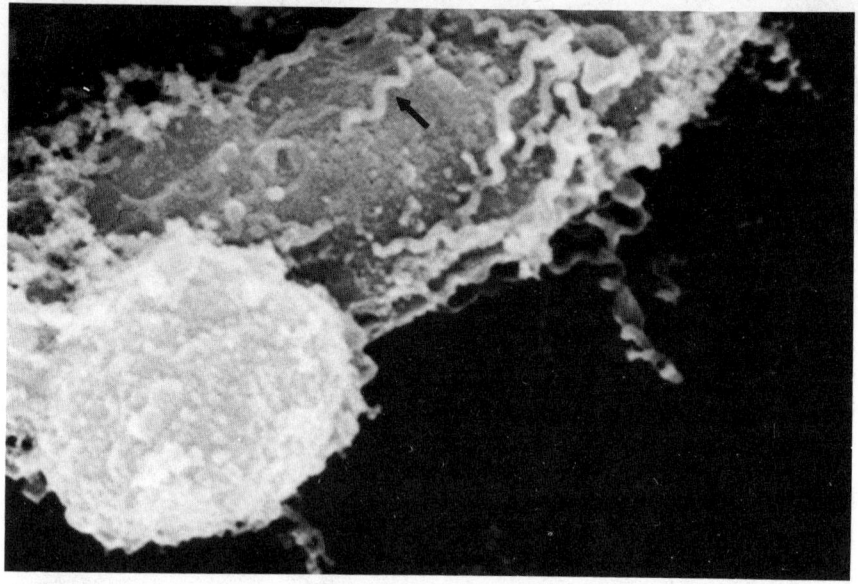

Figure 11 Portion of a half-treponeme at the surface of a capillary (×11,000). (From Ref. 6.)

treponemal, testicular, and inflammatory products, but not treponemes, did not damage the cultured cells; and third, cultured cells incubated inverted in chambers with viable organisms were not morphologically altered, indicating that treponemal damage is not due to the release of soluble mediators by viable organisms.

Repesh et al. (3,4), using cultured nerve cells, reported for the first time treponemal disruption of tissue culture cells. Morphologic damage initially involved holes in the nerve cell membrane, accompanied by a flattening of the typical elevated morphology. Further disruption of cellular integrity was characterized by condensation of the nucleus and an outlining of cellular boundaries by fibrous cytoskeletal remnants. Similar morphologic alterations have been shown in cells treated with Triton X (polyethylene glycol p-isoctylphenyl ether), a detergent that solubilizes the plasma membrane (11,12), or EGTA, a Ca^{2+} specific chelator. Cells treated with EGTA become round and detach from the substratum, leaving cellular retraction fibers that are associated with areas of cell substratum attachment. These processes can be easily broken by gentle manipulation and separated from material that remains attached to the substratum. This substrate-attached material mediates cell adhesion and is principally composed of fibronectin, glycosaminoglycans, and cytoskeletal proteins (13). A transmembrane association between extracellular fibronectin and internal actin-containing stress fibers has been demonstrated (14). These areas are important in cell attachment and appear to be more resistant to degradation by *T. pallidum*.

Similar treponeme-mediated damage has been observed using rabbit testicular cells, human foreskin cells, Hep-2 cells derived from human laryngeal tissue, rat cardiac muscle cells, and rat skeletal muscle cells. Since damage to the cultured cells is not mediated through soluble constituents of host or treponemal origin, it is probable that the initial cellular lesion occurs at the point of attachment of treponemes. Some type of treponemal toxin may exert a membrane lytic effect that degrades these different cell types.

Treponema pallidum apparently possesses the ability to penetrate cells, as demonstrated by the partial entry of the organism into the muscle cells. Treponemes appear to attain intracellular residence in vivo within a variety of host cells (15-18) and in vitro within cultured rabbit testicular cells (19). Penetration of treponemes may result from the membrane lytic action of the treponemal toxin that produces small holes in the membrane. If few organisms attach, cells may be able to repair the damage. If large numbers of organisms attach, membrane damage with eventual morphologic disruption may occur.

These findings give further insight into pathologic mechanisms in syphilis. Damage could emanate from host inflammatory reactions and from host defenses that clear the organisms and release treponemal components (20). This mechanism is supported by the minimal tissue pathology early in infection and by the rebound phenomenon in rabbits treated with cortisone (1,2). A second mechanism of tissue pathology may be related to the ability of *T. pallidum* to penetrate cells, thereby damaging mammalian cells, and/or to produce toxins. Both mechanisms of tissue pathology may be operative in syphilis. In the primary stage, early manifestations of erythema and induration may be attributed to degradation of host tissues by specific treponemal toxins. Later manifestations of necrosis and ulceration may be related to host defenses and clearance of organisms. This dual mechanism of tissue pathology may also apply to the much more severe clinical manifestations in tertiary and congenital syphilis.

Two preliminary reports (21,22) have indicated that *T. pallidum* is associated with nerve fibers within lesion material. Our in vitro observations involving cultured nerve cells may explain two characteristic findings in syphilitic infection. First, after attachment of treponemes to nerve cells, the ability of these cells to generate an action potential was impaired. This nerve cell dysfunction may be the basis for the painless nature of many of the clinical manifestations of primary, secondary, tertiary, and congenital syphilis. Second, with extended incubation, treponemes disrupted the morphologic integrity of the cultured neuronal cells. This pronounced effect may be the basis for the central nervous system damage that occurs in tertiary and congenital syphilis. Both syndromes involve severe nerve degeneration in the cerebral cortex, spinal cord, and peripheral nerves.

Capillary preparations provide a useful and convenient tool to investigate some of the aspects of treponemal pathogenesis because they represent intact tissues and probably reflect in vivo conditions more accurately than tissue culture cells. In primary, secondary, tertiary, and congenital syphilis, *T. pallidum* localized perivascularly. The half-treponeme observed on the capillary surface in our studies indicates that the organisms penetrate through endothelial cells or penetrate between endothelial cell junctions. *Treponema pallidum* possesses a mucopolysaccharidase enzyme (23) which could degrade the mucopolysaccharide ground substance between endothelial cells (Chapter 11). This would explain the entry of organisms into the bloodstream from the initial site of infection. *Treponema pallidum* associates with mucopolysaccharides on the surface of tissue culture cells (24); a similar association may occur in vivo. The interaction of treponemes with capillary ground substance could damage capillary integrity and inhibit blood supply, causing necrosis and ulceration of infected tissues. Furthermore, immune rabbit serum prevents treponemal attachment to tissue culture cells (7,25, Chaps. 11 and 12). Similar findings were reported using isolated capillary tissues (6). If these in vitro findings apply to in vivo infection, blockage of attachment to tissues may be one important aspect of the host immune response that results in healing. Unattached organisms could then be cleared by other host defenses such as activated T lymphocytes (26), macrophages (20,27), or polymorphonuclear leukocytes. Blockage of attachment to host tissues by humoral factors may also partially explain the immunity that follows infection (28-31). If immune rabbits are challenged with *T. pallidum*, the organisms remain localized for a number of days at the site of injection and fail to disseminate to draining lymph nodes and to other tissues. This lack of dissemination may reflect the inability of treponemes to attach to the outer surface of capillaries and to penetrate through endothelial cells to enter the bloodstream.

Acknowledgement

We wish to thank the following collaborators, who are directly responsible for this research: Dr. Robert S. Pozos and Steven Oakes in the Department of Physiology, Dr. Eugene Quist and Robert Zeleznikar in the Department of Pharmacology at the School of Medicine, University of Minnesota at Duluth. We also express our gratitude for expert technical assistance to Eileen Gannon, Paul Lima, Anne Utyro, Bonnie Tyson, and Carolynn Gabriel. Without their help this research would not have been accomplished.

References

1. T. B. Turner and D. H. Hollander. Biology of the treponematoses. *WHO Monogr. Ser.* 35:1-277 (1957).
2. T. B. Turner. Syphilis and the treponematoses. In *Infectious Agents and Host Reactions* (S. Mudd, Ed.). W. B. Saunders, Philadelphia, 1970, pp. 346-390.
3. L. A. Repesh, T. J. Fitzgerald, S. G. Oakes, and R. S. Pozos. Scanning electron microscopy of the attachment of *Treponema pallidum* to nerve cells in vitro. *Br. J. Vener. Dis.* 58:211-219 (1982).
4. S. G. Oakes, L. A. Repesh, R. S. Pozos, and T. J. Fitzgerald. Electrophysiologic dysfunction and cellular disruption of sensory neurons during incubation with *Treponema pallidum*. *Br. J. Vener. Dis.* 58:220-227 (1982).
5. T. J. Fitzgerald, L. A. Repesh, and S. G. Oakes. Morphologic destruction of cultured cells by *Treponema pallidum*. *Br. J. Vener. Dis.* 58:1-11 (1982).
6. E. E. Quist, T. J. Fitzgerald, L. A. Repesh, and R. Zeleznikar. Capillary tissues as a biologic tool for characterizing pathogenesis and immunology of *Treponema pallidum*. *Br. J. Vener. Dis.* (accepted 7/82).
7. T. J. Fitzgerald, R. C. Johnson, J. N. Miller, and J. A Sykes. Characterization of the attachment of *Treponema pallidum* (Nichols strain) to cultured mammalian cells and the potential relationship of attachment to pathogenicity. *Infect. Immun.* 18:467-478 (1977).
8. T. J. Fitzgerald, J. N. Miller, J. A. Sykes, and R. C. Johnson. Tissue culture and *Treponema pallidum*. In *The Biology of Parasitic Spirochetes* (R. C. Johnson, Ed.). Academic, New York, 1976, pp. 57-64.
9. J. A. Sykes and E. B. Moore. A simple tissue culture chamber. *Tex. Rep. Biol. Med.* 18:288-297 (1960).
10. T. J. Fitzgerald. Pathogenesis and immunology of *Treponema pallidum*. *Annu. Rev. Microbiol.* 35:29-54 (1981).
11. P. B. Bell, M. M. Miller, K. L. Carraway, and J. P. Revel. SEM revealed changes in the distribution of the triton insoluble cytoskeleton of Chinese hamster ovarian cells induced by dibutryl cyclic AMP. In *Scanning Electron Microscopy*, Vol. 2 (R. P. Becker and O. Johari, Eds.). SEM, Inc. AMP, O'Hare, Illinois, pp. 899-906.
12. D. Gospodarowicz, D. Delgado, and I. Vlodvasky. Permissive effect of the extracellular matrix on cell proliferation in vitro. *Proc. Nat. Acad. Sci.* 77:4094-4098 (1980).

13. L. A. Culp, B. A. Murray, and B. J. Rollins. Fibronectin and proteoglycans as determinants of cell-substrate adhesion. *J. Supramol. Struct.* 11:401-427 (1979).
14. I. I. Singer. The fibronexus: A transmembrane association of fibronectin containing fibers and bundles of 5 nm microfilaments in hamster and human fibroblasts. *Cell* 16:675-685 (1979).
15. H. A. Azar, T. D. Pham, and A. K. Kurban. An electron microscopic study of a syphilitic chancre. *Arch. Pathol.* 90:143-150 (1970).
16. V. Lauderdale and J. N. Goldman. Serial ultrathin sectioning demonstrating the intracellularity of *T. pallidum*. *Br. J. Vener. Dis.* 48:87-99 (1972).
17. J. A. Sykes and J. N. Miller. Intracellular location of *Treponema pallidum* (Nichols strain) in the rabbit testis. *Infect. Immun.* 4:307-314 (1971).
18. J. A. Sykes, J. N. Miller, and A. J. Kalan. *Treponema pallidum* within cells of a primary chancre from a human female. *Br. J. Vener. Dis.* 50:40-44 (1974).
19. T. J. Fitzgerald, J. N. Miller, and J. A. Sykes. *Treponema pallidum* (Nichols strain) in tissue cultures: Cellular attachment, entry, and survival. *Infect. Immun.* 11:1133-1140 (1975).
20. P. H. Hardy, D. J. Graham, E. E. Nell, and A. M. Dannenberg. Macrophages in immunity to syphilis: Suppressive effect of concurrent infection with *Mycobacterium bovis* BCG on the development of syphilitic lesions and growth of *Treponema pallidum* in tuberculin-possitive rabbits. *Infect. Immun.* 26:751-763 (1979).
21. P. S. Gregoriew. Uchebnik venericheskich i kojnich beleznej. Biomedgriz. NKA USSR, 1938.
22. N. M. Ovcinnikov and V. V. Delektorskij. *Treponema pallidum* in nerve fibers. *Br. J. Vener. Dis.* 51:10-18 (1974).
23. T. J. Fitzgerald and R. C. Johnson. Mucopolysaccharidase of *Treponema pallidum*. *Infect. Immun.* 24:261-268 (1979).
24. T. J. Fitzgerald, R. C. Johnson, and D. M. Ritzi. Relationship of *Treponema pallidum* to acidic mucopolysaccharides. *Infect. Immun.* 24:252-260 (1979).
25. N. S. Hayes, K. E. Muse, A. M. Collier, and J. B. Baseman. Parasitism by virulent *Treponema pallidum* of host cell surfaces. *Infect. Immun.* 17:174-186 (1977).
26. S. A. Lukehart, S. A. Baker-Zander, R. M. C. Lloyd, and S. Sell. Characterization of lymphocyte responsiveness in early experimental syphilis. II. Nature of cellular infiltration and *Treponema pallidum* distribution in testicular lesions. *J. Immunol.* 124:461-467 (1980).
27. S. A. Lukehart and J. N. Miller. Demonstration of the in vitro phagocytosis of *Treponema pallidum* by rabbit peritoneal macrophages. *J. Immunol.* 121:2014-2024 (1978).

28. A. M. Chesney and J. E. Kemp. Studies in experimental syphilis. VI. On variations in the response of treated rabbits to reinoculation; and on cryptogenetic reinfection with syphilis. *J. Exp. Med.* 44:589-606 (1926).
29. M. C. Cumberland and T. B. Turner. The rate of multiplication of *T. pallidum* in normal and immune rabbits. *Am. J. Syph.* 33:201-212 (1949).
30. F. W. Reynolds. The fate of *Treponema pallidum* inoculated subcutaneously into immune rabbits. *Johns Hopkins Hosp. Bull.* 69:53-60 (1941).
31. G. W. Waring and W. L. Fleming. The effect of partial immunity on the dissemination of infection in experimental syphilis. *Am. J. Syph.* 36:268-375 (1952).

11
Attachment of Treponemes to Cell Surfaces

T. J. FITZGERALD
University of Minnesota
School of Medicine
Duluth, Minnesota

Experimental Observations   196
Perspectives   214
Summary   220
References   221

Until recently, little was known about the pathogenic capabilities of *Treponema pallidum*. Turner and Hollander (1,2) compared strains of *T. pallidum* that exhibited different degrees of virulence. The Chicago strain was highly virulent; it produced extensive necrotic lesions, with rapid spread of *T. pallidum* to other tissues. In contrast, strain C and strain H were not as virulent; they produced less extensive lesions, with minimal spread to other tissues. The Nichols strain, Truffi strain, and strain F were intermediate in virulence. One potential virulence factor emanated from these studies. The more virulent strains consistently produced, or at least were associated with, larger amounts of mucoid material within lesions. This review will summarize recent findings on the interaction between *T. pallidum* and tissue cultures and discuss their relation to the pathogenesis of syphilis. Emphasis will be placed upon the treponemal mucopolysaccharide capsule and treponemal mycopolysaccharidase.

Experimental Observations

Attachment of *T. pallidum* to Cells In Vitro

The incubation of *T. pallidum* with tissue culture cells results in rapid attachment of treponemes to the surface of the cultured cells. This is demonstrated via phase-contrast microscopy (3) in Fig. 1 and scanning electron microscopy (4) in Fig. 2. This phenomenon of attachment was initially observed by Wright (5) in 1962, but she minimized its importance, attributing it to "fortuitous collision with a sticky surface." In 1975, Fitzgerald, Miller, and Sykes (6) demonstrated that atttachment to cultured cells prolonged treponemal survival, as shown by increased times of retention of both motility and virulence. Virulent organisms were detected after 24 hr of incubation with cultured cells derived from rabbit testis or from a human cervical carcinoma; in contrast, without cultured cells, virulent organisms were not detected after 9 hr of incubation. In subsequent experiments (7), improved conditions extended retention of virulence to 7 days in the presence of cultured cells; virulence was lost in 4 to 5 days in the absence of cultured cells. The beneficial effect of cultured cells on treponemal survival was also apparent within the individual tissue culture vessels. Not all organisms attached to the tissue cells, and the unattached organisms consistently lost motility before the attached organisms.

The number of organisms that attach to cultured cells is directly related to the quantity inoculated. With initial inocula of 10^6, 10^7, or 10^8 treponemes per milliliter from a 10-day testicular infection, a relatively consistant 50 to 60% of the organisms attached (3). This suggests that some of the treponemes, although actively motile, are unable to attach. Attached organisms do not exhibit a predilection for specific areas on the individual cultured cells but, rather, are randomly distributed over the entire surface. Furthermore, within the culture vessels, treponemes attach in equal numbers to all of the cultured cells.

Attachment is mediated by the interaction between the tip of the treponemes and the cultured cell surface. The remaining portion of the organism is actively motile. Most organisms attach only at one end; a few (5 to 10%) attach at both ends. Scanning electron microscopy revealed no detectable physical disruption such as swelling or indention of the cultured cell surface at the site of treponemal attachment (4). In addition, no attachment organelles are observed at the tip of the organism and each end is morphologically identical to the other end. Hayes et al. (8) suggested that the nosepiece of the tip of *T. pallidum* (9) serves as a specific attachment organelle, and it might seem likely that a specialized organelle mediates treponemal attachment; both scanning and transmission electron microscopy have failed to demonstrate such an organelle.

11. Attachment of Treponemes to Cell Surfaces

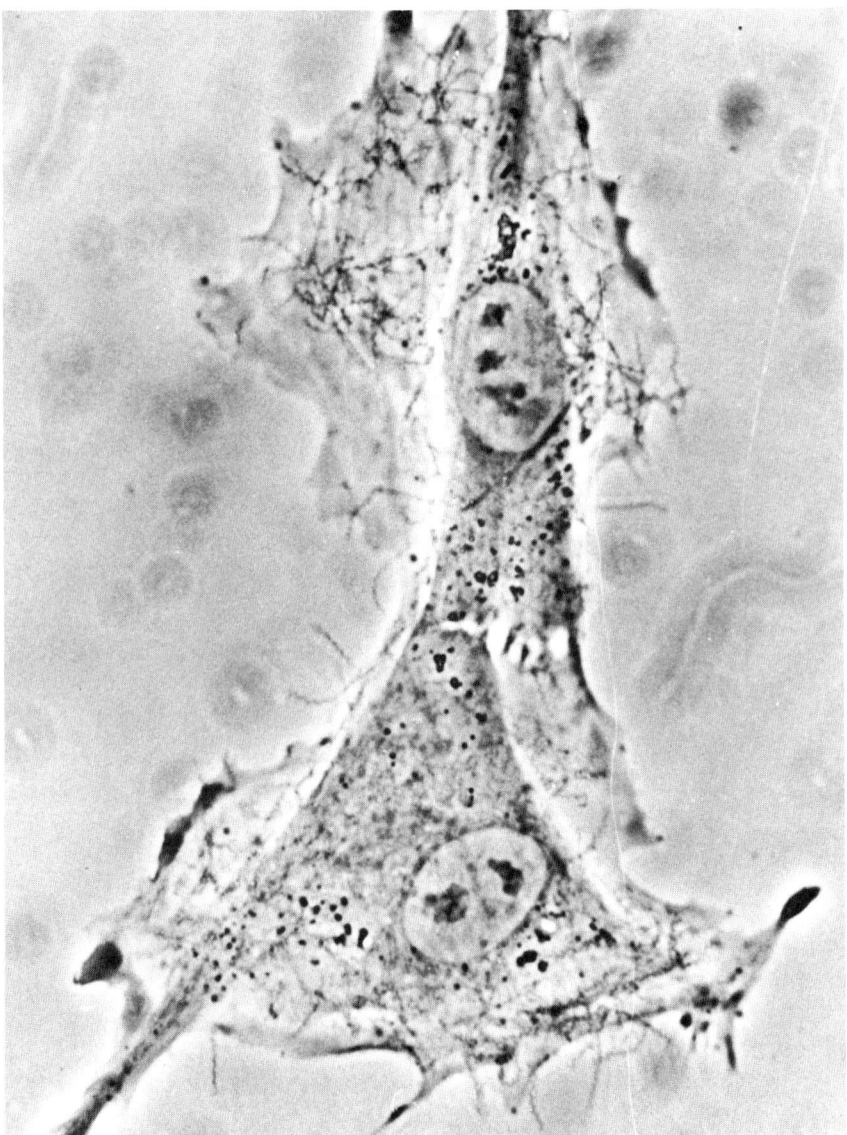

Figure 1 Phase-contrast micrograph of cultured cells derived from rabbit testis showing numerous attached treponemes (×1000). (From Ref. 3.)

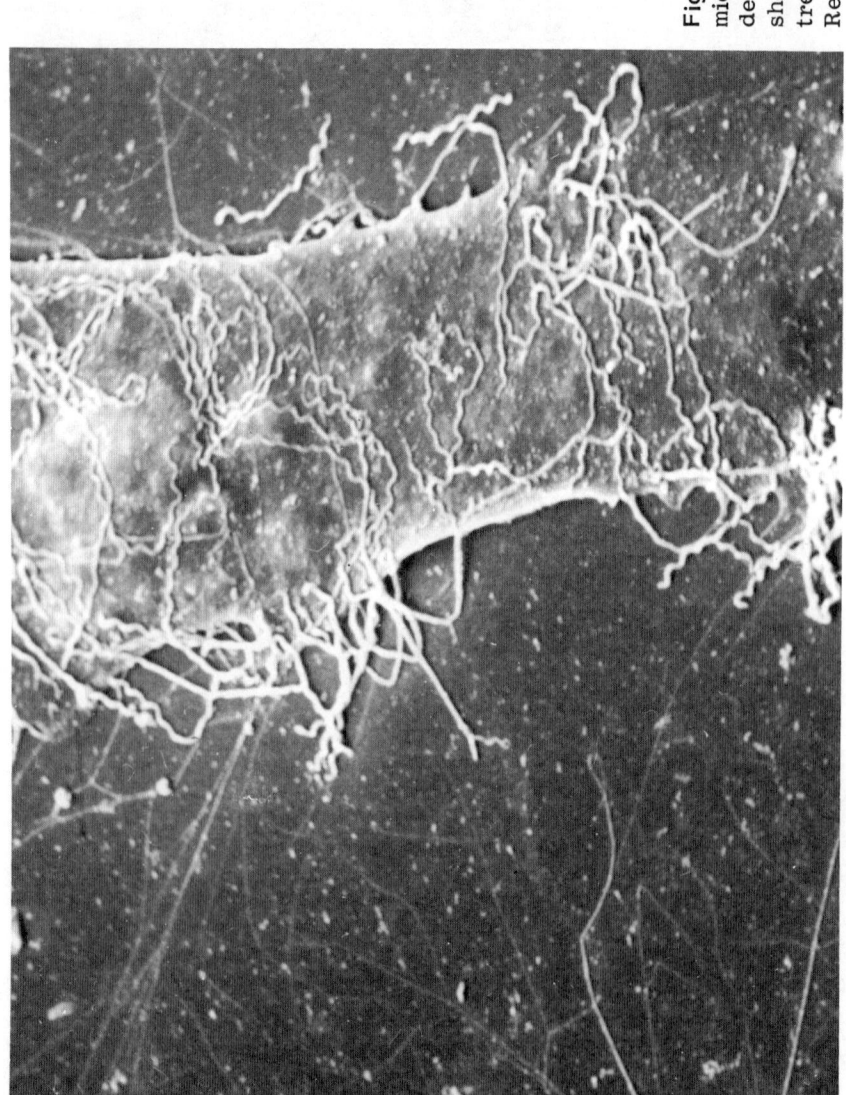

Figure 2 Scanning electron micrograph of cultured cells derived from rabbit testis showing numerous attached treponemes (×4000). (From Ref. 4.)

11. Attachment of Treponemes to Cell Surfaces

The attachment of treponemes may represent a balanced host-parasite interaction, occurring without harm to the cultured cells (3; see Chapter 10). In some experiments treponemes remain attached and actively motile for 6 to 7 days of incubation. Trypan Blue staining shows that attachment is not associated with loss of viability of the tissue culture cells. The only exception to this balanced host-parasite interaction was seen with large inocula of *T. pallidum*. In this situation, as many as 200 treponemes were attached per cultured cell; within 1 or 2 days some of the cultured cells lysed, leaving behind ghost remnants.

The following additional observations apply to the interaction of *T. pallidum* with tissue culture cells. First, attachment requires the viability of *T. pallidum*. When the organisms are rendered nonmotile by mild heat (50°C for 10 min) or exposure to air, they do not attach (6). Second, attachment is temperature dependent. As the temperature decreases from 37 to 4°C, the number of attached organisms decreases (8). These observations suggest that attachment is an active treponemal process, not a passive one. Third, *T. pallidum* is able to attach to a wide variety of cultured cells. In 20 published reports since 1975, treponemes attached to over 40 different cultured cell types, with consequent augmentation of the time of treponemal survival. Fourth, attachment of *T. pallidum* is also related to the viability of the cultured cells (3). When rabbit testis or rabbit kidney cultured cells were rendered nonviable by freeze-thaw cycles, far fewer organisms attached. Fifth, treponemes attach just as well to both actively growing and stationary-phase cultured cells (3). Lastly, the treponeme-cultured cell interaction is not adversely affected by different cell passages. Numbers of attached organisms and beneficial influences on treponemal survival were similar using rabbit testis cells that were primary cultures or cultures that were passaged two to nine times (3).

Nonpathogenic treponemes commonly associated with the human oral cavity or genital tract do not attach to tissue culture cells. This observation, initially reported by Fitzgerald et al. (6) using *T. denticola* and *Treponema phagedenis* biotype Reiter and rabbit testis cultured cells, has been confirmed in experiments using nine other nonpathogenic treponemes and six different cultured cell types (3). The authors proposed (1) that attachment of *T. pallidum* to cultured cells reflected a specific virulence determinant lacking in the nonpathogenic treponemes and (2) that attachment was an important initial step in the syphilitic disease process.

Mucopolysaccharide Capsule

The inability to detect antigen-antibody interactions in certain serologic tests that employ freshly isolated *T. pallidum* has been recognized for some time. It has been postulated that the treponemes possess an outer protective layer that has to be removed or altered prior to demonstrating seroreactivity (1,2,10-13). The electron micrographs of Schmerold and Deubner (14) and Swain (15) first suggested that *T. pallidum* had a capsular structure. Subsequently, a surface layer was demonstrated using ruthenium red and transmission or scanning electron microscopy (4,16). Figure 3 shows treponemes attached to cultured cells with (Fig. 3A) and without (Fig. 3B) exposure to ruthenium red. The amount of precipitate was variable. Some treponemes were heavily coated with a uniform layer; others exhibited an amorphous uneven distribution; while still others failed to react with ruthenium red. Using acidified bovine serum albumin (acid BSA), which produces a precipitate in the presence of acidic mucopolysaccharides, identical observations of variability relative to mucopolysaccharide distribution over the length of the organism were made (17). Furthermore, the total percentage of freshly harvested treponemes within individual preparations that reacted with acid BSA was highly variable. With some preparations, as many as 90% were at least partially acid BSA positive, whereas with others only 5% were. The treponemes were agglutinated by wheat germ and soybean agglutinins, indicating the presence of surface-associated N-acetyl-D-glucosamine and N-acetyl-D-galactosamine. The two mucopolysaccharides, hyaluronic acid and chondroitin sulfate, are long, straight-chain polymers compromised of N-acetyl-D-glucosamine and N-acetyl-D-galactosamine bound to D-glucuronic acid. It thus seems likely that the capsule of *T. pallidum* is comprised of hyaluronic acid, chondroitin sulfate, or mucopolysaccharides that are closely related to these two substances (17).

The occurrence of mucoid material within syphilitic lesions is characteristic of infection with *T. pallidum*. Observations on degeneration of tissue with mucoid accumulation were made in the early part of this century (18-23) and extended by Scott and Dammin (24-26). At various times after inoculation with *T. pallidum*, infected tissues were excised and stained with toluidine blue, a stain which changes from blue to violet purple in the presence of acidic mucopolysaccharides. The change in color, termed metachromasia, correlated with increasing numbers of organisms. Prior treatment of infected tissue with bovine hyaluronidase abolished the metachromasia, suggesting that the predominant mucopolysaccharide was hyaluronic acid and/or chondroitin sulfate. Turner and Hollander (27,28) reported greatly increased numbers of treponemes within lesions, and increased amounts of mucoid material in animals treated with cortisone; the accumulation of mucoid material was most apparent in the early stages of rapidly progressing dermal and testicular lesions.

A comparable phenomenon occurs during incubation of *T. pallidum* with culture cells (29). As shown in Figs. 4A,B, a randomly distributed amorphous material accumulates at the surface of the cultured cells during incubation at 30°C. Deposition of this amorphous material requires attachment of treponemes to the cultured cells. The amount deposited is related to the number of treponemes attached per cell, as demonstrated by altering the number of organisms initially inoculated or the number of cultured cells present within the culture vessels. Amorphous material does not accumulate if the organisms are inactivated prior to inoculation. In addition, the accumulation of amorphous material is not due to a soluble component from host testicular tissue or to a soluble component developing during treponemal infection; membrane-filtered preparations of *T. pallidum* failed to induce the deposition at the surface of the cultured cells. This material is composed of acidic mucopolysaccharide, as indicated by its metachromatic staining properties, its stainability with ruthenium red, and its partial degradation by bovine and streptomyces hyaluronidase. The amorphous material may be attributed to the dissipation of the treponemal capsule during attachment to the cultured cell.

In experiments performed to further investigate these acidic mucopolysaccharides (17), low concentrations of the polycations ruthenium red and toluidine blue were shown to enhance survival of *T. pallidum*. These polycations may have stabilized the treponemal capsule through interaction with highly charged polyanionic mucopolysaccharides. In addition, exogenous sources of acidic mucopolysaccharides (commercial preparation of hyaluronic acid and the mucoid material obtained from syphilitic lesions) were assessed for influence on the in vitro survival of *T. pallidum*. In the presence of both of these preparations, pronounced clumping of organisms occurred within 24 hr of incubation. These clumps of treponemes contained mucopolysaccharides, as shown by reaction with acid BSA, by metachromatic staining with toluidine blue, and by partial degradation by hyaluronidase. It was suggested that these clumps resulted from enhanced synthesis of the treponemal capsule in the presence of exogenous mucopolysaccharides.

Attempts were made to examine the immunogenicity of mucoid material from syphilitic testes (30). Surprisingly, this material appeared to be immunosuppressive. This fluid was injected intramuscularly 30 days before intradermal inoculation of rabbits with *T. pallidum*; the subsequent incubation periods were considerably shortened relative to the corresponding controls not injected with the mucoid fluid (Fig. 5). Lesions in both sets of animals began to heal about 35 days after inoculation of *T. pallidum*. At this time, the test animals were again injected intramuscularly with mucoid testicular fluid. This resulted in interruption of the healing process and reactivation of the healing lesions (Fig. 5). Within a few weeks the reactivated lesions again began to heal. When the rabbits were injected intramuscularly with a third preparation of mucoid fluid on day 84 after inoculation of *T. pallidum*, reactivation of lesions was again observed (Fig. 5). These lesions eventually healed approximately 115 days after inoculation of

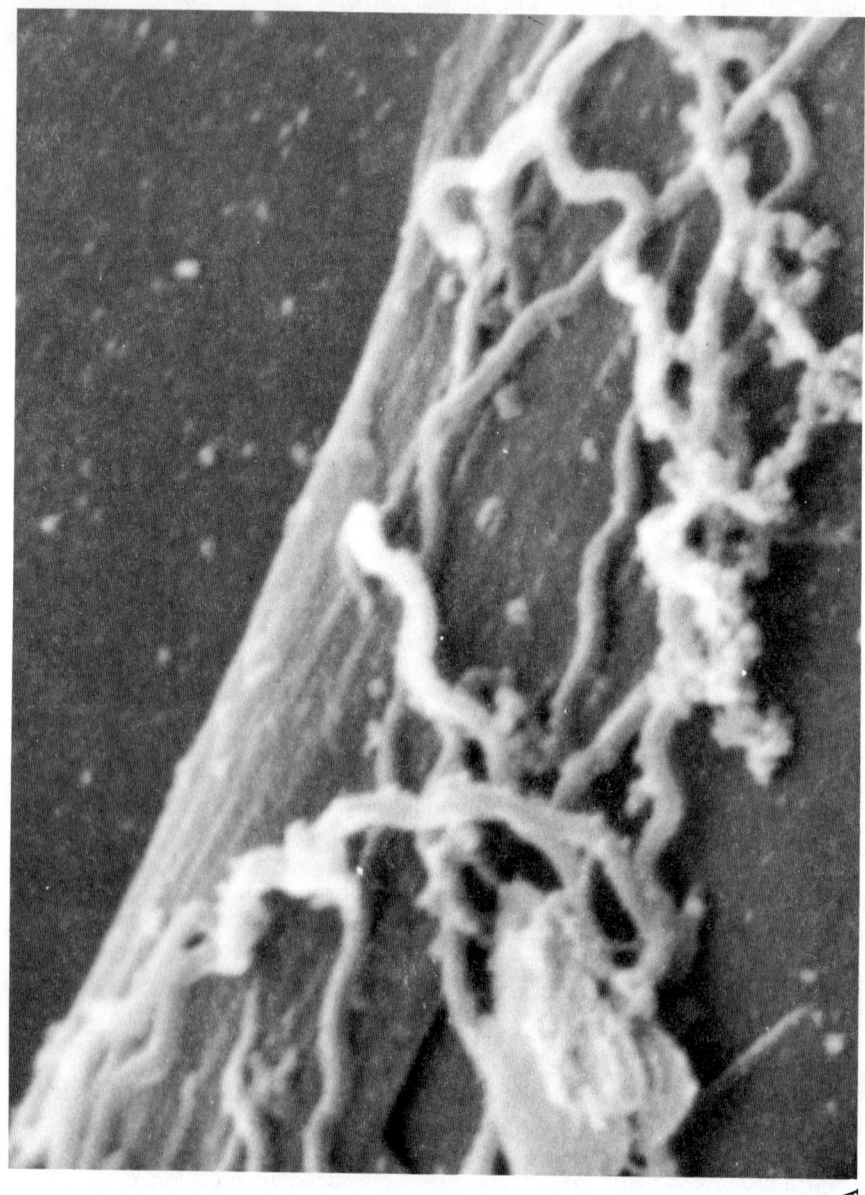

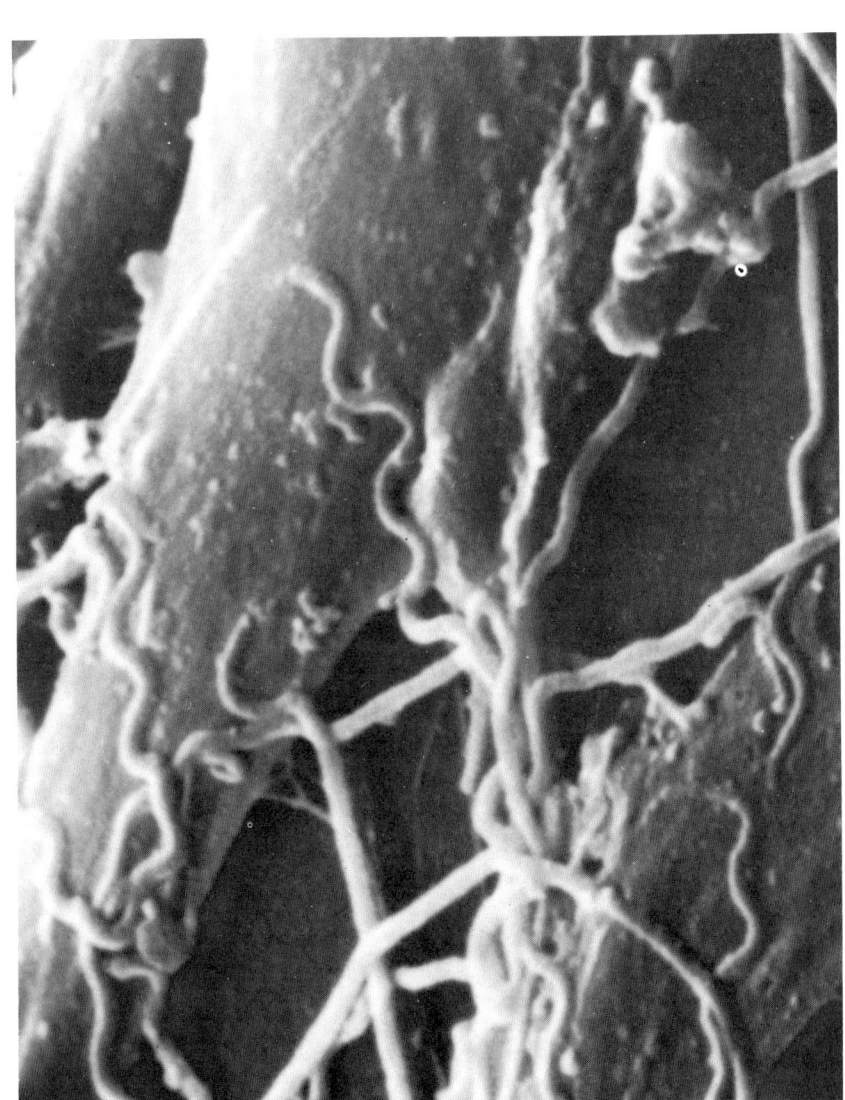

Figure 3 Scanning electron micrographs of treponemes (A) exposed to ruthenium red to demonstrate surface-associated mucopolysaccharides and (B) not exposed to ruthenium red (×10,000). (From Ref. 4.)

B

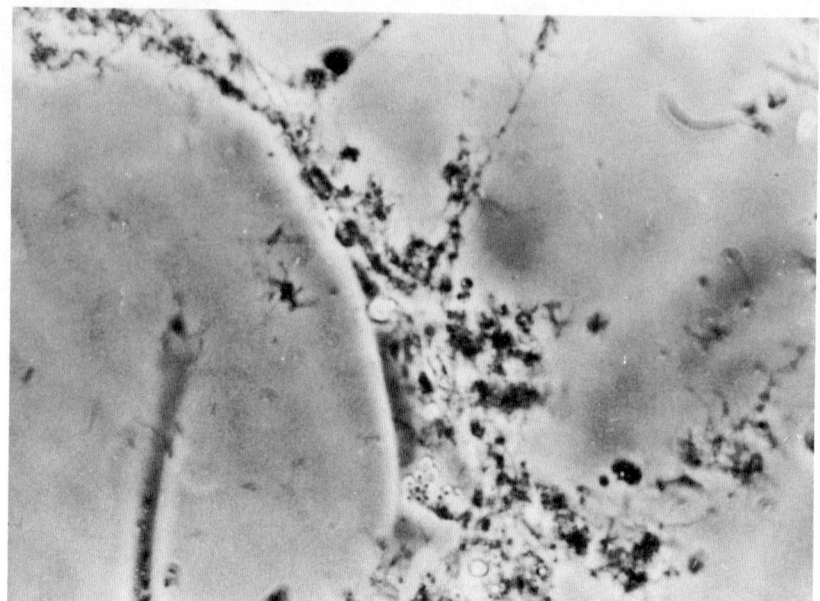

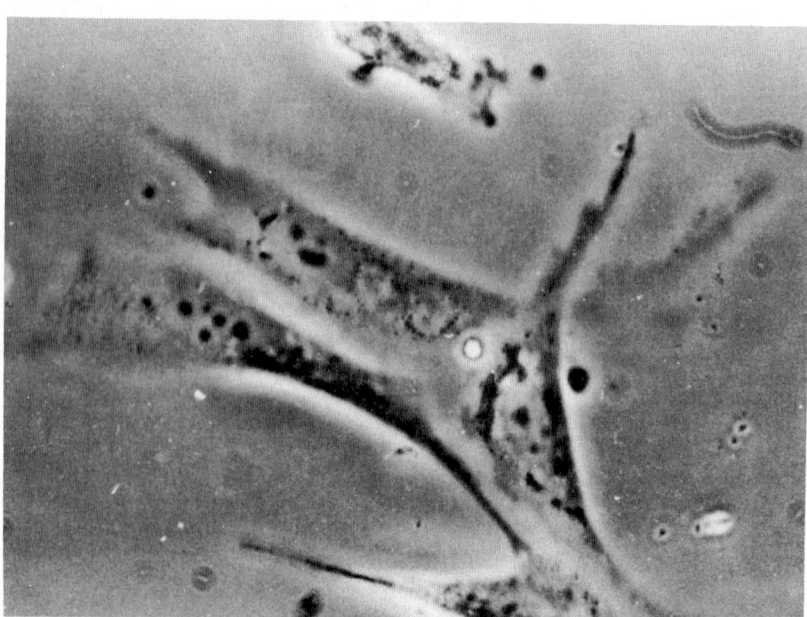

Figure 4 Phase-contrast micrographs of cultured cells derived from rabbit testis after incubation for 5 days (A) without and (B) with treponemes (×800). (From Ref. 29.)

11. Attachment of Treponemes to Cell Surfaces

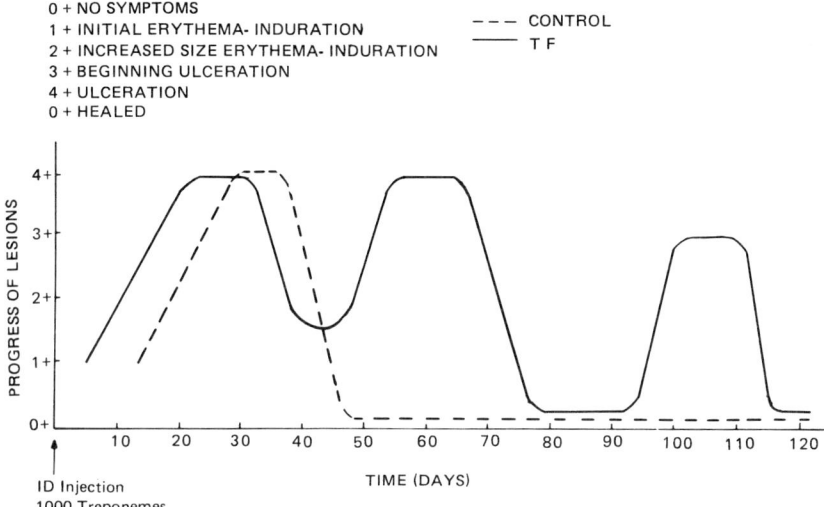

Figure 5 Two rabbits were inoculated interdermally on day 0 with 10^3 treponemes per site at four separate sites. The test rabbit (TF) was injected intramuscularly with infected testis fluid 30 days prior to day 0, and also on days 36 and 84. (From Ref. 30.)

T. pallidum. These in vivo observations suggest that the treponemal mucopolysaccharide capsule may act as an immunosuppressive agent. Other substances, such as cephaloridine or neoarsenobenzol, have been reported to cause reactivation of lesions (31).

The recent report of Bey et al. (32) provides further evidence that treponemal mucopolysaccharides are involved in the suppression of host responses. In this work, blast transformation of peripheral blood lymphocytes from uninfected rabbits was induced by incubation with Concanvalin A (ConA). Mucoid testicular fluid and sera from syphilitic rabbits were used as sources of treponemal capsular material; both of these preparations contain acidic mucopolysaccharides (30,33), presumably of treponemal origin. One set of experiments is summarized in Table 1. Mucoid testicular fluid inhibited the ConA induced blast transformation. This inhibition was abolished by prior treatment of the testicular fluid with commercial preparations of hyaluronidase. Sera from syphilitic rabbits also inhibited Con A induced blast transformation of lymphocytes, an effect that was abolished by pretreating the sera with hyaluronidase (Table 2). The presence of mucopolysaccharides in the infected sera paralleled the infective process. The inhibitory mucopolysaccharides were initially observed 3 days after inoculation of 1×10^7 to 3×10^7 treponemes per testis and remained detectable until day 35. With this inoculum, maximum numbers

Table 1 Inhibition of Blast Transformation by Infected Testis Fluid

Preparation	Mean CPM[a] per 0.2 ml culture
Control	1,100
ConA	252,100
Testis fluid	1,200
Testis fluid + ConA	1,800
Hyaluronidase-treated testis fluid	1,300
Hyaluronidase-treated testis fluid + ConA	251,000

[a]Counts per minute.
Source: Reference 32.

of treponemes occurred on days 9 to 11; thereafter, host defenses evolved that resulted in rapid decreases in treponemal numbers, and by day 24 few organisms were present (34,35).

Although immunosuppression in syphilis has been suggested in a large number of studies, these findings represent the initial demonstration of a specific treponemal component, the mucopolysaccharide capsule, that is immunosuppressive. Fitzgerald and Johnson (17) had shown that *T. pallidum* contained capsular mucopolysaccharides that were hyaluronic acid and chondroitin sulfate, or closely related substances. Bey et al. (32) indicated that blast transformation was

Table 2 Inhibition of Blast Transformation by Infected Serum

Preparation	Mean CPM[a] per 0.2 ml culture
Control (Preinfection Serum)	1,300
ConA	283,000
Infected serum	1,600
Infected serum + ConA	5,200
Hyaluronidase-treated infected serum	5,500
Hyaluronidase-treated infected serum + ConA	246,700

[a]Counts per minute.
Source: Reference 32.

11. Attachment of Treponemes to Cell Surfaces

inhibited by a commercial preparation of hyaluronic acid. Unless this commercial hyaluronic acid was somewhat degraded during preparation, this observation suggests that the treponemal mucopolysaccharides were not identical to hyaluronic acid.

Mucopolysaccharidase Enzyme

Fitzgerald and Johnson (33) documented the presence of a hyaluronidase-like enzyme, termed mycopolysaccharidase, in preparations of *T. pallidum*. The degradation of mucopolysaccharides was determined in the presence of viable *T. pallidum*, heat-inactivated (48°C, 10 min) *T. pallidum*, and a membrane filtrate of viable *T. pallidum*. Degradation was far more rapid in the preparation containing viable organisms. The presence of mucopolysaccharidase within treponeme preparations was also demonstrated by Ouchterlony immunodiffusion techniques.

During infection, antibody develops against the mucopolysaccharidase in parallel with the infective process. After intratesticular injection of 6×10^7 treponemes per testis, this antibody is apparent at 9, 16, and 32 days; antibody is no longer detected after 64 days. Antibodies against the treponemal mucopolysaccharidase enzyme apparently retard the activity of this enzyme. Uninfected rabbits were hyperimmunized with a commercial preparation of bovine hyaluronidase. The ability of *T. pallidum* to degrade mucopolysaccharides was then assessed in the presence of normal serum, syphilitic serum that contained antibodies to the commercial preparation of hyaluronidase, and antihyaluronidase serum. The greatest curtailment of mucopolysaccharide degradation was observed in the syphilitic serum (Table 3). It is interesting to note that the natural mode of presenting the enzyme to the host, i.e., during the course of syphilitic infection, enabled a seemingly more vigorous response than artificial sensitization.

Mechanism of Attachment

Attachment to host tissues appears to be an important step in initiating syphilitic disease (3,6,38). Two receptors are involved: the surface receptor on the host cells to which *T. pallidum* attaches, and the surface receptor on *T. pallidum* that interacts with the tissue receptor. Each will be discussed in turn.

Surface Receptors in Cultured Cells

As was noted above, treponemes appear to attach diffusely to cultured cells. Experiments were performed to determine whether the cultured cells used in adherence studies could be shown to contain surface mucopolysaccharides. Trypsinized cultured cells derived from rabbit testis were agglutinated by wheat germ agglutinin and soybean agglutinin. When wheat germ agglutinin was added to a monolayer of

Table 3 Treponemal Degradation of Mucopolysaccharides in the Presence of Normal; Immune; and Antihyaluronidase Sera

	Mucopolysaccharide concentration (µg/ml)					
	Experiment 1[a]			Experiment 2[b]		
Time (days)	Normal	Immune	Antihyaluronidase	Normal	Immune	Antihyaluronidase
0	250	250	250	125	125	125
1	62	250	250	<8	125	31
2				<8	125	31
3	62	250	125	<8	31	<8
6	16	125	50	<8	8	<8

[a]Mucopolysaccharide obtained from infected testis fluid.
[b]Mucopolysaccharide obtained from uninfected testicular tissue.
Source: Reference 33.

cultured cells for 1 hr and unbound lectin was removed by washing with culture medium, rabbit red blood cells (RBCs) which contain receptors for wheat germ agglutinin reacted with the lectin bound at the surface of the cultured cells and were not removed by subsequent washing. In a further experiment, the cultured cells were exposed to a commercial preparation of hyaluronidase before addition of lectin and RBCs. The results are shown in Fig. 6. The top micrograph (Fig. 6A) depicts cultured cells incubated with lectin, followed by RBCs; many of the RBCs were firmly bound to the tissue cells. The middle micrograph (Fig. 6B) depicts cultured cells pretreated with hyaluronidase, then incubated with lectin followed by RBCs; very few RBCs were bound. The bottom micrograph (Fig. 6C) depicts cultured cells incubated only with RBCs and not with lectin; nonspecific binding of RBCs did not occur.

These studies indicate that cultured testicular cells contain surface acidic mucopolysaccharides, and also that hyaluronidase under these laboratory conditions effectively removed the mucopolysaccharides. When similar procedures of enzyme incubation were performed, with treponemes being added to the tissue cells instead of wheat germ agglutinin and RBCs (Table 4), approximately half as many organisms were attached per cultured cell. This observation suggests that the cultured cell receptor mediating treponemal attachment is the surface layer of mucopolysaccharide (39).

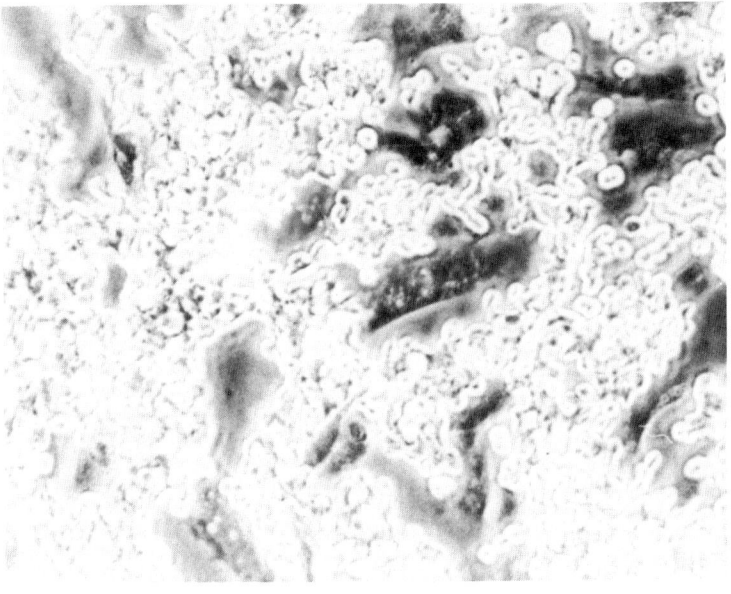

A

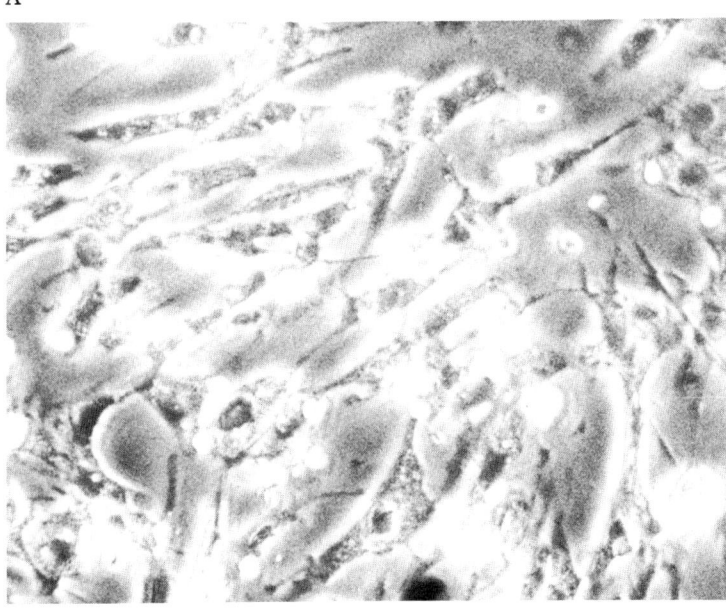

B

Figure 6 Cultured cells derived from rabbit testis treated as follows: (A) incubated with wheat germ agglutinin, followed by rabbit RBC; (B) pretreated with hyaluronidase, then incubated with wheat germ agglutinin, followed by rabbit RBC; and (C) incubated only with rabbit RBC (×400). (From Ref. 39.)

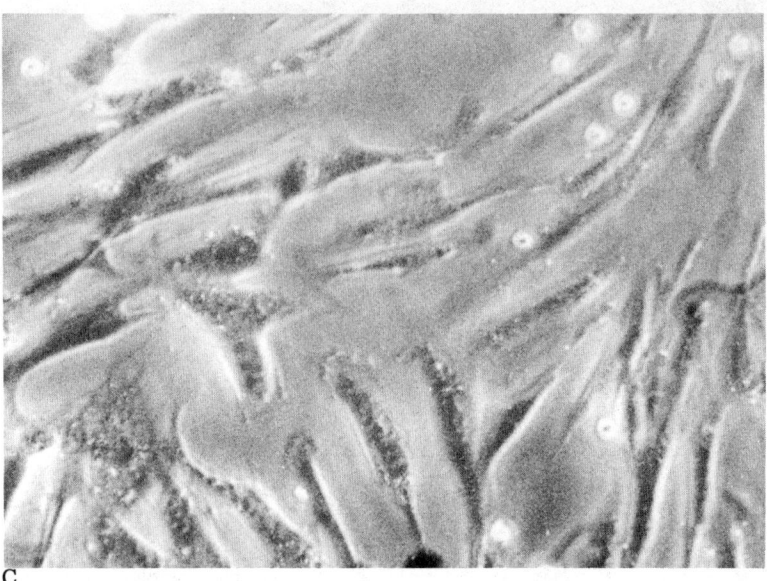

C

Figure 6 (Continued)

Treponemal Receptor

The attachment of *T. pallidum* to cultured cells usually does not physically alter these cells (3,4,6,38). The organisms attach at their distal end and remain actively motile. As shown by scanning electron microscopy (4), attachment seems to involve only a close physical proximity of treponemes to cultured cells; at the point of attachment, no morphological alterations in the cultured cell surface (swelling or indentation) were detected. Additionally, no attachment organelles were apparent at the tips of the organism (4).

Immune rabbit serum contains a factor, presumably antibody, that specifically blocks treponemal attachment to cultured cells (3). This ability to block attachment was demonstrated by preincubating *T. pallidum* for 22 hr in immune serum and then incubating them with cultured cells. After 1.5 to 3 hr the numbers of attached organisms were counted. Inhibition of attachment ranged from 73 to 100% in five separate experiments (Table 5). Using slightly different techniques Hayes et al. (8) observed approximately 50% inhibition of attachment. Preincubation of treponemes in immune serum for 22 to 33 hr followed by intradermal injection into rabbits caused a reduction in virulence, as shown by prolonged incubation periods when compared to similar preincubation in normal serum (Table 6). In seven experiments an average 2 log decrease in the numbers of virulent treponemes was observed after exposure to immune sera. This procedure was similar to

11. Attachment of Treponemes to Cell Surfaces

Table 4 Treponemal Attachment After Pretreatment of Cultured Cells with Hyaluronidase to Remove Cultured Cell Mucopolysaccharides

	Treponemes per culture cell	
Time (hr)	Control	Hyaluronidase treated
1	2-4	1
4	15-20	3-5
6	20-30	10-15
19	20-60	10-40
43	20-40	10-20

Source: Reference 39.

that previously used by Bishop and Miller (40) to demonstrate neutralizing activity in syphilitic rabbit serum. If blocking the attachment to mammalian cells is responsible for the decrease in virulence, this reaction is still not the same as other antigen-antibody interactions because of the long time required to bring it about. Perhaps other alterations in the *T. pallidum* must first occur during the in vitro incubation before the reaction can take place.

It is conceivable that the treponemal receptor is the mucopolysacharidase and that attachment is due to enzymatic reaction of the

Table 5 Blockage of Treponemal Attachment to Cultured Cells by Factors Within Immune Serum

	Preincubation with serum for 22-23 hr		Incubation with cultured cells for 1.5 to 3 hr		
	Percentage motile		Attached treponemes per 100 cultured cells		
Experiment	Normal	Immune	Normal	Immune	Percentage
1	76	76	600	165	73
2	68	60	100	20	80
3	92	76	400	0	100
4	52	64	350	0	100
5	98	98	750	125	83

Source: Reference 3.

Table 6 Reduction in Virulence of *Treponema pallidum* During Incubation with Immune Serum

Experiment	Incubation (hr)	Percentage motile		Sites positive sites inoculated		Day of appearance of EI[a]	
		Normal	Immune	Normal	Immune	Normal	Immune
1	22	52	64	2/2	2/2	8.0	11.5
2	26	92	80	4/4	4/4	6.0	12.5
3	26	98	84	4/4	4/4	6.5	14.5
4	33	10	20	4/4	4/4	6.9	10.2
5	24	96	96	4/4	3/4	5.2	10.0
6	26	98	94	4/4	4/4	6.2	13.5
7	24	88	92	3/3	3/3	11.7	18.0
Average						7.2	12.9
Estimated treponemes per milliliter						6×10^5	6×10^3

[a]Erythema and induration.

treponemal mucopolysaccharidase with the cultured cell mucopolysaccharide substrate. If the organisms attach enzymatically through their mucopolysaccharidase, and if blockage of attachment by immune serum is due to antibodies to this enzyme, then it should be possible to absorb these antibodies with commercial preparations of mucopolysaccharidase and abrogate immune serum blocking activity. Normal and immune sera without treponemes were exposed to bovine hyaluronidase (mucopolysaccharidase) for 17 hr; treponemes were then added to both sera and preincubated for 18 hr to sensitize the organisms. These preparations were then incubated with cultured cells for 3 hr to assess attachment of treponemes. As shown in Table 7, the immune serum blocking factor that prevents treponemal attachment was absorbed by prior incubation with hyaluronidase. This finding suggests that (1) the treponemal receptor interacting with the cultured cell mucopolysaccharide receptor involves the mucopolysaccharidase enzyme and (2) the blocking factor in immune serum is antibody directed against the treponemal mucopolysaccharidase.

Four other comments are relevant. First, inasmuch as the treponemes attach only at their distal end, it is probable that most of the mucopolysaccharidase is located at the outer tip of the organism. Second, since nonpathogenic treponemes do not attach to culture cells, they should not contain the mucopolysaccharidase enzyme. Some of these nonpathogens, however, do exhibit mucopolysaccharidase

Table 7 Absorption of Attachment-Blocking Factor from Immune Serum by Pretreatment with Bovine Hyaluronidase

Experiment	Pretreatment	Preincubation with serum for 18 hr (Percentage motile)		Incubation with cultured cells for 3 hr (treponemes per 100 cultured cells)		Percentage blockage
		Normal	Immune	Normal	Immune	
1	Untreated	88	76	600	100	83
	Hase[a] treated	76	72	600	600	—
2	Untreated	98	92	700	50	93
	Hase treated	96	92	650	700	—
3	Untreated	92	80	600	750	83
	Hase treated	96	86	700	750	—

[a]Hyaluronidase.
Source: Reference 33.

activity (41). It is possible that this enzyme is not localized at the outer tips of the nonpathogens, thereby explaining the inability to attach. Third, during attachment of *T. pallidum,* the mucopolysaccharidase might be expected to gradually degrade cultured cell surface mucopolysaccharides. These cultured cells respond to the loss of surface mucopolysaccharides by synthesizing new surface mucopolysaccharides (T. J. Fitzgerald, unpublished results). The finding that attachment of over 200 treponemes per cultured cell causes cell lysis suggests that mucopolysaccharide synthesis by the cultured cells may be overwhelmed by the large number of attached organisms. Fourth, Hayes et al. (8) suggested that attachment of treponemes to cultured cells altered the surface of the cultured cells; subsequent inoculation of additional treponemes resulted in fewer attached organisms. Also, far fewer treponemes were able to attach at 4°C. Both of these observations are explainable in terms of the treponemal mucopolysaccharidase mechanism of attachment.

Perspectives

Role of Capsule and Mucopolysaccharidase
in Pathogenesis of Syphilis

Treponema pallidum exhibits a distinct predilection for the ground substance mucopolysaccharides that are generally distributed throughout the body. This predilection is reflected by four observations of the infective process. First, *T. pallidum* attaches to tissues in vivo in identical fashion to attachment to cultured cells (3). In vitro attachment appears to be mediated through a layer of acidic mucopolysaccharides at the surface of the cultured cells (39). The ability of *T. pallidum* to infect almost every tissue of the body suggests that mucopolysaccharides are generally distributed throughout the body. Ground substance is the gel-like matrix between tissue cells that is found in almost every tissue of the body (42), including nerve tissue (43-46). It is comprised of proteins complexed with acidic mucopolysaccharides. Thus the potential receptors for treponemal attachment are widespread, and the ability of *T. pallidum* to infect so many different tissues could reflect the presence of ground substance mucopolysaccharides within these tissues.

Secondly, syphilis is a generalized rather than a localized infection. Preferred tissues, as shown by human infection and rabbit inoculation, include the dermis, testis, aorta, eye, placenta, and umbilical cord, tissues that are known to have higher concentrations of mucopolysaccharide ground substance. A further implication of the interaction of treponemes with ground substance involves the transmission of treponemes from an infected mother to her developing fetus, which does not occur until the 18th week of gestation. At this time the

11. Attachment of Treponemes to Cell Surfaces

placenta and umbilical cord are fairly well developed, and both tissues contain high amounts of mucopolysaccharide material.

Thirdly, syphilitic infection is associated with vascular components, specifically involving perivascular lesions. Inasmuch as mucopolysaccharides provide structural integrity for vessels, relatively high concentrations of mucopolysaccharide are prevalent immediately surrounding vessels (44,46,47).

Fourthly, *T. pallidum* is maintained in the laboratory by rabbit testicular passage. The organisms multiply only within the interstitial tissue, which possesses most of the mucopolysaccharide material of the testis, not in sperm tissue. Young animals with immature testes are far less susceptible to testicular infection. A major change associated with maturation of the testis is the deposition of much larger amounts of ground substance mucopolysaccharide.

The question remains as to whether the treponeme-associated mucopolysaccharides are part of a capsular layer or are host-derived tissue constituents. Three observations suggest that the mucopolysaccharides are synthesized by the organisms. First, during lesion development, the accumulation of mucopolysaccharides within lesions closely parallels the increase in treponemal numbers (1,2). These mucopolysaccharides differ from those found within host tissues, as shown by distinct metachromatic changes that are associated with treponemal multiplication (24). Second, during incubation of *T. pallidum* with cultured cells, acidic mucopolysaccharides accumulate at the surface of the cultured cells (29). This accumulation requires attachment of viable organisms and the amount of mucopolysaccharide is dependent on the number of organisms attached. Third, the immunological evidence of Bey et al. (32) suggests that the treponemal mucopolysaccharides are not identical to the hyaluronic acid found within host tissues.

Acidic mucopolysaccharides are extremely water soluble and should readily dissipate from the surface of *T. pallidum*. Zeigler et al. (16) demonstrated that when treponemes were harvested from infected tissue and immediately fixed for electron microscopy, the majority exhibited ruthenium red precipitate. However, when the tissue was extracted for 30 min and then fixed, far fewer treponemes exhibited ruthenium red precipitate. The constant dissipation of the treponemal capsular material would require continuous resynthesis by the organisms to replace this material. The accumulation of mucopolysaccharides that occurs at the surface of cultured cells during incubation with *T. pallidum* could be attributed to dissipation of the mucopolysaccharide treponemal capsule (29). *Streptococcus pneumoniae, Hemophilus influenzae,* and *Neisseria meningitidis* provide comparable precedents. Broth cultures of these bacteria yield large amounts of soluble capsular polysaccharides that dissipate from the surface of the organisms during in vitro growth. The dissipation of the treponemal capsule would also explain the occurrence of mucopolysaccharides within syphilitic lesions and syphilitic sera (32,33).

Acidic mucopolysaccharides are long, straight-chain polymers with a strong polyanionic charge. Toluidine blue and ruthenium red, which have a polycationic charge, enhance treponemal survival. By binding to the polyanionic treponemal mucopolysaccharides, these polycations may stabilize the treponemal capsule. This finding suggests an important concept: An intact mucopolysaccharide layer is vital to treponemal survival (17).

The treponemal mucopolysaccharide capsule could benefit the organisms by restricting the access of antitreponemal antibodies (1,2,10-13, 28). Mucopolysaccharides have an excluded volume which limits the penetration of large molecules such as antibodies (48). Furthermore, the addition of lysozyme to *T. pallidum* enhances seroreactivity (12). It was assumed that this enzyme degraded surface mucopeptides, thereby facilitating antibody reactions. An alternative possibility is related to the ability of lysozyme to precipitate acidic mucopolysaccharides (42). This phenomenon could result in removal of the treponemal surface mucopolysaccharides, which in turn would facilitate antibody reactions (17). The treponemal capsule may also be protective by retarding phagocytosis (1).

Another concept that may apply to treponemal mucopolysaccharides involves oxygen sensitivity (49-55; see Chapter 4 and 5). Acidic mucopolysaccharides irreversibly depolymerize in the presence of oxygen and reducing agents (56,57). This reaction is termed oxidative-reductive depolymerization (ORD). The oxygen sensitivity of *T. pallidum* may be due to the depolymerization of treponemal surface mucopolysaccharides. The ability of sulfhydryl reagents such as dithiothreitol, cysteine, glutathione, and sodium thioglycollate to enhance the in vitro survival of *T. pallidum* may be mediated through neutralization of the ORD reaction (7,53,58).

Turner (2) suggested that the mucoid material within lesions was the forerunner of the indurated hard chancre that is characteristic of primary syphilis. He postulated that the firmness was due to sulfation of hyaluronic acid to chondroitin sulfate. Alternatively, the mucopolysaccharides within lesions may gradually depolymerize via the ORD reaction, and this in turn may be responsible for the firmness of the chancre.

The predilection for host mucopolysaccharides by *T. pallidum* conceivably involves its requirement for an intact capsule. Canole-Parola (59) has stated that host-associated spirochetes lack the ability to synthesize N-acetyl-D-glucosamine. If this generalization can be extended to the spirochete of syphilis, it provides a most important correlation. The mucopolysaccharide capsule of *T. pallidum* contains N-acetyl-D-glucosamine (17). If *T. pallidum* cannot synthesize this compound, it would have to rely on an exogenous source. The treponemal mucopolysaccharidase would provide this source by breaking down host mucopolysaccharide ground substance which contains hyaluronic acid, a polymer of N-acetyl-D-glucosamine • D-glucuronic acid. Since acidic mucopolysaccharides are extremely water soluble, they should readily dissipate from the surface of the organisms. This constant capsular dissipation would require continuous resynthesis by the treponemes. This would account for the dependence of *T. pallidum* on relatively large amounts of ground substance within host tissue in order to multiply extensively. Furthermore, capsular dissipation would explain the source of the mucoid material within syphilitic lesions.

The influences of treponemal mucopolysaccharidase might be the basis for syphilitic histopathology. Early in syphilitic infection, large numbers of treponemes occur without overt damage to the tissues, indicating that *T. pallidum* lacks the potent toxins that some other bacteria possess. As the infection progresses, however, damage occurs. There is a striking similarity between the histopathology that develops within syphilitic lesions and the effects of hyaluronidase on normal tissue. In research not related to *T. pallidum*, attempts were made to determine the mechanism of tumor cell growth within tissues (37,60-65). It was postulated that tumor cells elaborated a "spreading factor" that destroyed ground substance to make room for tumor cell growth. Experiments were performed to assess the histological influences of hyaluronidase ("spreading factor") on normal tissue. The following changes occurred: degeneration of ground substance, evolution of amorphous embryonic-like tissue, alterations in metachromatic staining, rupture of endothelial cells with extravasation of blood into the surrounding tissues, marked vascular changes, hyperplasia of fibroblasts, degranulation of mast cells, intravascular thrombosis, and ulceration. Each of these changes is associated with syphilitic histopathology (1,21,22,24,25,28,36).

Within infected tissue *T. pallidum* localizes perivascularly. Bondareff (44), Gersch and Catchpole (46), and Luft (47) demonstrated relatively large amounts of mucopolysaccharide ground substance immediately surrounding capillary and lymph vessels. The rapid dissemination of *T. pallidum* through the bloodstream and lymphatics may be associated with attachment to the mucopolysaccharides present on the inner capillary walls. In support of this, Lauderdale and Goldman (66) and Ovcinnikov and Delektorskij (67) demonstrated that *T. pallidum* is intimately associated with (? attached to) the inner walls of capillary vessels. The attached organisms could then break down the mucopolysaccharide material, eventually splitting apart the tight junctions between the endothelial cells. This would provide the organisms with access to the perivascular areas, which contain relatively large amounts of mucopolysaccharide material. Ovcinnikov and Delektorskij (67) first suggested that *T. pallidum* in some undefined way reached perivascular areas by passing through endothelial cell junctions. As the organisms multiply in the perivascular areas, their mucopolysaccharidase would destroy the integrity of the mucopolysaccharide support material surrounding capillaries, resulting in inward or outward collapse of the vessels. This, in turn, would inhibit blood supply and explain the characteristic obliterative endarteritis, periarteritis, necrosis, and eventual ulceration. Thus mucopolysaccharidase activity is conceivably a prime factor responsible for the histopathology of syphilis. In addition, congenital syphilis results in birth defects that include interstitial keratitis, tooth deformation, eighth-nerve deafness, osteochondritis, cardiovascular and neurological problems, and bone deformation of the legs, nose septum, and hard palate. These birth defects may result from treponemal interference with ground substance mucopolysaccharide production during the very active fetal growth period.

One other observation is explainable in terms of the treponemal mucopolysaccharidase. Various strains of *T. pallidum* exhibit different degrees of virulence (2). The Chicago strain is highly virulent in terms of its ability to rapidly spread to other tissues and to produce extensive lesions with large necrotic areas. Strains C and H are less virulent; strain F and the Nichols and Truffi strains are intermediate in virulence. Turner (2) found that the more virulent isolates produced lesions containing larger amounts of mucoid material, and suggested that excess mucoid accumulation was a virulence factor. The more virulent isolates may have increased mucopolysaccharidase activity, enabling them to attach more readily to host tissues. Better attachment would provide increased accessibility to the exogenous source of N-acetyl-D-glucosamine for enhanced capsular biosynthesis, enhanced multiplication, and increased accumulations of mucoid material.

Zeigler et al. (16) were unable to demonstrate mucopolysaccharides at the surface of two nonpathogenic treponemes. Their lack of a capsule similar to *T. pallidum* may be the basis for their inability to cause disease. These nonpathogens may not possess surface mucopolysaccharidase activity. If this is the case, overt tissue histopathology emanating from mucopolysaccharidase degradation of host mucopolysaccharides would not occur.

Healing Response

Relative to healing and immunity, lymphocytes and plasma cells characteristically infiltrate syphilitic lesions. Healing of lesions is probably dependent on a number of factors. One that may be especially important is the serum factor, presumably antibody, that blocks treponemal attachment to host tissues. These putative antibodies may be directed against the treponemal receptor, the mucopolysaccharidase enzyme. The primary effect of blockage of attachment would be reduced accessibility to host tissue mucopolysaccharides. As a consequence, less N-acetyl-D-glucosamine would be available, resulting in

11. Attachment of Treponemes to Cell Surfaces

defective capsular biosynthesis and demise of the organisms. It is known that, shortly after the injection into nonimmune rabbits, *T. pallidum* rapidly disseminates to draining lymph nodes and to most tissues of the body. Dissemination apparently involves not only passive transport via the blood and lymphatics, but also attachment of organisms within tissues. Dissemination, however, does not occur in immune animals (68-71). The immune serum factor that blocks attachment may be primarily responsible for preventing dissemination (3,33).

This hypothesis does not exclude the role of T lymphocytes, which appear to be important mediators of the healing process (34,72-75). It is conceivable that activated T cells interact with the organisms after antibody interferes with tissue attachment and capsular biosynthesis. "Defective treponemes" may then be inactivated by the T cells.

Immunosuppression in Syphilis

Immunity in syphilis is a complex phenomenon. It evolves slowly over a relatively prolonged period. The healing of the primary chancre is the initial sign of an effective immune response. In experimental syphilis in the rabbit, healing may begin as early as 2 to 3 weeks after injection of *T. pallidum*. Solid immunity, however, as demonstrated by resistance to treponemal challenge, does not fully develop until 3 months after infection. A key question remains unresolved: Is the slowly evolving immunity due to poor immunogenicity of the important immunogens or to immunosuppression of the normal response to potent immunogens?

After healing of the primary stage has occurred, there is an exacerbation of the infective process that produces the secondary stage of syphilis. The specific factors involved in this exacerbation are unknown. The earlier hypothesis involved a "waxing and waning" of host immune responses. This simplistic view fails to explain the apparent lack of the usual anamnestic response. If the secondary stage of syphilis is due to a waning of host defenses, the subsequent reexposure of *T. pallidum* antigens should elicit an anamnestic response that would rapidly eradicate the secondary stage. This does not occur.

As discussed in other chapters in this book, a more recent hypothesis to explain the emergence of the secondary stage involves immunosuppression, supported by the fact that syphilis is a chronic infection lasting as long as 30 years.

Cortisone treatment of syphilitic rabbits results in increased numbers of organisms within lesions and significant delays in the usual healing responses (1,27). Metzger's group (76,77) reported that cyclophosphamide, 5-fluorouracil, and methotrexate greatly decreased the number of lymphocytes and macrophages within lesions. Disseminated dermal lesions in rabbits that are similar to secondary syphilitic lesions in humans usually occur in 5 to 10% of the rabbits inoculated intradermally (unpublished results). Interestingly, Metzger's group reported a much higher incidence of disseminated lesions in the immunosuppressed rabbits relative to the control rabbits. This suggests that immunosuppression may be directly involved in the secondary stage of syphilis.

Fitzgerald and Johnson (30) postulated that the immunosuppressive agent was the treponemal mucopolysaccharide capsular material. Several reports (32,78-81) have identified an immunosuppressive factor in the blood of syphilitic humans and rabbits that interferes with lymphocytic blast transformation. In experimental syphilis in rabbits, this factor was detected within 9 to 11 days after intratesticular infection (32,80,81). Mucopolysaccharides, which may result from treponemal capsular dissipation (17,33), are present within the serum of syphilitic rabbits (32,33). Bey et al. (32) showed that pretreatment of syphilitic serum with hyaluronidase effectively removed the immunosuppressive factor. This important finding suggests that the mucopolysaccharide capsular material is the immunosuppressive component of *T. pallidum*. Other biological precedents include *Streptococcus pneumoniae* (82), *Eikenella corrodens* (83), and *Pseudomonas aeruginosa* (84); their polysaccharide capsules or slime layers are also immunosuppressive.

Secondary syphilis could result from immunosuppression of the host defenses responsible for healing of primary syphilis. The treponemal mucopolysaccharide capsular material may inactivate lymphocytes (including T cells), plasma cells, or macrophages, thereby interfering with the production of antibodies to the treponemal mucopolysaccharidase. In syphilitic infection, treponemes are found primarily extracellularly. A few treponemes, however, attain an intracellular residence within various host tissue cells (66,85,86). These intracellular organisms may then exit and begin to multiply extracellularly, leading to the secondary stage. The cycle is again repeated. The host responds with an infiltration of lymphocytes and plasma cells at sites of treponemal infection. These cells overcome the immunosuppressive affects and antibodies evolve that block treponemal attachment to host tissues. Healing results. This hypothesis of immunosuppression during the early phases of the primary and secondary stages would explain the lack of the expected anamnestic response that should lead to a more rapid resolution of the secondary stage.

Summary

These observations conceivably explain the primary and secondary stages of syphilis. It is difficult, however, to apply similar findings to latency and the tertiary stage. Many questions remain unanswered: Why is latency so prolonged? Are the organisms protected against host defenses by an intracellular residence? What is the role of mucopolysaccharides within nerve tissue (43-45)? How does *T. pallidum* pass the blood-brain barrier? What host or treponemal component leads to hypersensitivity and gumma formation?

This overall picture of primary and secondary syphilis leans heavily on humoral factors, specifically antibodies to the mucopolysaccharidase enzyme. The cellular immune response plays some important but as yet undefined role. Could it be that this response, besides inactivating antibody-coated treponemes within lesions, is directed toward removing intracellular treponemes? It is well established that the cellular response is important in eradicating other intracellular organisms such as listerias, salmonellas, brucellae, and mycobacteria. In the Oslo study (87) only 25% of the patients developed secondary syphilis. If intracellularity is important to syphilitic infection, the remaining 75% that did not progress beyond the primary stage may have possessed effective cellular immune responses that killed the intracellular treponemes.

Lastly, an effective and practical vaccine is of paramount importance in controlling syphilis (13). Metzger and Smogor (88) and Miller (89) have demonstrated that an effective vaccine is feasible. If the newly emerging concepts about pathogenesis can be further substantiated, the treponemal mucopolysaccharidase may assume a prominent role in the disease process.

Acknowledgment

I would like to thank the following people for constructive criticism and valuable assistance in the preparation of this manuscript: Dr. Arthur Johnson, University of Minnesota (Duluth); Dr. James Miller, University of California at Los Angeles; and Dr. Dwayne Savage, University of Illinois (Urbana). The comments of each were most helpful. I also wish to thank Virginia Fitzgerald for evaluating the grammatical expression and context of this manuscript.

References

1. T. B. Turner and D. H. Hollander. Biology of the treponematoses. *WHO Monogr.* 35:1-277 (1957).
2. T. B. Turner. Syphilis and the treponematoses. In *Infectious Agents and Host Reactions* (S. Mudd, Ed.), W. B. Saunders, Philadelphia, 1970, pp. 346-390.
3. T. J. Fitzgerald, R. C. Johnson, J. N. Miller, and J. A. Sykes. Characterization of the attachment of *Treponema pallidum* (Nichols strain) to cultured mammalian cells and the potential relationship of attachment to pathogenicity. *Infect. Immun.* 18:467-478 (1977).

4. T. J. Fitzgerald, P. Cleveland, R. C. Johnson, J. N. Miller, and J. A. Sykes. Scanning electron microscopy of *Treponema pallidum* (Nichols strain) attached to cultured mammalian cells. *J. Bacteriol.* 130:1333-1344 (1977).
5. M. I. Wright. Exploratory studies in tissue culture of *T. pallidum*. *Proc. XII Int. Congr. Dermatol.* 2:884-887 (1962).
6. T. J. Fitzgerald, J. N. Miller, and J. A. Sykes. *Treponema pallidum* (Nichols strain) in tissue culture: Cellular attachment, entry, and survival. *Infect. Immun.* 11:1133-1140 (1975).
7. T. J. Fitzgerald, R. C. Johnson, J. A. Sykes, and J. N. Miller. Interaction of *Treponema pallidum* (Nichols strain) with cultured mammalian cells: Effects of oxygen, reducing agents, serum supplements, and different cell types. *Infect. Immun.* 15:444-452 (1977).
8. N. S. Hayes, K. E. Muse, A. M. Collier, and J. B. Baseman. Parasitism by virulent *Treponema pallidum* of host cell surfaces. *Infect. Immun.* 17:174-186 (1977).
9. S. E. Wiegand, P. L. Stobel, and L. H. Glassman. Electron microscopic anatomy of pathogenic *Treponema pallidum*. *J. Invest. Dermatol.* 58:186-204 (1972).
10. S. Christiansen. Protective layer covering pathogenic treponemata. *Lancet* 1:423-425 (1963).
11. P. H. Hardy and E. E. Nell. Study of the antigenic structure of *Treponema pallidum* by specific agglutination. *Am. J. Hyg.* 66:160-172 (1957).
12. M. Metzger, P. H. Hardy, and E. E. Nell. Influence of lysozyme upon the treponeme immobilization reaction. *Am. J. Hyg.* 73:236-244 (1961).
13. J. N. Miller. Development of an experimental syphilis vaccine. *Med. Clin. North Am.* 56:1217-1220 (1972).
14. W. Schmerold and B. Deubner. Elektronenmikroskopische Untersuchungen an Reiter-Spirochaetales und Nichols-treponemen. *Hautarzt* 5:511-513 (1954).
15. R. H. A. Swain. Electron microscopic studies of the morphology of pathogenic spirochaetes. *J. Pathol. Bacteriol.* 69:117-128 (1955).
16. J. A. Zeigler, A. M. Jones, R. H. Jones, and K. M. Kubica. Demonstration of extracellular material at the surface of pathogenic *T. pallidum* cells. *Br. J. Vener. Dis.* 52:1-8 (1976).
17. T. J. Fitzgerald and R. C. Johnson. Surface mucopolysaccharides of *Treponema pallidum*. *Infect. Immun.* 24:244-251 (1979).
18. P. Uhlenhuth, P. Mulzer, and M. Koch. Uber die histopathologischen veranderungen bei der experimentellen kaninchen syphilis. *Dtsch. Med. Wochenschr.* 38:1079-1981 (1912).
19. F. Graetz and E. Delbanco. Beitrage zum studien der Histpathologie der experimentellen kaninchen syphilis. *Med. Klin.* 10:375-420 (1914).

20. F. Graetz and E. Delbanco. Wetere beitrage zum studien der Histopathologie der experimentellen kaninchen syphilis. *Dermatol. Wochenschr.* 58:6-28 (1914).
21. A. Akutsu. Histopathy of the scrotal chancre. *Z. Jpn. Mikrobiol. Ges.* 15:205-210 (1921).
22. P. S. Gregoriew and K. G. Jarisheva. The histological structure of syphilitic lesions of rabbits. *Am. J. Syph.* 12:67-81 (1928).
23. R. Strempel and G. Armuzzi. Histobiologie der ersten Inkubationsperiode der kaninchensyphilis. *Exp. Untersuch. Dermatol. Z.* 46:267-288 (1926).
24. V. Scott and G. J. Dammin. Hyaluronidase and experimental syphilis. III. Metachromasia in syphilitic orchitis and its relation to hyaluronic acid. *Am. J. Syph.* 34:501-514 (1950).
25. V. Scott and G. J. Dammin. Morphologic and histochemical sequences in syphilitic and tuberculous orchitis in the rabbit. *Am. J. Syph.* 38:189-202 (1954).
26. V. Scott and G. J. Dammin. Experimental syphilis in the rabbit. The relationship of metachromasia to fibrinoid degeneration of collagen and the localization of spirochaetes in the testis. *J. Lab. Clin. Med.* 34:1748-1755 (1949).
27. T. B. Turner and D. H. Hollander. Cortisone in experimental syphilis. *Johns Hopkins Hosp. Bull.* 87:505-509 (1950).
28. T. B. Turner and D. H. Hollander. Studies on the mechanism of action of cortisone in experimental syphilis. *Am. J. Syph.* 38:371-387 (1954).
29. T. J. Fitzgerald, R. C. Johnson, and E. T. Wolff. Mucopolysaccharide material resulting from the interaction of *Treponema pallidum* (Nichols strain) with cultured mammalian cells. *Infect. Immun.* 22:575-584 (1978).
30. T. J. Fitzgerald and R. C. Johnson. Influence of *Treponema pallidum* infected testicular fluid on intradermal lesions. *Br. J. Vener. Dis.* 56:125-128 (1980).
31. K. Ito. A model of experimental syphilitic re-induratio. *Euph. Cacoph.* 4:16-40 (1977).
32. R. F. Bey, R. C. Johnson, and T. J. Fitzgerald. Suppression of lymphocyte response to concanavalin A by mucopolysaccharide material from *Treponema pallidum* infected rabbits. *Infect. Immun.* 26:64-69 (1979).
33. T. J. Fitzgerald and R. C. Johnson. Mucopolysaccharidase of *Treponema pallidum*. *Infect. Immun.* 24:261-268 (1979).
34. S. A. Lukehart, S. A. Baker-Zander, and S. Sell. Characterization of lymphocyte responsiveness in early experimental syphilis. In vitro response to mitogens and *Treponema pallidum* antigens. *J. Immunol.* 124:454-460 (1980).
35. N. Yeagle, C. Kalinka, S. Nakeeb, V. Wicher, and K. Wicher. Immunopathology of rabbit testes infected with *Treponema pallidum*. *Abstr. Annu. Meet. Am. Soc. Microbiol.* 78:17 (1978).

36. E. D. Delamater, V. R. Saurino, and F. Urbach. Studies on the immunology of sirochetoses. I. Effect of cortisone on experimental spirochetoses. *Am. J. Syph.* 36:127-139 (1952).
37. E. Cameron. *Hyaluronidase and Cancer*, Pergamon Press, Oxford, 1966, pp. 1-245.
38. T. J. Fitzgerald, J. N. Miller, J. A. Sykes, and R. C. Johnson. Tissue culture and *Treponema pallidum*. In *The Biology of Parasitic Spirochetes* (R. C. Johnson, Ed.). Academic Press, New York, 1976, pp. 57-64.
39. T. J. Fitzgerald, R. C. Johnson, and D. Ritzi. Relationship of *Treponema pallidum* to acidic mucopolysaccharides. *Infect. Immun.* 24:252-260 (1979).
40. N. B. Bishop and J. N. Miller. Humoral immunity in experimental syphilis. I. The demonstration of resistance conferred by passive immunization. *J. Immunol.* 117:191-196 (1976).
41. M. S. Hussey and W. W. Nowinski. Hyaluronidase activity in the Reiter strain of *Treponema pallidum*. *Tex. Rep. Biol. Med.* 7:73-81 (1949).
42. J. S. Brimacombe and J. M. Weber. *Mucopolysaccharides, Chemical Structure, Distribution, and Isolation*, Elsevier, Amsterdam, 1964, p. 68.
43. L. G. Abood and S. K. Abul-Haj. Histochemistry and characterization of hyaluronic acid in axons of peripheral nerve. *J. Neurochem.* 1:119-125 (1956).
44. W. Bondareff. An intercellular substance in rat cerebral cortex: Submicroscopic distribution of ruthenium red. *Anat. Rec.* 157:527-536 (1967).
45. J. H. Luft. Ruthenium red and violet. II. Fine structural localization in animal tissues. *Anat. Rec.* 171:369-416 (1971).
46. I. Gersch and H. R. Catchpole. The organization of ground substance and basement membrane and its significance in tissue injury, disease and growth. *Am. J. Anat.* 85:457-521 (1949).
47. J. H. Luft. Fine structure of capillary and endocapillary layer as revealed by ruthenium red. *Fed. Proc. Fed. Am. Soc. Exp. Biol.* 25:1773-1783 (1966).
48. T. C. Laurent and A. G. Ogstand. The interaction between polysaccharides and other macromolecules. 4. The osmotic pressure of mixtures of serum albumin and hyaluronic acid. *Biochem. J.* 89:249-253 (1963).
49. C. D. Cox and M. K. Barber. Oxygen uptake by *Treponema pallidum*. *Infect. Immun.* 10:123-127 (1974).
50. A. H. Fieldsteel, F. A. Becker, and J. G. Stout. Prolonged survival of virulent *Treponema pallidum* (Nichols strain) in cell free and tissue culture systems. *Infect. Immun.* 18:173-182 (1977).

51. A. H. Fieldsteel, J. G. Stout, and F. A. Becker. Comparative behavior of virulent strains of *Treponema pallidum* and *Treponema pertenue* in gradient cultures of various mammalian cells. *Infect. Immun.* 24:337-345 (1979).
52. K. Kiraly and I. Horvath. Survival of *T. pallidum* under microaerophilic conditions in cell and tissue cultures. *Zentralbl. Bakteriol. Parasitenk. Infecktskr. Hyg. Abt. 1 Orig. Reihe A* 235: 500-505 (1976).
53. S. J. Norris, J. N. Miller, J. A. Sykes, and T. J. Fitzgerald. Influence of oxygen tension, sulfhydryl compounds, and serum on the motility and virulence of *Treponema pallidum* (Nichols strain) in a modified tissue culture medium. *Infect. Immun.* 22: 689-697 (1978).
54. P. L. Sandok, H. M. Jenkin, H. M. Matthews, and M. S. Roberts. Unsustained multiplication of *Treponema pallidum* (Nichols virulent strain) in vitro in the presence of oxygen. *Infect. Immun.* 19: 421-429 (1978).
55. S. Graves and T. Billington. Optimum concentration of dissolved oxygen for the survival of virulent *Treponema pallidum* under conditions of low oxidation-reduction potential. *Br. J. Vener. Dis.* 55:387-393 (1979).
56. W. Pigman and S. Rizvi. Hyaluronic acid and the ORD reaction. *Biochem. Biophys. Res. Commun.* 1:39-43 (1959).
57. B. Skanse and L. Sundblad. Oxidative breakdown of hyaluronic acid and chondroitin sulfuric acid. *Acta Physiol. Scand.* 6:37-51 (1943).
58. T. J. Fitzgerald, R. C. Johnson, and E. T. Wolff. Sulfhydryl oxidation using procedures and experimental conditions commonly employed for *Treponema pallidum*. *Br. J. Vener. Dis.* 56:129-136 (1980).
59. E. Canale-Parola. Physiology and evolution of spirochetes. *Bacteriol. Rev.* 41:181-204 (1977).
60. R. G. Williams. The effects of continuous local injection of hyaluronidase on skin and subcutaneous tissue in rats. *Anat. Rec.* 122:349-361 (1955).
61. S. H. Bensley. Histological studies of the reactions of cells and intercellular substances of loose connective tissue to the spreading factor of testicular extracts. *Ann. N. Y. Acad. Sci.* 52: 983-988 (1950).
62. G. Szabo and S. Magyar. Effect of hyaluronidase on capillary permeability, lymph flow and the passage of dye labelled protein from plasma to lymph. *Nature London* 182:377-379 (1958).
63. G. Asboe-Hansen. The origin of synovial mucin. Erlich's mast cell—A secretory element of the connective tissues. *Ann. Rheum. Dis.* 9:149-158 (1950).

64. E. F. Lascano. Mast cells in human tumors. *Cancer (Philadelphia)* 11:1110-1114 (1958).
65. B. W. Zweifach and R. Chambers. The action of hyaluronidase extracts on the capillary wall. *Ann. N. Y. Acad. Sci.* 52:1047-1051 (1950).
66. V. Lauderdale and J. N. Goldman. Serial ultrathin sectioning demonstrating the intracellularity of *T. pallidum*. *Br. J. Vener. Dis.* 48:87-99 (1972).
67. N. M. Ovcinnikov and V. V. Delektorskij. Electron microscopy of phagocytosis in syphilis and yaws. *Br. J. Vener. Dis.* 48:227-248 (1972).
68. A. M. Chesney and J. E. Kemp. Studies in experimental syphilis VI. On variations in the response of treated rabbits to reinoculation; and cryptogenetic reinfection with syphilis. *J. Exp. Med.* 44:589-606 (1926).
69. M. C. Cumberland and T. B. Turner. The rate of multiplication of *T. pallidum* in normal and immune rabbits. *Am. J. Syph.* 33:201-212 (1949).
70. F. W. Reynolds. The fate of *Treponema pallidum* inoculated subcutaneously into immune rabbits. *Johns Hopkins Hosp. Bull.* 69:53-60 (1941).
71. G. W. Waring and W. L. Fleming. The effect of partial immunity on the dissemination of infection in experimental syphilis. *Am. J. Syph.* 36:368-375 (1952).
72. S. M. Maret, J. B. Baseman, and J. D. Folds. Cell mediated immunity in *Treponema pallidum* infected rabbits: In vitro response of splenic and lymph node lymphocytes to mitogens and specific antigens. *Clin. Exp. Immunol.* 39:38-43 (1980).
73. R. E. Baughn and D. M. Musher. Altered immune responsiveness associated with experimental syphilis in the rabbit: Elevated IgM and depressed IgG responses to sheep erythrocytes. *J. Immunol.* 120:1691-1695 (1978).
74. J. K. Chan, R. F. Schell, and J. L. Lefrock. Ability of enriched immune T cells to confer resistance in hamsters to infection with *Treponema pertenue*. *Infect. Immun.* 26:448-452 (1979).
75. V. Wicher and K. Wicher. In vitro cell response of *Treponema pallidum* infected rabbits. I. Lymphocyte transformation. *Clin. Exp. Immunol.* 24:480-486 (1977).
76. M. Metzger. The role of immunologic responses in protection against syphilis. In *The Biology of Parasitic Spirochetes* (R. C. Johnson, Ed.). Academic, New York, 1976, pp. 327-337.
77. J. M. Pacha, M. Metzger, W. Smogor, E. Michalska, J. Podwinska, and J. Ruczkowska. Effect of immunosuppressive agents on the course of experimental syphilis in rabbits. *Arch. Immunol. Ther. Exp.* 27:45-51 (1979).
78. F. S. Kantor. Infection, anergy, and cell mediated immunity. *N. Engl. J. Med.* 292:629-634 (1975).

79. G. M. Levene, J. L. Turk, D. L. Wright, and A. G. S. Grimble. Reduced lymphocyte transformation due to a plasma factor in patients with active syphilis. *Lancet* 11:246-247 (1969).
80. V. Wicher and K. Wicher. In vitro cell response of *Treponema pallidum* infected rabbits. II. Inhibition of lymphocyte response to phytohaemagglutinin by serum of *T. pallidum* infected rabbits. *Clin. Exp. Immunol.* 29:487-495 (1977).
81. J. L. Ware, J. D. Folds, and J. B. Baseman. Serum of rabbits infected with *Treponema pallidum* (Nichols) inhibits in vitro transformation of normal rabbit lymphocytes. *Cell. Immunol.* 42:363-372 (1979).
82. L. D. Felton. The significance of antigen in animal tissues. *J. Immunol.* 61:107-117 (1949).
83. A. H. Behling, P. H. Pham, and A. Nowtony. Biological activity of the slime and endotoxin of the periodontopathic organism *Eikenella corrodans*. *Infect. Immunol.* 26:580-584 (1979).
84. G. L. Floersheim, J. F. Borel, D. Wiesinger, J. Brundell, and Z. Kis. Antiarthritic and immunosuppressive effects of *Pseudomonas aeruginosa*. *Agents Actions* 2:231-235 (1972).
85. J. A. Sykes and J. N. Miller. Intracellular location of *Treponema pallidum* (Nichols strain) in the rabbit testis. *Infect. Immunol.* 4:307-314 (1971).
86. H. A. Azar, T. D. Pham, and A. K. Kurban. An electronmicroscopic study of a syphilitic chancre. *Arch. Pathol.* 90:143-150 (1970).
87. T. Gjestland. The Oslo study of untreated syphilis. *Acta Derm. Venereol. Suppl.* 34:1-365 (1955).
88. M. Metzger and W. Smogor. Artificial immunization of rabbits against syphilis. I. Effect of increasing doses of treponemes given by the intramuscular route. *Br. J. Vener. Dis.* 45:308-312 (1969).
89. J. N. Miller. Immunity in experimental syphilis. VI. Successful vaccination of rabbits with *Treponema pallidum*, Nichols strain, attenuated by gamma irradiation. *J. Immunol.* 110:1206-1215 (1973).

12

The Parasitic Strategies of *Treponema pallidum*

JOEL B. BASEMAN and JOHN F. ALDERETE
University of Texas
Health Science Center
San Antonio, Texas

Syphilis is a unique disease associated with a complex host response and accompanied by intermittent periods of latency and classical stage development. Neither protective immunogens nor mechanisms of host resistance have been clearly demonstrated. We have attempted to define biologic properties of *Treponema pallidum*, the causative infectious agent, that might be categorized as virulence determinants. This experimental dissection of *T. pallidum* could lead to ways of interrupting or controlling the development of disease.

During our initial attempts to manipulate virulent treponemes freshly extracted from infected rabbit tissue, we observed the predilection of these spirochetes for eukaryotic cell surfaces (1). Additional evidence (1,2) reinforced the concept of a selective and specific interaction which appeared to be mediated by the treponemal tiplike organelle, suggesting a ligand-receptor mechanism of recognition (Table 1). So we set out to fractionate *T. pallidum* in order to characterize the apparent surface molecule(s) responsible for attachment. We initially found that intact treponemes were coated with loosely associated host macromolecules (3). Also, avidly bound host proteins were detected at the outer envelope of treponemes, and these host-derived components could be released only after extensive trypsin treatment resulting in the concomitant loss of *T. pallidum* proteins (3). Additional

Table 1 Preliminary Evidence for Putative Ligand-Receptor Interaction

1. *Treponema pallidum*
   a. Specific orientation via tiplike organelle.
   b. Requirement for active metabolism; heat-killed or glutaraldehyde-fixed treponemes do not attach.
   c. Reduced attachment after pretreatment with proteases or specific antitreponemal antibody.
   d. Inability of avirulent treponemes to attach, suggesting a relationship between virulence and adherence.
2. Host cell
   a. Degree of attachment determined by eukaryotic cell type (per unit membrane, fibroblasts accommodate more treponemes than do epithelial cells and peritoneal macrophages; red blood cells lack "receptors").
   b. Brief periodate or trypsin treatment prevents attachment.
   c. Negative cooperativity or refractoriness of host cell surface after initial surface parasitism (1).
   d. Lack of treponemal attachment to diversely charged and chemically modified substrates or surfaces unless lectin mediated (6).

surface properties have been described (4,6). A schematic representation of the treponemal surface topography appears in Fig. 1.

The obstacle posed by host contaminants in complicating the identification and characterization of treponemal surface components was circumvented by employing biosynthetically radiolabeled *T. pallidum*. Experimental conditions were established to permit extensive [^{35}S]-methionine incorporation into proteins by treponemes with retained virulence as determined by injecting rabbits intradermally with matched, unlabeled test samples. Figure 2 displays the extensive protein profiles of [^{35}S]methionine-labeled *T. pallidum* based upon two-dimensional gel electrophoresis (7). The establishment of a binding assay (Table 2) permitted detection of treponemal macromolecules that selectively and avidly adhered to the host cell surface. As seen in Fig. 3, only three [^{35}S]-labeled *T. pallidum* proteins remained bound to HEp-2 cells after extensive washing (8). Additional information supported the biologic specificity of these proteins as potential mediators of host cell surface parasitism (Table 3).

We then investigated the immunogenicity of these proteins during infection by combining the highly sensitive techniques of radioimmunoprecipitation, *Staphylococcus aureus* protein A (Staph A) adsorption, SDS-acrylamide gel electrophoresis, and fluorography (8). This strategy could clarify the role of these antigens in relation to disease

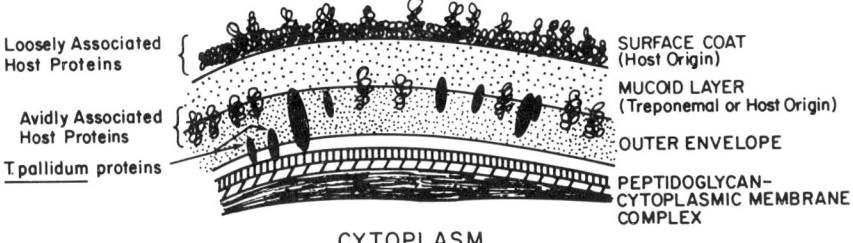

Figure 1 Schematic representation of the interaction between host macromolecules and the outer envelope of *T. pallidum*. Both loosely and avidly associated serum proteins have been detected on the treponemal surface. (*Source*: Ref. 3.)

progression and as potential protective immunogens. Sera from syphilitic humans and experimentally infected rabbits were preincubated with detergent-solubilized, [^{35}S]methionine-labeled *T. pallidum*, and the radioactive immune complexes were selectively removed with Staph A. Data revealed the highly antigenic nature of the putative ligands, proteins 1, 2, and 3, as well as other exposed treponemal outer-envelope proteins (8-10). In Fig. 4 representative sera from rabbits infected via intratesticular and intradermal routes are compared for the presence of antibody against these treponemal proteins. Several relevant findings should be addressed: (1) the host IgG response against proteinaceous components of *T. pallidum* is preferentially directed at treponemal surface proteins; (2) the height of the response occurs at approximately 50 days postinfection when antibodies are readily detected against each surface component; (3) high levels of antibody against a spectrum of proteins can be measured in the sera of infected animals at 4 months; and (4) a noticeable host discrimination in the IgG profile is seen at 6 months postinfection when the humoral response is directed at *T. pallidum* proteins 2 and 3, previously implicated as ligands along with protein 1. In the latter case, this highly selective immunogenic response is consistent with the idea of long-term *in vivo* retention of these ligandlike proteins possibly bound to host cell membrane receptors, thus promoting preferential and/or prolonged antigenic processing. It might also be caused by a type of host immunologic imprinting arising early in the infection. Further reinforcement as to the surface-directed nature of the IgG response is presented in Fig. 5. Here washed, intact [^{35}S]-labeled *T. pallidum* were exposed to test sera obtained from infected rabbits bled at specific intervals. Agglutination was measured by selective immunoprecipitating with Staph A, washing, and determining radioactivity in the readily precipitable treponeme-antibody-staphyloccus complex. Note

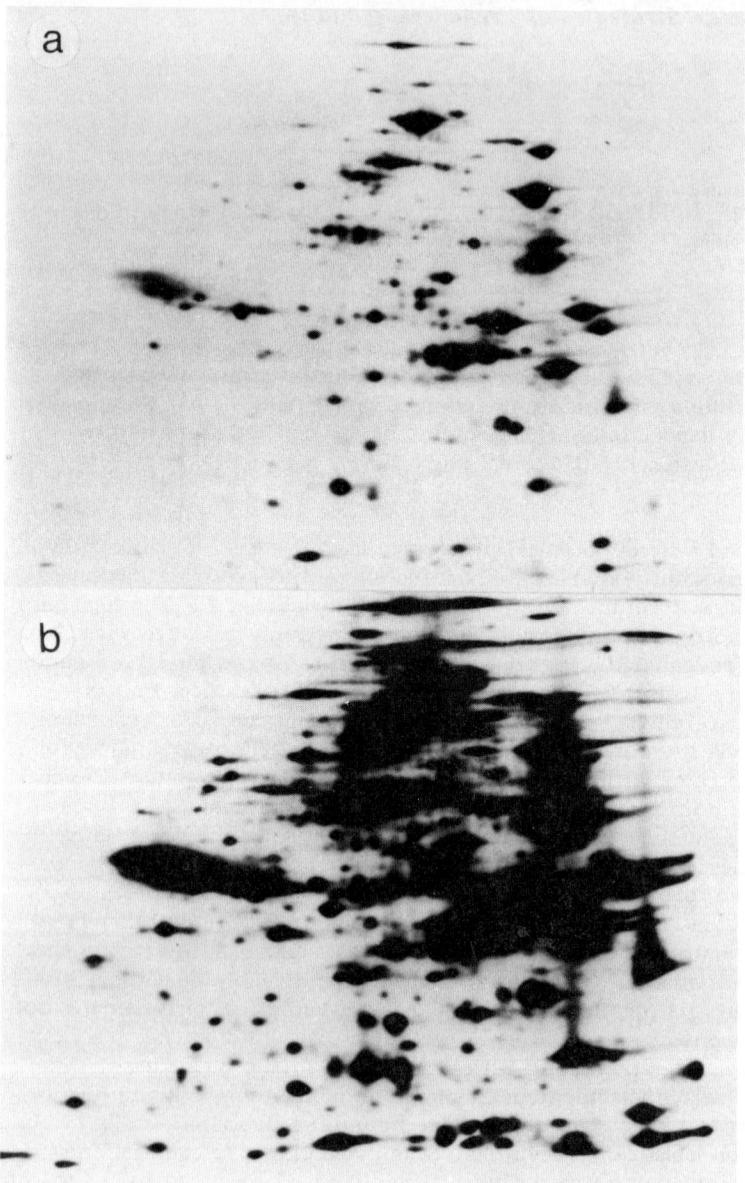

Figure 2 Two-dimensional gel-electrophoretic analysis of proteins from virulent *Treponema pallidum*. Each fluorogram represents the identical protein pattern following nonequilibrium pH gradient – sodium dodecylsulfate – polyacrylamide gel electrophonesis. Treponemes were radiolabeled for 16 hr with [^{35}S]methionine (8,9), and x-ray film exposure was for 20 hr (fluorogram a) and 8 days (fluorogram b).

Table 2 Analysis of *Treponema pallidum* Ligands

1. Mix detergent-soluble [^{35}S]methionine-labeled *T.pallidum* preparation with formaldehyde-fixed eukaryotic cells (HEp-2).
2. Incubate 1 hr at 34°C with intermittent mixing.
3. Wash HEp-2 cells four times with buffer containing 0.05% Triton X-100 to remove nonspecifically bound material.
4. Release tightly bound radioactive material with buffer containing 1% sodium dodecylsulfate.
5. Identify treponemal macromolecules by acrylamide gel electrophoresis and fluorography.

the direct correlation between the extent of agglutination and the fluorograms. These data offer a chemical-molecular explanation of earlier reports (1,11) describing reduced attachment to host cells of *T. pallidum* previously exposed to rabbit syphilitic sera. Antibody that blocks treponemal binding proteins and/or complexes with accessible outer-membrane proteins could effectively reduce the ability of virulent treponemes to parasitize targeted host cells.

An additional finding has further established the structural and functional relatedness of *T. pallidum* ligand proteins 1 and 2. Antibody raised against either protein 1 or 2 using specific excised acrylamide gel bands as immunizing agents reacts with both proteins, indicating that these molecules share antigenic homology (9). This could then explain the similarities in the selective and avid binding of these proteins to putative host cell receptors. Also, *T. pallidum* preexposed to antibody directed against these proteins or to sera containing antiprotein 1 and 2 IgG show markedly reduced attachment to HEp-2 cells (Table 4). It is equally interesting that sera obtained from individuals with yaws, a treponemal infection caused by *Treponema pertenue*, also react strongly with *T. pallidum* proteins 1, 2 and 3 (4). This observation is consistent with the report of Fieldsteel et al. (12), that *T. pertenue* attach to tissue culture cells. Furthermore, if *T. pertenue* are passaged in rabbits and radiolabeled with [^{35}S]methionine as described for *T. pallidum* (8,10), radioimmune complexes formed between syphilitic sera and the detergent-soluble *T. pertenue* preparation contain major outer-envelope proteins closely related or identical to those of *T. pallidum* (Z. Zachar and J. Baseman, unpublished data). It seems that *T. pallidum* and *T. pertenue* possess common antigens and that these specific macromolecules correlate with virulence; the Reiter treponeme, an avirulent spirochete, which does not attach to eukaryotic cells, lacks these components.

It should be emphasized that *T. pallidum* is capable of circumventing the humoral immune response, since infection continues in certain individuals in spite of high-titered antibody directed against

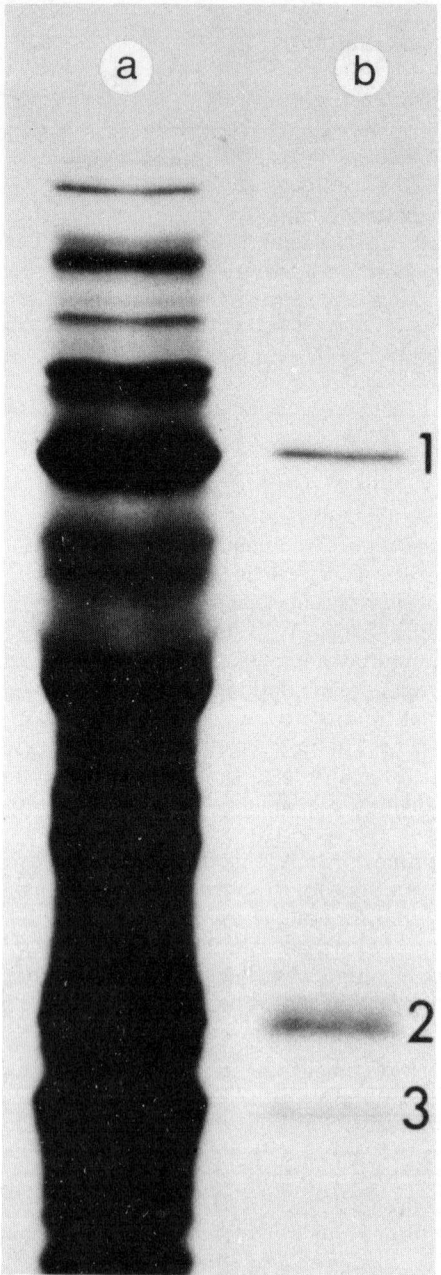

Figure 3 Identification of potential treponemal ligands mediating host cell surface parasitism. Washed, formaldehyde-fixed HEp-2 cells in suspension were incubated with [^{35}S]methionine-labeled,

Table 3 Characterization of *Treponema pallidum* Binding Proteins

1. Kinetics of binding to HEp-2 cells is linear as a function of time.
2. Reduced binding of treponemal proteins occurs after trypsin treatment of host cells, suggesting proteinaceous host membrane "receptors."
3. Competitive binding of [^{35}S]proteins to host cell surfaces is observed in the presence of unlabeled *T. pallidum* extract, but not with soluble extract from avirulent treponemes.
4. Surface location of *T. pallidum* proteins 1, 2 and 3 is established by lactoperoxidase-catalyzed iodination of intact treponemes and release of specific proteins by high salt and octyl glucoside treatment (9).

treponemal surface proteins. This apparent inconsistency is resolvable if one considers the biological properties of *T. pallidum* and of the host response to infection. As previously discussed, these spirochetes are coated with host macromolecules. This host-derived encasement may disguise the infectious agent from immune surveillance as well as sterically prevent antitreponemal antibody from reaching the appropriate antigenic sites on *T. pallidum*. It may limit phagocytosis by reducing access to specific ligands on the pathogen. We had earlier described the difficulty that rabbit peritoneal macrophages displayed when attempting to ingest treponemes adhering to the macrophage surface, even in the presence of syphilitic sera (2). It seems likely that among a given population of virulent treponemes, subgroups exist in vivo that are more or less resistant to host defense mechanisms as determined by physical attributes such as the acquisition of a host macromolecular coat, the dimension and shape of individual spirochetes, and/or their specific tissue location. Each or all of these properties may be influenced by the molecular organization of treponemal outer-membrane proteins. The possibility that treponemes can regulate the external exposure of ligandlike macromolecules such as proteins 1 or 2, which was suggested by us earlier (9), permits *T. pallidum* parasitism of and release from host cells with accompanying dissemination and redistribution. The establishment of latency could reflect these biological properties along with a balance between host response and the

detergent-solubilized *T. pallidum* proteins as previously published (8). After incubation and extensive washing, putative ligands selectively and avidly bound, as indicated by gel electrophoresis-fluorography (8). (A) An aliquot of total [^{35}S]radiolabeled treponemal proteins in the reaction mixture. (B) Proteins 1, 2, and 3 bound to HEp-2 cells. Evidence of the surface localization of these ligands appears in Ref. 9. (*Source*: Ref. 8.)

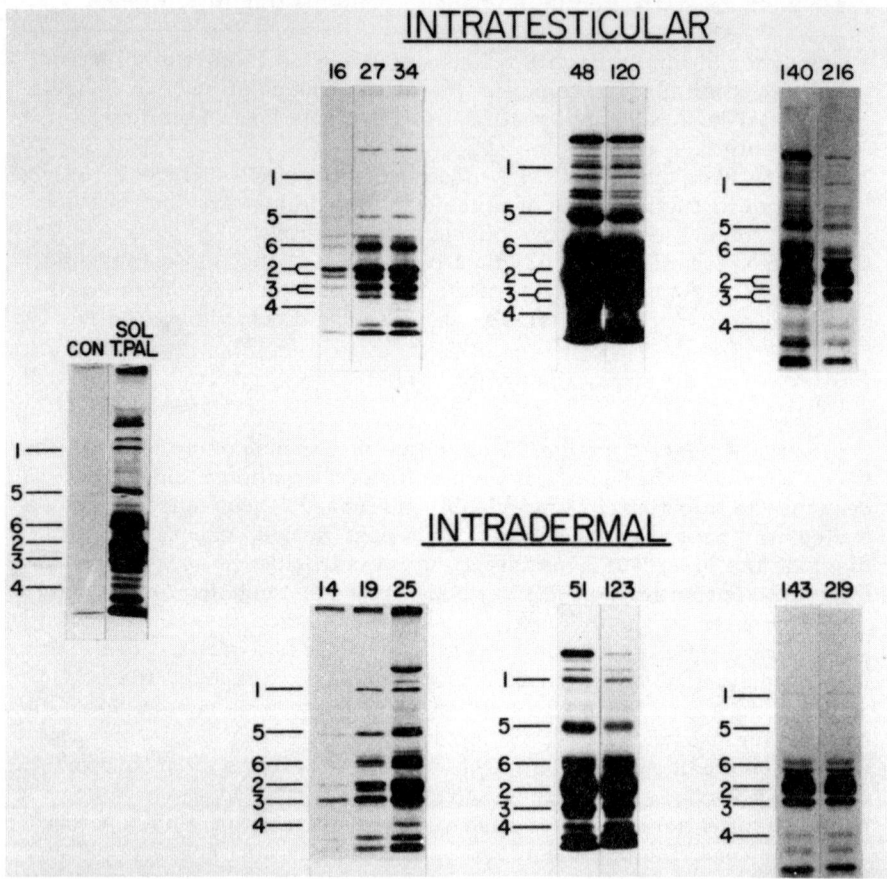

Figure 4 Radioimmunoprecipitation (RIP) patterns of [^{35}S]methionine-labeled T. pallidum proteins reactive with syphilitic sera from rabbits challenged by intratesticular and intradermal routes. Numbers indicate the day postinfection when sera were collected. Control normal rabbit serum (CON) was obtained from each animal prior to infection. Total [^{35}S]-labeled, detergent-solubilized treponemal antigens (SOL T. PAL) shows the labeled, detergent-solubilized treponemal antigens present in the total reaction mixture. The final serum concentration used to obtain each fluorogram was 10% (see Ref. 10). The methodology for the RIP has been published elsewhere (8,9). (Source: Ref. 10.)

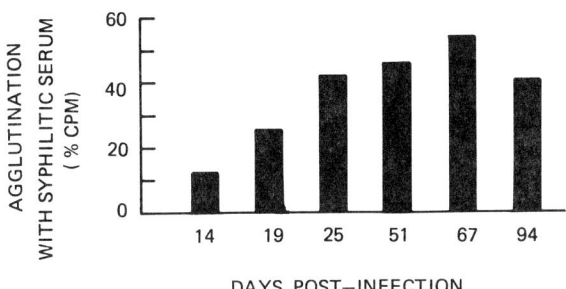

Figure 5 Staphylococcus protein A-mediated agglutination of [^{35}S]methionine-labeled *T. pallidum*. Radiolabeled treponemes were washed and preincubated with serum obtained at various days after intradermal infection. Serum reactivity against specific antigens for the days indicated (14, 19, 25, and 51 days) is shown in Fig. 4. The extent of agglutination of the treponeme-antibody-staphylococcus complex is expressed as the percentage of counts per minute of specific agglutination subtracted from the number of counts per minute obtained using prebled normal rabbit serum (NRS) (10). Control values never exceeded 30% of the reported test values, and all sera were diluted 1:100 in a NaCl-EDTA-Tris HCl buffer as previously described (9). (From Ref. 10.)

Table 4 Effect of Antiserum and IgG Fraction on Attachment of *Treponema pallidum* to Hep-2 Cells

Antiserum	Concentration	Number of Treponemes per Cell[a]
NRS[b]	25%	22 ± 3
RSS[c] (day 48)	25%	8 ± 2
IgG Fraction[d]		
NRS[b]	1 mg/ml	22 ± 3
RSS[c] (day 48)	1 mg/ml	6 ± 2
Antiprotein 1 or protein 2	1 mg/ml	6 ± 2

[a]Percentage of cells with adherent treponemes for all samples = 100%.
[b]Normal rabbit serum.
[c]Rabbit syphilitic serum.
[d]Purified by protein A-Sepharose affinity chromatography.

predilection of treponemes for privileged target sites. Also, autoimmune reactions (13) could result from the intimate association between either surface-associated host proteins and virulent *T. pallidum* or the treponemal ligand-host membrane receptor complex. In addition, evidence that cellular immune mechanisms undergo a transitory period of delayed responsiveness during early infection (14-16) further contributes to the pathophysiology of syphilis.

The success story of *T. pallidum* as a bacterial parasite can be credited to the numerous properties discussed above. It appears that virulent treponemes promote their survival in vivo by avoiding or compromising host defense mechanisms. At the same time perturbation of host cell function is sufficient to enable the establishment of infection. In so doing, this pathogen has become a rather brilliant strategist with remarkable specialization for maintaining a parasitic existence.

References

1. N. S. Hayes, K. E. Muse, A. M. Collier, and J. B. Baseman. Parasitism by virulent *Treponema pallidum* of host cell surfaces. *Infect. Immun.* 17:174-186 (1977).
2. J. B. Baseman, N. S. Hayes, J. K. Spitznagel, and E. C. Hayes. Virulence determinants among the spirochetes. In *Microbiology – 1979* (D. Schlessinger, Ed.). American Society for Microbiology, Washington, D.C., pp. 203-208.
3. J. F. Alderete and J. B. Baseman. Surface-associated host proteins on virulent *Treponema pallidum*. *Infect Immun.* 26:1048-1056 (1979).
4. J. A. Ziegler, A. M. Jones, R. H. Jones, and K. M. Kubica. Demonstration of extracellular material at the surface of pathogenic *T. pallidum* cells. *Br. J. Vener. Dis.* 52:1-8 (1976).
5. T. J. Fitzgerald and R. C. Johnson. Surface mucopolysaccharide of *Treponema pallidum*. *Infect. Immun.* 24:244-251 (1979).
6. J. B. Baseman, Z. Zachar, and N. S. Hayes. Concanavalin A-mediated affinity film for *Treponema pallidum*. *Infect. Immun.* 27:260-263 (1980).
7. P. Z. O'Farrell, H. M. Goodman, and P. H. O'Farrell. High resolution two-dimensional electrophoresis of basic as well as acidic proteins. *Cell* 12:1133-1142 (1977).
8. J. B. Baseman and E. C. Hayes. Molecular characterization of receptor binding proteins and immunogens of virulent *Treponema pallidum*. *J. Exp. Med.* 151:573-586 (1980).
9. J. F. Alderete and J. B. Baseman. Surface characterization of virulent *Treponema pallidum*. *Infect. Immun.* 30:814-823 (1980).

10. J. F. Alderete and J. B. Baseman. Analysis of serum IgG against *Treponema pallidum* protein antigens in experimentally infected rabbits. *Br. J. Vener. Dis.* 57(5):302-308 (1981).
11. T. J. Fitzgerald, R. C. Johnson, J. N. Miller, and J. A. Sykes. Characterization of the attachment of *Treponema pallidum* (Nichols strain) to cultured mammalian cells and the potential relationship of attachment to pathogenicity. *Infect. Immun.* 18:467-478 (1977).
12. A. H. Fieldsteel, J. G. Stout and F. A. Becker. Comparative behavior of virulent strains of *Treponema pallidum* and *Treponema pertenue* in gradient cultures of various mammalian cells. *Infect. Immun.* 24:337-345 (1979).
13. R. E. Baughn, K. S. K. Tung, and D. M. Musher. Detection of circulating immune complexes in the sera of rabbits with experimental syphilis: Possible role in immunoregulation. *Infect. Immun.* 29:575-582 (1980).
14. C. S. Pavia, J. D. Folds, and J. B. Baseman. Cell-mediated immunity during syphilis. *Br. J. Vener. Dis.* 54:144-150 (1977).
15. J. L. Ware, J. D. Folds, and J. B. Baseman. Serum of rabbits infected with *Treponema pallidum* (Nichols) inhibits in vitro transformation of normal rabbit lymphocytes. *Cell Immunol.* 42:363-372 (1979).
16. S. M. Maret, J. B. Baseman, and J. D. Folds. Cell-mediated immunity in *Treponema pallidum*-infected rabbits: In vitro response of spleens and lymphocytes to mitogens and specific antigen. *Clin. Exp. Immunol.* 39:38-43 (1980).

13

Humoral Immune Mechanisms in Acquired Syphilis

NANCY H. BISHOP
California State University
Northridge
Northridge, California

JAMES N. MILLER
UCLA School of Medicine
Los Angeles, California

Role of the Humoral Immune Response in Pathogenesis   242
The Role of the Humoral Immune Response in Acquired Resistance to
  Challenge   248
Summary   260
References   261

The continuing increase in the prevalence of syphilis throughout the world together with the severity of the late clinical manifestations point not only to the importance of more effective control measures but also to the necessity for a clear understanding of the pathogenesis and immunology of the disease. Several investigators have explored the immunological events resulting from host-treponeme interaction following introduction of the organism into either humans or experimental animals. However, during the past decade, efforts have been directed mainly toward elucidating the potential role of cellular immune mechanisms with little attention being focused upon the humoral response. It is our intention to present several lines of evidence which support the hypothesis that humoral immune mechanisms are operative during the pathogenesis of syphilis and in the development of acquired resistance to challenge. This in no way implies that such mechanisms are at play to the exclusion of cell-mediated factors; indeed, it is becoming apparent that both are operative. Emphasis will be placed upon the human disease utilizing data provided by both animal and human studies.

Role of The Humoral Immune Response in Pathogenesis

Natural Resistance

It has been known for some time that humans exert some degree of natural resistance to *Treponema pallidum* infection (1,2). Hanff (3), extending the early suggestive studies of Turner and co-workers (4), Fribourg-Blanc (5), and Hederstedt (6-9), demonstrated that normal human serum contains a heat-stable, cross-reactive treponemicidal* antibody elicited by the nonpathogenic, host-indigenous *Treponema phagedenis*, biotype Reiter (TPR). He has presented the hypothesis that the relatively low attack rate may be dose dependent and influenced by these factors (1,2).

Primary Stage

Within a short time after treponemes have established themselves in the host, local multiplication and dissemination occur. Although early replication is primarily extracellular, evidence has been presented that at least some treponemes establish intracellular residence following attachment and penetration (10-16). The inflammatory response to primary infection in both the human and experimental rabbit disease consists essentially of a lymphocytic, plasma cell, and macrophage infiltration, with distribution depending upon the stage of lesion development versus healing (17). There is an influx of plasma components, including complement (C) and immunoglobulin (Ig), and the exudate is somewhat mucoid in nature. It has been proposed that perturbations or disturbances occur in immunoregulatory function as a consequence of primary infection resulting in suppressor T-cell subsets which may act to suppress treponemicidal antibody formation and thus allow progression of the disease (18,19). However, one must use caution in equating events which occur during the syphilitic process with data derived from plaque-forming assays in which splenic lymphocytes from *T. pallidum*-infected rabbits are suppressed in their ability to produce antibody to sheep erythrocytes. Baughn, Tung, and Musher (20) have demonstrated the presence of circulating immune complexes in the serum of rabbits with primary disease and have presented data which they interpret as supporting the hypothesis that complexes contribute to humoral immunosuppression (Chap. 14).

---

*Unless otherwise noted, use of the term *treponemicidal* refers to activity against *T. pallidum*. The terms *treponemicidal* and *neutralizing* are used interchangeably.

13. Humoral Immune Mechanisms in Acquired Syphilis

Again, such conclusions remain speculative inasmuch as they are based upon the observation that complex-containing serum suppresses the Ig response of normal rabbit spleen cells to sheep erythrocytes. Several investigators have shown that the specific responsiveness of lymphocytes to *T. pallidum* antigens during primary syphilis may be decreased by humoral factors in the serum or plasma of infected animals and humans (21-30). However, this may simply reflect a normal shutdown mechanism of the specific immune response rather than a specific immunosuppressive mechanism (30). Thus it would appear that a convincing case for immunosuppression or impairment has not been made. Rather, it seems more compelling that treponemal survival and proliferation may occur due to the relatively slow mobilization and activation of functional humoral and cellular components necessary to cope with the organisms. When the immune response is mobilized and activated (in contrast to suppressed), healing occurs with survival of a limited number of treponemes. There is an abundance of evidence that implicates humoral immune mechanisms in the healing process:

1. Normal human serum (and presumably serum present in exudates) has been shown to exhibit treponemicidal activity (3,5-9),
2. The presence of specific IgG antibody directed against *T. pallidum* is demonstrable in the serum of 9-day infected rabbits immune or partially immune to challenge, as measured by a radioiodinated staphylococcal protein A anti-*T. pallidum* (SPA-TP) assay (31),
3. *T. pallidum* present late in the course of experimental primary lesions is coated with specific Ig (32, J. N. Miller, unpublished observations that *T. pallidum* from late rabbit orchitis is immobilized in the presence of C alone),
4. Numerous plasma cells infiltrate the infected tissues at the height of early lesion development and during healing (33-35),
5. The number of IgG-bearing lymphoid cells is significantly increased in patients with primary syphilis (36),
6. Significant in vitro phagocytosis of *T. pallidum* by proteose peptone-induced and *T. pallidum*-induced rabbit peritoneal macrophages is demonstrable in the presence of immune rabbit serum (37) (R. H. Doe and J. N. Miller, unpublished studies), and
7. Peak infiltration of both macrophages and lymphocytes occurs just prior to the initiation of *T. pallidum* disappearance in the early lesions of rabbits (38).

These findings lend credence to the concept that healing may occur due to (1) inactivation of *T. pallidum* by treponemicidal antibody in concert with C and/or (2) opsonization of *T. pallidum* by specific antibody with resultant enhanced phagocytosis and destruction by macrophages.

The reason(s) for survival of limited numbers of treponemes following the healing process remains an enigma. However, several hypotheses have been proposed in an effort to explain this event; these include (1) a normal shutdown of immune mechanisms (39), (2) *T. pallidum* alteration through an "antigenic shift" or "host antigen acquisition" mechanism (38-40), (3) coating of *T. pallidum* by "blocking antibody" which prevents destruction of the organisms by immune factors (39-42), (4) a mucopolysaccharide-containing or host protein "outer coat" surrounding *T. pallidum* which prevents destruction of the organism by immune factors (35,37,39,40,43-55), (5) location within immunologically privileged sites such as the brain and aorta (38,40), and (6) protection from host immune mechanisms by virtue of an intracellular location (11,14,56). In our opinion, the last hypothesis has the greatest appeal.

Secondary Stage

The reason(s) for the events leading to the secondary stage of the disease are not well understood. It is difficult, for example, to explain the healing of local lesions at the precise time that the infectious process is continuing to proceed at widely disseminated sites. Indeed, continued proliferation of the organisms elicits a mobilization and activation of the immune process which makes it equally difficult to accept an hypothesis for tissue destruction based upon immune suppression, depletion, and/or impairment as postulated by several investigators on the basis of their findings (23,57-62).

Sølling and co-workers (63), Piette and co-workers (64), and Hanff (3) have presented evidence which strongly suggests the presence of circulating treponemal immune complexes in the sera of patients with secondary syphilis. Additionally, it has been shown that the nephropathy of secondary syphilis is caused by immune complex deposition (65,66). These complexes are present in most if not all patients with secondary disease, including those without nephritic involvement (63), and their role is presently unknown. However, an immunosuppressive mechanism seems unlikely in view of the relatively high treponemicidal antibody activity ($\geqslant 1:128$) demonstrable in untreated secondary syphilitic serum containing treponemal immune complexes (3). It seems more plausible that treponemal proliferation may be a function of relatively slow and inadequate mobilization and activation of the immune process. When the immune response level necessary to inactivate the organism is reached, healing again results with the survival of limited numbers of organisms by the potential mechanisms already described. Once more, the evidence that humoral immune mechanism(s) operative in the healing process may be summarized as follows: (1) in preliminary studies, C-dependent serum treponemicidal activity is demonstrable during the secondary stage in relatively high titers ranging from $\geqslant 1:16$ to $\geqslant 1:128$ (3); (2) plasma cell and macrophage infiltration occurs within secondary lesions during the active disease process and during healing (17); and (3) phagocytosis by macrophages is demonstrable in the presence of immune syphilitic rabbit serum (37). As in primary syphilis, specific killing of treponemes by antibody and C and/or the phagocytosis and destruction of opsonized *T. pallidum* by macrophages become a distinct possibility.

Despite the fact that relatively high treponemicidal antibody levels are demonstrable in the face of what appears to be treponemal proliferation, it is also conceivable that healing of the observed clinical manifestations is underway, due either partly or completely to these high antibody titers, and that endogenous resistance may, indeed, be a function of the *quantitative* level of treponemicidal antibody. Humoral immune factors may simply be present at levels too low to cause treponeme destruction during the proliferative process; but when adequate concentrations are reached, healing with limited survival of treponemes in an intracellular or extracellular environment, or latency, results. Conversely, high levels of humoral factors may be present and may form circulating immune complexes which bind and deplete serum C; if the C concentration falls below that level necessary for C-dependent treponemicidal activity, proliferation of the organisms could then provoke secondary lesions. Furthermore, it is conceivable that secondary lesions may recur as a result of treponemal antigenic alteration. This would then require antibody directed against new determinants in order for healing to occur.

Latency

The maintenance of latency may well be governed by humoral immune factor(s) in which the organism is literally "bathed." Evidence for this hypothesis stems from the following observations: (1) During latency relatively high serum levels of neutralizing (NZ) antibody active against *T. pallidum* are demonstrable in rabbits at titers of 1:16 to 1:128 (51), as well as in humans at titers of 1:8 to $\geqslant 1:128$ (3). (2) Relatively high levels of *T. pallidum*-specific IgG antibody ranging from 19.9 to 91.0 ng are demonstrable in rabbits with latent syphilis by the in vitro SPA-TP microassay (31). (3) A close quantitative correlation exists between the immune state and both neutralizing (NZ) and SPA-TP antibodies (31,51, Tables 1 and 2). (4) Blockage of attachment of *T. pallidum* to cultured mammalian cells by immune serum from rabbits with latent syphilis has been accomplished (16,56). (5) Immune serum from rabbits with latent syphilis contains sufficient anti-*T. pallidum* activity to confer upon normal recipients partial passive protection against homologous challenge (67,68); the specific antibody resides principally if not entirely in the IgG fraction (69). (6) Partial resistance to homologous challenge can be achieved in normal inbred hamsters by passive transfer of immune serum from syngeneic hamsters infected with endemic *T. pallidum* or with *Treponema*

Table 1 A Comparison of Antibody Responses During the Development and Persistence of Immunity in Experimental Syphilis

Characterization of IRS[a] pools

Pool number	Duration of infection	Immune status of donor rabbits	Neutralizing end point[b] (NEP)	Serologic response	
				TPI[b]	VDRL[b]
1	9 days	Susceptible[c,d]	0	NR[a]	1
2	9 days	Partially resistant[c,d]	0	NR	8
3	9 days	Partially resistant[c,d]	0	NR	4
4	9 days	Resistant[c,d]	0	NR	4
5	1 month	Resistant	<1	55	32
6	3 months	Resistant	16	279	4
8	7 months	Resistant	128	557	2
9	17 months	Resistant	64	484	1

[a]IRS = immune rabbit serum; NR = nonreactive.
[b]Neutralizing end point (NEP) = reciprocal of the highest dilution of immune serum which prevents lesion development at 50% of rabbit dermal sites inoculated with 10^3 $T.$ $pallidum$ incubated 16 hr in vitro with the serum dilution; TPI ($Treponema$ $pallidum$ immobilization) = reciprocal of the highest dilution of serum immobilizing 50% of the treponemes; VDRL (Venereal Disease Research Laboratory) = reciprocal of the highest dilution of serum exhibiting reactivity.
[c]Determined 11 days postinfection.
[d]Susceptible = developed typical, ulcerative, darkfield positive lesions from challenge with 10^3 $T.$ $pallidum$ at each of four sites on the clipped back; partially resistant = developed atypical, delayed, non-ulcerative lesions, either dark field positive (pool 2) or negative (pool 3), following challenge; resistant = developed no dermal lesions following challenges.
Source: Data from Ref. 51.

Table 2 The Staphylococcal Protein A-IgG (SPA-TP) Antibody Response of Individual Rabbits During the Development and Persistence of Immunity in Experimental Syphilis

Rabbit number	Immune status[a]	Time after infection	SPA-TP[b]
2	Susceptible[c]	9 days	9 (0.1)
1	Partially resistant[c]	9 days	370 (2.6)
3	Resistant[c]	9 days	227 (1.6)
7	Resistant[c]	9 days	391 (2.7)
4	Resistant	1 month	5,927 (42.5)
5	Resistant	1 month	7,787 (54.5)
6	Resistant	1 month	5,878 (41.2)
1	Resistant	3 months	7,225 (50.6)
2	Resistant	3 months	4,984 (34.9)
3	Resistant	3 months	12,996 (91.0)
4	Resistant	3 months	8,480 (59.4)
5	Resistant	3 months	4,800 (33.6)
6	Resistant	3 months	5,670 (39.7)
7	Resistant	3 months	7,064 (49.5)
1	Resistant	7 months	4,292 (30.0)
2	Resistant	7 months	6,267 (43.9)
3	Resistant	7 months	9,787 (68.5)
4	Resistant	7 months	5,721 (40.1)
5	Resistant	7 months	4,637 (32.5)
6	Resistant	7 months	2,856 (19.9)
7	Resistant	7 months	9,011 (63.1)
6	Resistant	17 months	5,802 (40.6)

[a]Immune status was determined by intradermal challenge with 10^3 *T. pallidum* at each of four sites on the clipped backs.
[b]SPA-TP values are expressed in counts per minute of radio-iodinated staphylococcal protein A bound to *T. pallidum*-IgG complexes less the counts per minute obtained with the individual preinfection sera; the numbers in parentheses are the numbers of nanograms of antibody bound to treponemes reacted with serum from *T. pallidum*-infected rabbits; 1000 counts per minute = 7 ng of bound antibody.
[c]Immune status was determined 11 days after infection.
Source: Data from Ref. 31.

pertenue (70,71). (7) In vitro phagocytosis of *T. pallidum* by rabbit peritoneal macrophages induced by either proteose peptone or *T. pallidum* is enhanced in the presence of immune serum from rabbits with latent infection (37).

Once again, the evidence is convincing for treponemicidal antibody in concert with C and/or phagocytosis of opsonized treponemes by macrophages as mediator(s) for maintenance of the latent state. Several investigators have expressed the view that failure to demonstrate complete protection of rabbits by passive transfer of immune serum discounts a role for humoral factors in the persistence of latency. This will be discussed later in this chapter. Thus, during latency we envision a host-parasite relationship in which intracellular and/or extracellular treponemes are held in check by the participation of humoral and cellular immune factors.

Tertiary Stage

One of the fascinating challenges to our understanding of the pathogenesis of syphilis is the explanation as to why the balance shifts in favor of the treponemes in some patients, remains in equilibrium for the lifetime of other patients, and seems to shift in favor of the host in still others (72,73). Is there a breakdown in humoral immune mechanisms operative during latency that allows the organisms to initiate the tertiary manifestations of the disease? It is conceivable that differences in neutralization or SPA-TP antibody titers may reflect the degree of endogenous resistance which influences the maintenance of latency; studies designed to test this hypothesis have been planned. It is pertinent to note that rabbits, whose resistance remains at a high level during latency, have relatively high neutralizing and SPA-TP titers (31,51, Tables 1 and 2). Although a breakdown in the immune process could explain the onset of late manifestations, an "antigenic shift" or "host antigen acquisition" mechanism could also permit treponemal proliferation.

The Role of the Humoral Immune Response in Acquired Resistance to Challenge

Immunity Induced by Infection and Vaccination

The induction of acquired resistance by human syphilitic infection has been known since the 16th century. Early experimental investigations of immunity have been reviewed authoritatively in the monograph of Turner and Hollander (43). Of prime interest among the work reviewed are the studies of Chesney (74,75), Magnuson and Rosenau (76), and Turner and Nelson (77), who established the relationship between the level of immunity to reinfection and the duration of syphilitic infection in rabbits, and Magnuson, Rosenau, and Clark (78), who showed the persistence of established immunity despite elimination of the infection by antibiotic therapy. In past years, several attempts to immunize rabbits have failed with (1) T. pallidum inactivated by heat, merthiolate, lyophilization, or Mapharsen and (2) protein antigens and ultrasonic lysates prepared from T. pallidum or nonpathogenic treponemes (79-86). Partial protection of rabbits against homologous challenge was reported with time-inactivated T. pallidum, Nichols strain, stored at 4°C for 6 to 10 days (87), but this has not been confirmed as yet in our laboratory. Miller (49) reported complete protection of rabbits against homologous challenge, utilizing a total of 3.71×10^9 freshly isolated T. pallidum, Nichols strain, inactivated by γ irradiation; the vaccine was administered over a 37-week period in a total of 60 intravenous injections. While the vaccine is far from practical, it provides a tool for assessing immune mechanisms responsible for acquired resistance following vaccination.

Humoral Mechanisms of Resistance

Until recent suggestive evidence became available, potential mechanisms of resistance in both the acquired experimental and human diseases were virtually unknown. Earlier attempts to relate reagin, Reiter protein, and T. pallidum complement fixing, fluorescent treponemal antibody absorbed (FTA-ABS), and TPI antibodies, per se, as the fundamental "protective" immune response following infection and vaccination were unsuccessful (47,80,82-84,87-91).

The pioneering investigations of Turner and his associates (4,92) provided a basis for the concept that humoral immune factors are associated with the development and persistence of host resistance following infection. In his initial experiment with serum from "infection-immune" rabbits, Turner (92) combined three, four, and nine parts of whole immune serum with one part of spirochete suspension each; the mixtures were incubated for 6 hr at 37°C and inoculated intradermally into the clipped backs of normal rabbits. The protective power of the serum was demonstrated by its ability to inhibit lesion development, increase the incubation period, or decrease the lesion size; higher concentrations of immune serum afforded greater protection, whereas normal serum exerted no effect. In similar investigations conducted by Turner and co-workers (4) serum from patients with secondary, latent, or tertiary syphilis showed marked protection by the same criteria of inhibition or modulation of the lesions. The addition of guinea pig complement to the incubation mixture in these experiments led to the development of the TPI test (32, 93,94).

Turner and Hollander (43) criticized the protection test on the basis of subsequently acquired knowledge of the biology of T. pallidum. They concluded that the incubation conditions and temperature may have reduced the viability of the treponemes; furthermore, a requirement for complement and the incubation period of only 6 hr may have precluded specific antibody immobilization. Regardless of criticisms of technical problems in the experiments, the authors provided a valid experimental approach to the assessment of humoral immunity in syphilis.

Efforts to elucidate the contribution of humoral factors to mechanisms of immunity to reinfection have concentrated primarily on experiments designed to demonstrate (1) a quantitative relationship between treponemicidal factor (immunoglobulin) and/or SPA-TP antibody and acquired resistance to challenge, and (2) passive protection. Studies relating to blockage of attachment of *T. pallidum* to cultured mammalian cells by immune rabbit serum and to phagocytosis of opsonized *T. pallidum* by macrophages provide additional evidence of the role of humoral factors in resistance to reinfection (see Chap. 11 and 18).

Treponemicidal Factors

The development of the in vitro-in vivo neutralization (NZ) test by Bishop and Miller (51) for the measurement of serum treponemicidal factors in experimental syphilis in rabbits has opened additional avenues of approach to the study of humoral immune mechanisms in both the acquired experimental and human diseases. In contrast to the TPI test, the assay utilizes rabbit serum as the source of C and thus provides a more accurate assessment of the relationship between treponemicidal antibody and acquired resistance. Immune serum is permitted to react with virulent *T. pallidum* in vitro under conditions favoring treponemal survival, and the virulence of the treponemes after incubation is determined by inoculation into normal, susceptible rabbits. Evidence obtained by the use of the NZ test in the experimental disease in rabbits has established the following: (1) immune serum contains factor(s) that specifically inactivate *T. pallidum*; (2) in vitro treponemal inactivation begins within 4 hr of incubation and becomes complete within 16 hr; (3) the killing of treponemes depends upon both a heat-stable factor present only in immune serum (immunoglobulin) and upon a heat-labile factor present in both immune and nonimmune sera (presumably complement); (4) a relatively close correlation exists between the neutralizing effect of the serum and the status of developing immunity during the course of infection; and (5) a close qualitative and quantitative correlation exists between the development and maintenance of resistance to symptomatic reinfection and the appearance and persistence of neutralizing factor(s) (Tables 1 and 3 and Fig. 1).

The neutralizing activity of syphilitic human sera has been investigated by Hanff (3) utilizing a test in which normal human serum is used as the suspending medium for the treponemes and as the source of complement. Two distinct treponemicidal serum components were identified, namely, a cross-reacting factor which occurs in the serum of nonsyphilitic individuals and a *T. pallidum*-specific factor present in the sera of individuals with secondary and late latent syphilis.

Table 3 Neutralizing Effect of Immune Rabbit Serum on *T. pallidum* Incubated In Vitro and Assessed In Vivo in Rabbits[a]

Serum	Incubation period (hr)	Lesion development	
		Lesions/total sites	Mean incubation time (days)
IRS[b], unheated	4	9/10	16.3 ± 5.3[c,d]
IRS, heated[e]	4	10/10	18.6 ± 6.4[d]
NRS[b], unheated	4	10/10	11.9 ± 1.3
NRS, heated	4	10/10	12.1 ± 1.3
IRS, unheated	16	0/10	
IRS, heated	16	9/10	16.8 ± 1.9[d]
NRS, unheated	16	10/10	13.3 ± 1.4
NRS, heated	16	10/10	13.2 ± 1.5

[a]Five rabbits were inoculated intradermally at duplicate sites on their clipped backs with 10^3 *T. pallidum* in each final mixture.
[b]IRS = pooled immune serum; NRS = pooled nonimmune serum.
[c]Mean ± standard deviation.
[d]$p < 0.05$
[e]56°C for 30 min.
Source: Data from Ref. 51.

The treponemicidal activity of normal human serum (NHS) was demonstrated against both *T. pallidum* and *T. phagedenis* biotype Reiter (TPR), was shown to require heat-stable and heat-labile factors, and could be removed from serum by absorption with TPR. Furthermore, the binding of immunoglobulins to the treponemes used for absorption correlated with the removal of anti-TPR activity as measured in a plaque assay (3). Although not conclusive, these results suggest that the heat-stable serum factor is, indeed, immunoglobulin. As indicated previously, the presence of treponemicidal activity in the sera of nonsyphilitic individuals may be an important factor in innate human resistance to syphilitic infection. Whether this immune mechanism could be exploited in vaccine development remains to be determined.

The inactivation of *T. pallidum* by NZ factors present in NHS necessitated the development of a methodology which would allow the relationship of both specific and nonspecific NZ factors to immunity to be determined. Sera from nonsyphilitic normal individuals and from patients with primary, secondary, or late latent syphilis were then tested for treponemicidal factors by a modified quantitative neutralization assay in which the serum was tested both unabsorbed and absorbed

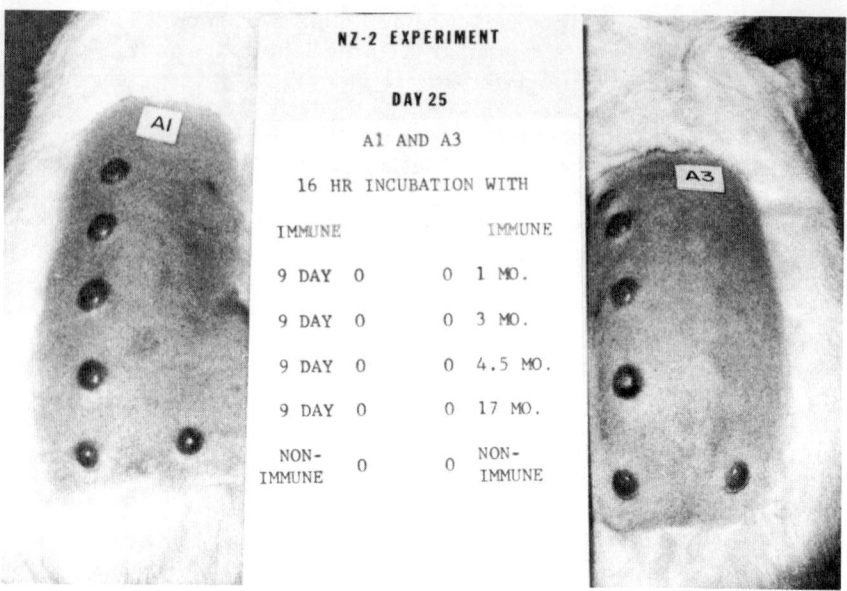

Figure 1 The results in duplicate rabbits after intradermal inoculation of 10^3 T. pallidum previously incubated in vitro for 16 hr with immune sera obtained from rabbits at intervals after infection. Note (1) the relationship between the capacity of immune serum to neutralize T. pallidum and the duration of infection and (2) the delayed lesion development of the site on rabbit A1 inoculated with treponemes incubated with serum obtained 1 month postinfection. (Source: Reference 51.)

with TPR for removal of nonspecific antibody (3). The incubation mixtures contained nine parts of whole serum or serum dilutions and one part of T. pallidum suspension, such that the final concentration was 10^7 treponemes per milliliter. After suitable incubation the mixture was diluted to 10^4 organisms per milliliter and injected into rabbits as previously described (51).

Preliminary results have revealed the presence of neutralizing activity in the sera of three patients with secondary and latent disease; this activity was not present in the sera of two patients with primary syphilis but was demonstrable at a titer of $\geqslant 1:1$ in one serum from an individual previously infected (Table 4). The presence of relatively high levels of treponemicidal factors in the three untreated secondary syphilis patients ($\geqslant 1:16$, $\geqslant 1:128$, $\geqslant 1:128$) may be at least partly or completely responsible for exogenous resistance in this stage of the disease; on the basis of his observations, Chesney (95) concluded that patients with secondary syphilis were not only immune

Table 4 Neutralizing Antibody Levels in Syphilitic Human Sera

Serum	Neutralizing end point[a]					
	Primary[b]		Secondary[b]		Late latent[b]	
	Unabsorbed	Absorbed[c]	Unabsorbed	Absorbed[c]	Unabsorbed	Absorbed[c]
1	0	0	ND[d]	16	⩾128	64
2	1	0	⩾128	128	32	32
3	⩾1	⩾1	⩾128	128	8	4

[a] Neutralizing end point (NEP) = reciprocal of the highest serum dilution resulting in a significant delay in the mean time of dermal lesion development in rabbits, as compared with heated serum controls; the inoculum at each site consisted of 10^3 $T.$ $pallidum$ incubated 16 hr in vitro with whole or diluted human syphilitic serum (10^7 treponemes per milliliter; 90% human serum), then diluted 1000-fold with 50% heat-inactivated normal rabbit serum in FTA-ABS buffer and injected intradermally into the clipped backs of normal rabbits.
[b] Diagnostic category.
[c] Serum absorbed for 30 min at 4°C with $T.$ $phagedenis$ biotype Reiter.
[d] Not determinable owing to the fact that the titers of specific neutralizing factor and anticomplementary activity were equivalent; however, the end point was considered to be ⩾16.

Source: Data from Ref. 3.

to chancre formation upon reexposure but may also be resistant to superimposed secondary lesion development. The quantitative data further showed that the serum from the untreated late latent patient in the study had an unabsorbed NZ titer of 1:8, whereas the sera from the treated late latents had titers of ≥1:4, 1:32, and ≥1:128. Magnuson and his co-workers (89) reported that each of 5 untreated late latents and 13 of 26 treated late latents were immune to challenge. Moreover, it is also known that a waning of the immune response occurs in one-third of patients with untreated latency, resulting in late manifestations of the disease (72,73). Thus NZ titers of 1:4 may reflect values close to the minimum required for both exogenous and endogenous resistance. If so, the treated patients with titers of 1:32 and ≥1:128 may be resistant to reinfection.

SPA-TP (Specific IgG) Antibodies

Zeltzer and his co-workers (96) have shown that an antitreponemal IgG response in acquired experimental syphilis can be measured utilizing radioiodinated staphylococcal protein A and killed *T. pallidum* in an in vitro microassay system (SPA-TP) capable of detecting less than 2 ng of antibody. The IgG response in intratesticularly infected rabbits was first detected at 9 days postinfection, reached a peak at 30 days, and remained elevated for 12 months. Absorption studies with an extract of TPR demonstrated that 65 to 85% of the total antitreponemal IgG response was specific for *T. pallidum* throughout the course of infection. Pepose and his co-workers (31) have presented evidence that the IgG detected by the SPA-TP technique correlates quantitatively with the onset and persistence of immunity to symptomatic reinfection (Table 2). Detection of the antibody at 9 days after infection paralleled the appearance of immunity. At 1 month the SPA-TP antibody level increased in correspondence with increasing resistance and remained elevated as immunity to symptomatic reinfection was maintained throughout the observed 17-month course of the disease. The SPA-TP assay may be a measurement of IgG directed against *T. pallidum* immunogens different from or the same as those which stimulate NZ antibody; yet the possibility exists that it may be applicable not only for assessment of the immune status of the host, but also as a potential marker or screening procedure in recombinant DNA, hybridoma, and molecular analysis studies for isolation of "protective" immunogens.

Passive Immunization

Passive immunization studies by several investigators have provided evidence for the protective role of factors present in the serum of rabbits previously infected with *T. pallidum*, Nichols strain, and

13. Humoral Immune Mechanisms in Acquired Syphilis

resistant to symptomatic reinfection (67,68,97-101, Fig. 2). In each instance partial but significant protection against homologous challenge was observed. The detailed methodology and results of each of these studies are summarized in Table 5. Resistance was achieved with both unheated and heat-inactivated serum from the donor animals, suggesting the potential immunoglobulin nature of the protective factor. Confirmatory evidence has been provided by Titus and Weiser (69), who demonstrated that the specific antibody responsible for passive protection by "infection-immune" serum resides principally, if not entirely, in the IgG fraction.

As indicated previously, several investigators have discounted a role for humoral factors in both endogenous and exogenous resistance during latency on the basis of incomplete protection of rabbits by

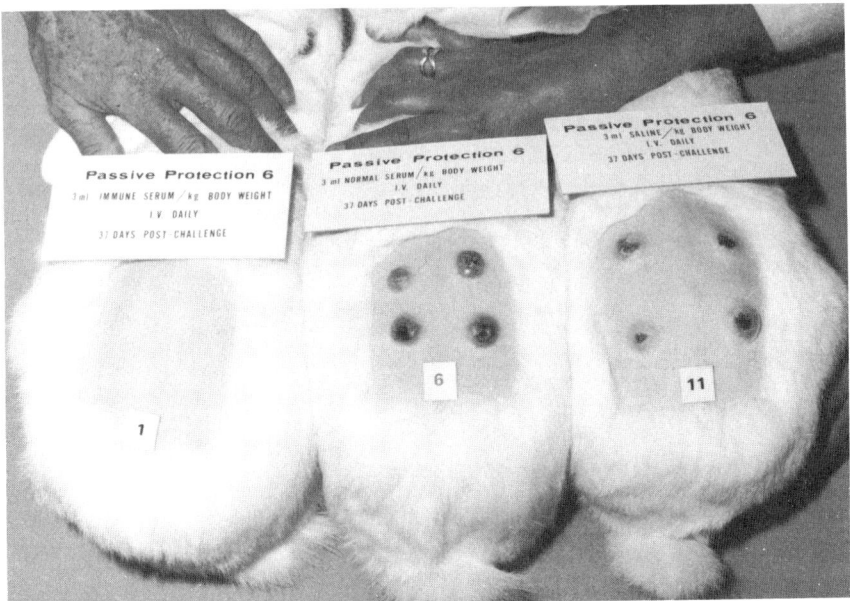

Figure 2 Results of intradermal challenge on the clipped backs of a passively immunized rabbit and two control rabbits at the termination of daily injections 37 days after challenge at each of four sites with 10^3 T. pallidum, Nichols strain, per site. To the left is rabbit 1 immunized with pooled immune rabbit serum; the center is rabbit 6 injected with pooled nonimmune rabbit serum; and to the right is rabbit 11 injected with saline. See Table 5 for methodology. (Source: Reference 67.)

Table 5 Summary of Passive Immunization Studies in Experimental Treponemal Disease

Authors	Number of animals immunized	Immunization schedule			Intradermal challenge		Characteristics of lesions	
		Number, volume, and route of serum injections		Time relative to challenge (days)	Dose per site	Number of sites	Delay in development (days)	Appearance

Treponema pallidum, Nichols strain

Authors	N	Injections	Route	Time	Dose/site	Sites	Delay (days)	Appearance
Bishop and Miller (67)	5	38 × 3 ml/kg	IV	0 to 37, daily	1.1×10^3	4	28	Small, atypical, non-ulcerative, dark-field negative, accelerated healing; complete absence of disseminated infection in one animal.
N. H. Bishop and J. N. Miller (unpublished data, 1972)	2	26 × 4.5 ml	IV	0 to 25, daily	1×10^3	4	21	Small atypical, non-ulcerative.
	4	38 × 5 ml	IV	0 to 37, daily	2×10^3	4	6	Small atypical, non-ulcerative.
Graves and Johnson (100)	3	6 × 10 ml	IV	0 to 10, 2-day intervals	1 to 10^4 in 10-fold increments	2 per dose, 10 total	9	Delay with 10^4 and 10^3 treponeme doses. No delay with 10^2 and 1 treponeme doses.

13. Humoral Immune Mechanisms in Acquired Syphilis

Reference		Dose	Day (4 or 5) (24 hr after lesion development)	Challenge		NA[a]	Effect
Perine et al. (98)	8	1 × 80 ml/kg IP		1 × 10^6	6		Temporary suppression of ulceration.
	4	1 × 80 ml/kg IP	−1	1 × 10^3	6	3	Accelerated healing.
Perine et al. (98)	1	5 × 80 ml/kg IP	−1 to 15	1 × 10^3	6		Delay until 4 to 12 days after immunization discontinued.
	1	7 × 80 ml/kg IP	−1 to 21	1 × 10^3	6		
Sepetjian et al. (97)	2	11 × 20 ml IV	0 to 14	8 × 10^5	6	2	Nonulcerative, darkfield negative, accelerated healing.
Turner et al. (99)	4	1 × 50 ml/kg IP	−1	1 × 10^4	4	2	Decreased severity.
	4	1 × 10 ml/kg IV	0	5 × 10^2	4	2	Decreased severity.
	6	1 × 10 ml/kg IV	−1	5 × 10^2	6	4	Decreased severity.
	5	1 × 10 ml/kg IV	7	5 × 10^2	6	3	Decreased severity.
	5	2 × 10 ml/kg IV	−1, 0	5 × 10^2	6	3	Decreased severity.
	3	1 × 50 ml/kg[b] IP	−1	5 × 10^2	4	5	Decreased severity.
	6	1 × 50 ml/kg[b] IP	−1	5 × 10^2	4	7	Decreased severity.
	6	2 × 25 ml/kg[b] IP	−1, 8	5 × 10^2	4	6	Decreased severity.

Table 5 (continued)

Authors	Number of animals immunized	Immunization schedule			Intradermal challenge		Characteristics of lesions	
		Number, volume, and route of serum injections	Time relative to challenge (days)		Dose per site	Number of sites	Delay in development (days)	Appearance
Weiser et al. (68)	3	8 × 7 ml/kg IV	-2 to 5, daily		1×10^3	8	9	Small, atypical, non-ulcerative.
	3	8 × 7 ml/kg IV	0 to 7, daily		1×10^3	8	0	Temporary suppression.
	1	14 × 30 ml/kg IP	-2 to 36, 3-day intervals		1×10^3	8	20	Temporary suppression.
	3	1 × 25 ml/kg IP 13 × 15 ml/kg IP	-2 1 to 36, 3-day intervals		1×10^3	8	10	Decreased severity.

Treponema pallidum, Melbourne 1 strain

Graves and Alden (101)	3c	5 × 10 ml	IV	-9, -7, -5, -2, 0	1 to 10^4 in 10-fold increments	2 per dose, 10 total		
	3d	5 × 10 ml	IV	-9, -7, -5, -2, 0				Delay in 10^4 treponeme dose only.
	3e	5 × 10 ml	IV	-9, -7, -5, -2, 0			4	Reduced numbers of 10 treponeme dose only.

Treponema pallidum, Bosnia A strain								
Schell et al. (70)	5	11 × 0.4 ml	IV	-3 to 25, 3-day intervals	1 × 10^4	1	∞^{f}	Complete prevention of skin lesions, lymph node infection of reduced severity.
Treponema pertenue, Haiti B strain								
Schell et al. (71)	5	8 × 0.5 ml	IV	-3 to 18, 3-day intervals	1 × 10^6	2	∞	Complete prevention of skin lesions, lymph node infection of reduced severity.

^{a}NA = not applicable.
^{b}plasma was used rather than serum.
^{c}Immune serum obtained from 3-month infected rabbits.
^{d}Immune serum obtained from 4-month infected rabbits.
^{e}Immune serum obtained from 6-month infected rabbits.
^{f}∞ = absence of dermal lesions.

passive transfer of immune serum. The protection achieved, though partial, is reproducible and provides supportive evidence for an operative humoral mechanism; it is relevant that in the study of Bishop and Miller (67) one rabbit was completely protected against homologous challenge as measured by the absence of both symptomatic and disseminated asymptomatic infection. The level and distribution of antibody achieved in the recipient animals cannot compare with those of the donor animals, whose resistance also happens to be at a significantly higher level; in studies conducted by Bishop and Miller (67) the mean TPI levels achieved by the recipient animals were significantly lower than those of the donor serum pools.

Similar studies have been conducted with other pathogenic strains and species of *Treponema* (Table 5). Graves and Alden (101) have presented data which they interpret as supporting a role for a limited protective humoral response to *T. pallidum* infection. Immune serum from rabbits infected with the newly isolated *T. pallidum*, Melbourne 1 strain, conferred partial protection upon normal recipient animals as evidenced by a delay of 3 to 4 days in lesion development compared to control animals. Differences in experimental procedures, however, prevent a direct comparison of the protection with that incited by *T. pallidum*, Nichols strain. Moreover, the reported protection conferred by nonimmune serum contrasts with the data of others in which untreated or saline-treated and nonimmune serum-treated rabbits showed similar response to challenge (67,97,98). Schell and his co-workers (70,71) have presented data to support the concept that protection of inbred hamsters against homologous challenge can be achieved by passive immunization with serum obtained from syngeneic animals immunized by infection with *T. pertenue*, Haiti B strain, and endemic *T. pallidum*, Bosnia A strain, respectively. In each instance partial protection was achieved. Schell's ability to confer similar protection by the adoptive transfer of immune splenic lymphocytes from these animals suggests a role for both humoral and cell-mediated immunity in the treponemal immune process.

Summary

A body of experimental evidence has been presented which supports a functional role for humoral immune mechanisms during the pathogenesis of syphilis and the development of acquired resistance to challenge. Evidence for the contribution of humoral immunity to the healing process in primary disease is provided by the presence of complement-dependent treponemicidal antibody in normal human serum, *T. pallidum*-specific IgG in serum early in the course of disease, and macrophages and plasma cells along with *T. pallidum* coated with specific Ig in late primary lesions. Although the mechanism of secondary lesion formation and the role of immune complexes in their pathogenesis are unknown, healing of these lesions may be effected partly or completely by opsonizing antibodies or by the relatively high treponemicidal antibody level which develops during this stage of the disease. The participation of humoral immune mechanisms in the maintenance of latency (endogenous resistance) and persistence of acquired resistance to reinfection (exogenous resistance) is supported by two major lines of evidence. The first is the demonstration of a *T. pallidum*-specific antibody response, measured by the NZ and SPA-TP assays and shown to correlate with resistance to challenge. The data which show the protective functions of immune serum components comprise the second line of evidence and include the demonstration of complement-dependent antibody-mediated treponemal killing, protection of normal hosts by passive immunization with serum from resistant animals, the requirement for immune serum (presumably opsonins) for macrophage engulfment of *T. pallidum*, and the capability of immune serum to prevent the attachment of treponemes to cultured cells. The mechanisms which erode the resistance present in latency and precipitate tertiary disease are unknown; explanations postulated include a breakdown in the immune process or "antigenic shift" in the treponemes.

Thus there is compelling evidence that syphilitic infection stimulates the production of specific immunoglobulin which is treponemicidal and protective to the host; these data contrast with much of the current evidence for cell-mediated mechanisms which depend upon in vitro tests as indicators of potential in vivo function and which, therefore, must be interpreted with a degree of caution (102). However, the evidence in no way precludes the possibility that resistance is mediated by humoral factors, particularly immunoglobulins, in concert with specifically stimulated immune cells. Understanding these mechanisms and their respective contributions to resistance remains the ultimate goal in all of these studies; eventually it may permit not only the assessment of the level of resistance of individual patients, but also the stimulation or modulation of the response to assure protective immunity.

References

1. M. B. Moore, E. V. Price, J. M. Knox, and L. W. Elgin. Epidemiologic treatment of contacts to infectious syphilis. *Public Health Rep.* 78:966-970 (1963).
2. A. L. Schroeter, R. H. Turner, J. B. Lucas, and W. J. Brown. Therapy for incubating syphilis. Effectiveness of gonorrhea treatment. *J. Am. Med. Assoc.* 218:711-713 (1971).
3. P. A. Hannf. Humoral immunity in human syphilis. Ph.D. dissertation, University of California, Los Angeles, California, (1980).

4. T. B. Turner, F. C. Kluth, C. McLeod, and C. P. Windsor. Protective antibodies in the serum of syphilitic patients. *Am. J. Hyg.* 48:173-181 (1948).
5. A. Fribourg-Blanc. Le pouvoir tréponémicide naturel du sérum humain. *Presse Med.* 64:1396-1397 (1956).
6. B. Hederstedt. *Treponema pallidum* immobilization in normal serum. *Acta Pathol. Microbiol. Scand.* 58:158 (1963).
7. B. Hederstedt. Studies of the *Treponema pallidum* immobilizing activity in normal human serum. I. A method. *Acta Pathol. Microbiol. Scand. Sect. B* 82:185-200 (1974).
8. B. Hederstedt. Studies on the *Treponema pallidum* immobilizing activity in normal human serum. 2. Serum factors participating in the normal serum immobilization reaction. *Acta Pathol. Microbiol. Scand. Sect. C* 84:135-141 (1976).
9. B. Hederstedt. Studies on the *Treponema pallidum* immobilizing activity in normal human serum. 3. The kinetics of the immobilization reaction of normal and immune sera. *Acta Pathol. Microbiol. Scand. Sect. C* 84:142-147 (1976).
10. H. A. Azar, T. D. Pham, and A. K. Kurban. An electron microscopic study of a syphilitic chancre. *Arch. Pathol.* 90:143-150 (1970).
11. J. A. Sykes and J. N. Miller. Intracellular location of *Treponema pallidum*, Nichols strain, in the rabbit testis. *Infect. Immun.* 4:307-314 (1971).
12. V. Lauderdale and J. N. Goldman. Serial ultrathin sectioning demonstrating the intracellularity of *T. pallidum*. An electron microscopic study. *Br. J. Vener. Dis* 48:87-96 (1972).
13. J. A. Sykes, J. N. Miller, and A. J. Kalan. *Treponema pallidum* within cells of a primary chancre from a human female. *Br. J. Vener. Dis.* 50:40-44 (1974).
14. T. J. Fitzgerald, J. N. Miller, and J. A. Sykes. *Treponema pallidum* (Nichols strain) in tissue cultures: Cellular attachment, entry, and survival. *Infect. Immun.* 11:1133-1140 (1975).
15. J. A. Sykes and J. Kalan. Intracellular *Treponema pallidum* in cells of a syphilitic lesion of the uterine cervix. *Am. J. Obstet. Gynecol.* 122:361-367 (1975).
16. N. S. Hayes, K. E. Muse, A. M. Collier, and J. B. Baseman. Parasitism by virulent *Treponema pallidum* of host cell surfaces. *Infect. Immun.* 17:174-186 (1977).
17. S. L. Robbins and R. S. Cotran. *Pathologic Basis of Disease*, 2nd ed. W. B. Saunders, Philadelphia, 1979, pp. 407-408.
18. R. E. Baughn and D. M. Musher. Altered immune responsiveness associated with experimental syphilis in the rabbit: Elevated IgM and depressed IgG responses to sheep erythrocytes. *J. Immunol.* 120:1691-1695 (1978).

19. R. E. Baughn and D. M. Musher. Aberrant secondary antibody responses to sheep erythrocytes in rabbits with experimental syphilis. *Infect. Immun.* 25:133-138 (1979).
20. R. E. Baughn, K. S. K. Tung, and D. M. Musher. Detection of circulating immune complexes in the sera of rabbits with experimental syphilis: Possible role in immunoregulation. *Infect. Immun.* 29:575-582 (1980).
21. G. M. Levene, J. L. Turk, D. J. M. Wright, and A. G. S. Grimble. Reduced lymphocyte transformation due to a plasma factor in patients with active syphilis. *Lancet* 2:246-247 (1969).
22. J. M. Dwyer, J. Thompson, R. Mangi, and R. Lee. Suppression of the lymphocyte response to PHA by serum from subjects with syphilis. *Fed. Proc. Fed. Am. Soc. Exp. Biol.* 34:996 (1975).
23. E. From, K. Thestrup-Pedersen, and H. Thulin. Reactivity of lymphocytes from patients with syphilis towards *T. pallidum* antigen in the leukocyte migration and lymphocyte transformation tests. *Br. J. Vener. Dis.* 52:224-229 (1976).
24. C. S. Pavia, J. D. Folds, and J. B. Baseman. Depression of lymphocyte response to concanavalin A in rabbits infected with *Treponema pallidum* (Nichols strain). *Infect. Immun.* 14:320-322 (1976).
25. C. S. Pavia, J. D. Folds, and J. B. Baseman. Selective *in vitro* response of thymus-derived lymphocytes from *Treponema pallidum*-infected rabbits. *Infect. Immun.* 18:603-611 (1977).
26. V. Wicher and K. Wicher. *In vitro* cell response of *Treponema pallidum*-infected rabbits. II. Inhibition of lymphocyte response to phytohemagglutinin by serum of *T. pallidum* infected rabbits. *Clin. Exp. Immunol.* 29:487-495 (1977).
27. P. S. Friedmann and J. L. Turk. The role of cell-mediated immune mechanisms in syphilis in Ethiopia. *Clin. Exp. Immunol.* 31:59-65 (1978).
28. J. L. Ware, J. D. Folds, and J. B. Baseman. Serum of rabbits infected with *Treponema pallidum* (Nichols) inhibits *in vitro* transformation of normal rabbit lymphocytes. *Cell. Immunol.* 42:363-372 (1979).
29. S. M. Maret, J. B. Baseman, and J. D. Folds. Cell-mediated immunity in *Treponema pallidum* infected rabbits: *In vitro* response of splenic and lymph node lymphocytes to mitogens and specific antigens. *Clin. Exp. Immunol.* 39:38-43 (1980).
30. S. A. Baker-Zander, S. A. Lukehart, and S. Sell. *In vitro* inhibition of antigen specific lymphocyte blast transformation by sera from *Treponema pallidum* infected rabbits. *Annu. Meet. Am. Soc. Microbiol.*, p. 57 (1981).

31. J. S. Pepose, N. H. Bishop, S. Feigenbaum, J. N. Miller, and P. M. Zeltzer. The humoral immune response in rabbits infected with *Treponema pallidum*: Comparison of antibody levels measured by the staphylococcal protein A-IgG (SPA-TP) microassay with VDRL, FTA-Abs, and TPI antibody responses during the development of acquired resistance to challenge. *Sex. Transm. Dis.* 7:125-129 (1980).
32. R. A. Nelson, Jr. and J. A. Diesendruck. Studies on immobilizing antibodies in syphilis. I. Technique of measurement and factors influencing immobilization. *J. Immunol.* 66:667-685 (1951).
33. P. S. Gregoriew and K. G. Jarisheva. The histologic structure of syphilitic lesions of rabbits. *Am. J. Syph.* 12:67-81 (1928).
34. V. Scott and G. J. Dammin. Hyalurouidase and experimental syphilis. III. Metachromasia in syphilitic orchitis and its relationship to hyaluronic acid. *Am. J. Syph.* 34:501-514 (1950).
35. P. H. Hardy, Jr., D. J. Graham, E. E. Nell, and A. M. Dannenberg, Jr. Macrophages in immunity to syphilis: Suppressive effect of concurrent infection with *Mycobacterium bovis* BCG on the development of syphilitic lesions and growth of *Treponema pallidum* in tuberculin-positive rabbits. *Infect. Immun.* 26:751-763 (1979).
36. J. D. Bos, F. Hamerlinck, and R. H. Cormane. Immunoglobulin-bearing lymphoid cells in primary syphilis. Quantitative and elution studies. *Br. J. Vener. Dis.* 56:69-73 (1980).
37. S. A. Lukehart and J. N. Miller. Demonstration of the in vitro phagocytosis of *Treponema pallidum* by rabbit peritoneal macrophages. *J. Immunol.* 121:2014-2024 (1978).
38. S. A. Lukehart, S. A. Baker-Zander, R. M. C. Lloyd, and S. Sell. Characterization of lymphocyte responsiveness in early experimental syphilis. II. Nature of cellular infiltration and *Treponema pallidum* distribution in testicular lesions. *J. Immunol.* 124:461-467 (1980).
39. S. Sell, S. A. Baker-Zander, and R. M. C. Lloyd. T-cell hyperplasia of lymphoid tissue of rabbits infected with *T. pallidum*: Evidence for a vigorous immune response. *Sex Transm. Dis.* 7:74-84 (1980).
40. S. Sell, D. Gamboa, S. A. Baker-Zander, S. A. Lukehart, and J. N. Miller. Host response to *Treponema pallidum* in intradermally-infected rabbits: Evidence for persistence of infection at local and distant sites. *J. Invest. Dermatol.* 75:470-475 (1980).
41. M. A. Medici. The immunoprotective niche - A new pathogenic mechanism for syphilis, the systemic mycoses and other infectious diseases. *J. Theor. Biol.* 36:617-625 (1972).

42. D. J. M. Wright and A. G. S. Grimble. Why is the infectious stage of syphilis prolonged? *Br. J. Vener. Dis.* 50:45-49 (1974).
43. T. B. Turner and D. H. Hollander. *Biology of the Treponematoses.* World Health Organization, Geneva, 1957.
44. P. H. Hardy and E. E. Nell. Study of the antigenic structure of *Treponema pallidum* by specific agglutination. *Am. J. Hyg.* 66:160-172 (1957).
45. M. Metzger, P. H. Hardy, Jr., and E. E. Nell. Influence of lysozyme upon the treponeme immobilization reaction. *Am. J. Hyg.* 73:236-244 (1961).
46. S. Christiansen. Protective layer covering pathogenic treponemata. *Lancet* 1:423-425 (1963).
47. J. N. Miller. Immunity in experimental syphilis. V. The immunogenicity of *Treponema pallidum* attenuated by γ-irradiation. *J. Immunol.* 99:1012-1016 (1967).
48. R. H. Jones, T. A. Nevin, W. J. Guest, and L. C. Logan. Lytic effect of trypsin, lysozyme, and complement on *Treponema pallidum*. *Br. J. Vener. Dis.* 44:193-200 (1968).
49. J. N. Miller. Immunity in experimental syphilis. VI. Successful vaccination of rabbits with *Treponema pallidum*, Nichols strain, attenuated by γ-irradiation. *J. Immunol.* 110:1206-1215 (1973).
50. L. C. Logan. Rabbit globulin and anti-globulin factors associated with *Treponema pallidum* grown in rabbits. *Br. J. Vener. Dis.* 50:421-427 (1974).
51. N. H. Bishop and J. N. Miller. Humoral immunity in experimental syphilis. II. The relationship of neutralizing factors in immune serum to acquired resistance. *J. Immunol.* 117:197-207 (1976).
52. J. A. Ziegler, A. M. Jones, R. H. Jones, and K. M. Kubica. Demonstration of extracellular material at the surface of pathogenic *T. pallidum* cells. *Br. J. Vener. Dis.* 52:1-8 (1976).
53. T. J. Fitzgerald, R. C. Johnson, and E. T. Wolff. Mucopolysaccharide material resulting from the interaction of *Treponema pallidum* (Nichols strain) with cultured mammalian cells. *Infect. Immun.* 22:575-584 (1978).
54. T. J. Fitzgerald and R. C. Johnson. Surface mucopolysaccharides of *Treponema pallidum*. *Infect. Immun* 24:244-251 (1979).
55. J. F. Alderete and J. B. Baseman. Surface-associated host proteins on virulent *Treponema pallidum*. *Infect. Immun.* 26:1048-1056 (1979).
56. T. J. Fitzgerald, R. C. Johnson, J. N. Miller, and J. A. Sykes. Characterization of the attachment of *Treponema pallidum* (Nichols strain) to cultured mammalian cells and the

potential relationship of attachment to pathogenicity. *Infect. Immun.* 18:467-478 (1977).
57. H. Noguchi. A cutaneous reaction in syphilis. *J. Exp. Med.* 14:557-568 (1911).
58. H. Noguchi. The luetin reaction. *J. Am. Med. Assoc.* 59:1262-1263 (1912).
59. L. C. Marshak and S. Rothman. Skin testing with a purified suspension of *Treponema pallidum*. *Am. J. Syph.* 35:35-41 (1951).
60. J. Thivolet, A. Simeray, M. Rolland, and F. Challut. Etude de l'intradermo-réaction aux suspensions de tréponèmes formolées (souche Nicholes pathogène) chez les syphilitiques et les sujets normaux. *Ann. Inst. Pasteur* 85:23-33 (1953).
61. D. M. Musher, R. F. Schell, and J. M. Knox. In vitro lymphocyte response to *Treponema refringes* in human syphilis. *Infect. Immun.* 9:654-657 (1974).
62. D. M. Musher, R. F. Schell, R. H. Jones, and A. M. Jones. An *in vitro* correlate of immune suppression *in vivo*? *Infect. Immun.* 11:1261-1264 (1975).
63. J. Sølling, K. Sølling, K. U. Jakobsen, and E. From. Circulating immune complexes in syphilis. *Acta Derm. Venereol.* 58:263-267 (1978).
64. F. Piette, W. Wattre, J. P. Dessaint, P. Devemy, and H. Bergoend. Les complexes immune circulants dans la syphilis primosecondaire et sérologique. *Ann. Dermatol. Venereol.* 106:967-972 (1979).
65. C. N. Gamble and J. B. Reardan. Immunopathogenesis of syphilitic glomerulonephritis. Elution of antitreponemal antibody from glomerular immune-complex deposits. *N. Engl. J. Med.* 292:449-454 (1975).
66. D. R. Tourville, L. H. Byrd, D. U. Kim, D. Zajd, I. Lee, L. B. Reichman, and S. Baskin. Treponemal antigen in immunopathogenesis of syphilitic glomerulonephritis. *Am. J. Pathol.* 82:479-492 (1976).
67. N. H. Bishop and J. N. Miller. Humoral immunity in experimental syphilis. I. The demonstration of resistance conferred by passive immunization. *J. Immunol.* 117:191-196 (1976).
68. R. S. Weiser, D. Erickson, P. L. Perine, and N. N. Pearsall. Immunity to syphilis: Passive transfer in rabbits using serial doses of immune serum. *Infect. Immun.* 13:1402-1407 (1976).
69. R. G. Titus and R. S. Weiser. Experimental syphilis in the rabbit: Passive transfer of immunity with immunoglobulin G from immune serum. *J. Infect. Dis.* 140:904-913 (1979).
70. R. F. Schell, J. K. Chan, and J. L. LeFrock. Endemic syphilis: Passive transfer of resistance with serum and cells in hamsters. *J. Infect. Dis.* 140:378-383 (1979).

71. R. F. Schell, J. L. LeFrock, and J. P. Babu. Passive transfer of resistance to frambesial infection in hamsters. *Infect. Immun.* 21:430-435 (1978).
72. E. Bruusgaard. Über das Schicksal der nicht spezifisch behandelten Luetiker. *Arch. Dermatol. Syph.* 157:309-332 (1929).
73. D. H. Rockwell, A. R. Yobs, and M. B. Moore, Jr. The Tuskegee study of untreated syphilis. The 30th year of observation. *Arch. Intern. Med.* 114:792-798 (1964).
74. A. M. Chesney. *Medicine Monographs. XII. Immunity in Syphilis.* Williams and Wilkins, Baltimore, Maryland, 1927.
75. A. M. Chesney. Acquired immunity in syphilis. *Harvey Lect.* 25:103-128 (1931).
76. H. J. Magnuson and B. J. Rosenau. The rate of development and degree of acquired immunity in experiment syphilis. *Am. J. Syph.* 32:418-436 (1948).
77. T. B. Turner and R. A. Nelson, Jr. The relationship of treponemal immobilizing antibody to immunity in syphilis. *Trans. Assoc. Am. Physicians* 63:112-117 (1950).
78. H. J. Magnuson, B. J. Rosenau, and J. W. Clark. The duration of acquired immunity in experimental syphilis. *Am. J. Syph.* 33:297-302 (1949).
79. H. J. Magnuson, S. P. Halbert, and B. J. Rosenau. Attempted immunization of rabbits against syphilis with killed *Treponema pallidum* and adjuvants. *J. Vener. Dis. Inform.* 28:267-271 (1947).
80. H. Eagle and R. Fleischman. The antibody response in rabbits to killed suspensions of pathogenic *T. pallidum*. *J. Exp. Med.* 87:369-384 (1948).
81. G. W. Waring and W. L. Fleming. Further attempts to immunize rabbits with killed *Treponema pallidum*. *Am. J. Syph.* 35:568-572 (1951).
82. C. P. McLeod and H. J. Magnuson. Production of immobilizing antibodies unaccompanied by active immunity to *Treponema pallidum* as shown by injecting rabbits and mice with killed organisms. *Am. J. Syph.* 37:9-22 (1953).
83. C. P. McLeod. Studies on *Treponema pallidum* complement fixation antigen. Antigenicity in rabbits and relation to immunity. *Public Health Rep.* 77:431-436 (1962).
84. J. N. Miller, S. J. Whang, and F. P. Fazzan. Studies on immunity in experimental syphilis. I. Immunologic response of rabbits immunized with Reiter protein antigen and challenged with virulent *Treponema pallidum*. *Br. J. Vener. Dis.* 39:195-198 (1963).
85. N. N. Izzat, W. G. Dacres. J. M. Knox, and R. Wende. Attempts at immunization against syphilis with avirulent *Treponema pallidum*. *Br. J. Vener. Dis* 46:451-453 (1970).

86. N. N. Izzat, J. M. Knox, W. G. Dacres, and E. B. Smith. Resistance and serological changes in rabbits immunized with virulent *Treponema pallidum* sonicate. *Acta Derm. Venereol.* 51:157-160 (1971).
87. M. Metzger and W. Smogór. Artificial immunization of rabbits against syphilis. I. Effect of increasing doses of treponemes given by the intramuscular route. *Br. J. Vener. Dis.* 45:308-326 (1969).
88. H. J. Magnuson, F. A. Thompson, and C. P. McLeod. Relationship between treponemal immobilizing antibodies and acquired immunity in experimental syphilis. *J. Immunol.* 67:41-48 (1951).
89. H. J. Magnuson, E. W. Thomas, S. Olansky, B. I. Kaplan, L. De Mello, and J. C. Cutler. Inoculation syphilis in human volunteers. *Medicine* 35:33-82 (1956).
90. J. N. Miller, F. P. Fazzan, and S. J. Whang. Studies on immunity in experimental syphilis. II. *Treponema pallidum* immobilization (TPI) antibody and the immune response. *Br. J. Vener. Dis.* 39:199-203 (1963).
91. M. Metzger, E. Michalska, J. Podwińska, and W. Smogór. Immunogenic properties of the protein component of *Treponema pallidum*. *Br. J. Vener. Dis* 45:299-304 (1969).
92. T. B. Turner. Protective antibodies in the serum of syphilitic rabbits. *J. Exp. Med.* 69:867-889 (1939).
93. R. A. Nelson, Jr. Factors affecting the survival of *Treponema pallidum in vitro*. *Am. J. Hyg.* 48:120-132 (1948).
94. R. A. Nelson, Jr. and M. M. Mayer. Immobilization of *Treponema pallidum in vitro* by antibody produced in syphilitic infection. *J. Exp. Med.* 89:369-393 (1949).
95. A. M. Chesney. Immunity in syphilis. *Medicine* 5:463-547 (1926).
96. P. M. Zeltzer, J. S. Pepose, N. H. Bishop, and J. N. Miller. Microassay for immunoglobulin G antibodies to *Treponema pallidum* with radioiodinated protein A from *Staphylococcus aureus*: Immunoglobulin G response in experimental syphilis in rabbits. *Infect. Immun.* 21:163-170 (1978).
97. M. Sepetjian, D. Salussola, and J. Thivolet. Attempt to protect rabbits against experimental syphilis by passive immunization. *Br. J. Vener. Dis* 49:335-337 (1973).
98. P. L. Perine, R. S. Weiser, and S. J. Klebanoff. Immunity to syphilis. I. Passive transfer in rabbits with hyperimmune serum. *Infect. Immun.* 8:787-790 (1973).
99. T. B. Turner, P. H. Hardy, Jr., B. Newman, and E. E. Nell. Effects of passive immunization on experimental syphilis in the rabbit. *Johns Hopkins Med. J.* 133:241-251 (1973).

100. S. R. Graves and R. C. Johnson. Effect of pretreatment with *Mycobacterium bovis* (strain BCG) and immune syphilitic serum on rabbit resistance to *Treponema pallidum*. *Infect. Immun.* 12:1029-1036 (1975).
101. S. Graves and J. Alden. Limited protection of rabbits against infection with *Treponema pallidum* by immune rabbit sera. *Br. J. Vener. Dis.* 55:399-403 (1979).
102. B. R. Bloom. The unspecificity of cellular reactions. *J. Immunol.* 124:2527-2529 (1980).

14

Immunoregulatory Effects in Experimental Syphilis

ROBERT E. BAUGHN
*Baylor College of Medicine and
Syphilis Research Laboratory
Houston Veterans Administration Medical Center
Houston, Texas*

Host-Parasite Relationships in Treponemal Infections 272
Impaired T-Lymphocyte Function During *Treponema pallidum*
 Infection 274
Immunosuppression to a Heterologous Antigen During *Treponema
pallidum* Infection 275
Attempts to Delineate the Nature of the Immunologic Unresponsiveness
 in Experimental Syphilis 279
Detection of Immune Complexes in the Sera of Rabbits with Experimental Syphilis 284
Conclusion 290
References 291

Despite years of intensive research on the immune response to infection with *Treponema pallidum*, the failure of host defense mechanisms to eradicate the infecting organism remains unexplained. We have proposed that aberrant immune responses, specifically the inability to produce a treponemicidal immunoglogulin, may be responsible. Since a humoral response can be detected shortly after infection, some investigators are reluctant to admit that anything could be wrong with the host's immune response. This reasoning may miss the mark for two reasons. First, the host may produce antibodies that are not relevant to the development of protection despite their importance in diagnosing the disease. As will be discussed below, several possible mechanisms may underlie the host's failure to produce an appropriate antibody. Secondly, immunity is often a double-edged sword with the development of certain antibodies and the subsequent formation of circulating immune complexes (IC) being detrimental to the host. The presence of antibody at a time when lesions are flourishing argues as much against the concept of a slowly developing humoral immune response (Chapter 13) as it does against a role for aberrant responses.

The mechanisms whereby IC can impair or augment humoral and cellular immune responses both in vivo and in vitro by interacting with F_c, complement (C), and/or antigen receptors on the surfaces of B and T cells have been reviewed recently (1,2). This chapter will present the arguments for and against the possible role of aberrations in humoral immune regulation in syphilis, and present evidence that IC may be, in part, responsible for altered states of immune responsiveness. Modulation of humoral immune responses is by no means limited to IC: In recent years several bacterial products have been shown to exert modulatory effects, although the actual mechanism(s) of enhancement or suppression remains unclear (3). Just as with IC, the modulatory effects of these substances depend on the dosage, route, and time of administration. The reader should therefore bear in mind that the in vivo situation is a dynamic one in which IC, bacterial products, and other undefined factors may be acting in concert or against one another to alter the immunoregulatory machinery. A comprehensive analysis is extremely difficult because of the complexity of the mammalian immune system and the equality complex antigenic mosaic of the infecting organisms, which at the present time is poorly defined.

Host-Parasite Relationships in Treponemal Infections

Laboratories engaged in studying host defense mechanisms to *T. pallidum* in the rabbit have utilized intratesticular (IT), intradermal (ID), and intravenous (IV) routes of infection. Accordingly, one might expect differences in the modulation of immune responses as they relate to factors such as the time of appearance, the extent and duration of lesions, the antigenic load or level of bacterial products, and the levels of immune complexes in the circulation and tissues. As we shall see, differences do exist and probably account, at least in part, for discrepancies in the literature concerning abnormal immune responses during early infection.

As noted in Chap. 7, rabbits develop a typical orchitis within 7 to 10 days of IT challenge, in the absence of other signs of disease. Animals infected via this route also appear to develop partial resistance to subsequent ID challenge as early as the 11th day. This so-called partial resistance is not associated with detectable serum levels

of treponemicidal antibodies, although immunoglobulins directed against
the organism exist within the testicular exudates of infected animals
at this time (4).

In contrast, ID inoculation of T. pallidum is followed by the appearance of a chancre within a time period of a few days to 3 weeks, depending on the inoculum size; in the absence of treatment the chancre regresses within the next 3 to 6 weeks. During this time, a number of circulating antibodies to T. pallidum appear, including T. pallidum immobilizing (TPI) antibody, which in the presence of complement immobilizes and inactivates the infecting organism in vitro (5-7); however, there is no necessary relationship between the regression of the chancre and the appearance of TPI antibody.

The IV route of infection, which has been studied extensively in our laboratory, results in experimental disease that in many ways mimics primary and secondary infection in the human (6). If rabbits are infected via the marginal ear vein with 4×10^7 T. pallidum and then shaved regularly, a small local lesion develops at the injection site in about 25% of animals. Circulating antibodies [Venereal Disease Research Laboratories (VDRL), fluoroscent treponemal antibody absorption (FTA-ABS), and TPHA] develop in all these rabbits by the 10th to 14th day, whether or not a chancre has appeared at the injection site. Subsequently, around the 17th day, a macular-papular rash develops over the shaven areas of the rabbits' backs; 4 to 8 days after that, discrete lesions appear, with marked erythema and induration. These lesions persist for several weeks, undergoing necrosis and eventual healing. Unlike human disease, a characteristic orchitis appears around day 28 or nearly 2 weeks after the initial detection of a humoral immune response. Overall, the appearance of treponemal and nontreponemal antibodies together with marked plasma cell proliferation in the lymphoid tissues during syphilitic infection might indicate that B-lymphocyte function is normal or enhanced. As will be discussed below, however, the biologic importance of this antibody response can certainly be questioned.

In the natural host (man), the progression of syphilis from localized (primary) to disseminated (secondary) infection, the persistence of disseminated disease for weeks to months, and the occurrence of relapses of secondary infection in up to 20% of untreated patients (6) suggest a failure on the part of the immune system to respond appropriately to the infecting organism. Although both treponemal and nontreponemal antibodies appear in syphilis, an appropriate and specific antibody which effectively limits the growth and spread of the organism is not produced, at least not in the early stages of infection (Chap. 13). Thus VDRL antibody, TPHA, and FTA-ABS are universally present early in secondary syphilis. In fact, antibody that inactivates T. pallidum in vitro (TPI) is present in one-third of the patients with primary syphilis (all of whom may be expected to develop secondary disease in the absence of treatment) and in two-thirds of secondary syphilitics whose lesions nevertheless contain abundant treponemes (6). Recurring crops of lesions in secondary syphilis argue further against effective containment.

Similarly, the early humoral immune responses in both the ID and IV rabbit models, as well as in the human host, do not appear to be suppressed; kinetically, the production of antibodies follows an active stage of induction and cellular proliferation. These initial events in human and experimental subjects restrict but do not eradicate the infecting organism. Thus *T. pallidum*, like many of the metazoan and protozoan parasites, appears to be a highly successful parasite (8); the organism is immunogenic and the initial immune responses (and/or natural host defenses) appear to maintain the treponemal burden at tolerable levels without eliminating it. The persistence of treponemes in active lesions long after the development of antibody has led a number of investigators to question the regulation and control of the host's immune response. Parallel with the advances in cellular immunology seen during the 1960s and 1970s many of these questions were aimed at the assessment of T-lymphocyte function in early and secondary syphilis.

Impaired T-Lymphocyte Function During *T. pallidum* Infection

Much of the evidence suggesting that syphilis is associated with impairment or modification of T-cell function is presented in Chap. 16 and 17. Basically, three divergent sets of observations support the thesis that transient immunosuppression in syphilis may result from modifications in T-cell function: (1) lymphocyte transformation in response to a variety of mitogens and treponemal and nontreponemal antigens is said to be suppressed during active infection (9-19); (2) thymus-dependent areas of spleens and lymph nodes from syphilitic subjects are hypoplastic (20,21); and (3) the onset of lymphokine production does not appear to begin until relatively late in the infection (22).

In general, the depressed lymphocyte responses (9-19) have been interpreted as being indicative of impaired cell-mediated immunity, presumably reflecting an effect on T cells which allows for development of an immunosuppressive state and in turn permits survival of the organism. Two very recent studies (23,24) have failed to substantiate depressed responses to Concanavalin A during the early and late stages of infection and argue that responsiveness of splenic and lymph node lymphocytes from infected animals to *T. pallidum* sonicate is enhanced compared with the responses of lymphocytes from uninfected rabbits. While it is important that the discrepancies in the literature concerning lymphocyte transformation be reconciled, an attempt to do so is beyond the scope of the present discussion. The bulk of the evidence argues favorably for a transitory state of immunosuppression in early syphilis. Moreover, certain other recent studies have provided evidence to suggest that plasma or serum factors (14,25,26), as well as factors in cell-free testicular extracts (14,27), present during syphilitic infection inhibits the in vitro reactivity of normal lymphocytes to mitogens.

In terms of cellular immunity, interference with T lymphocytes could account for impaired release of soluble mediators (lymphokines) necessary for activation of phagocytic cells during early *T. pallidum* infection, and contribute widespread dissemination and establishment of the treponemes in selected sites. We reasoned that another possibility might exist, namely, that stimulation or depletion of certain T-cell subpopulations or that interference with the regulatory functions of T lymphocytes during antigen processing could alter humoral immunity. Widespread dissemination of treponemal antigen(s) might induce B-cell precursors of low-affinity, IgM antibody-secreting cells and simultaneously cause tolerance in many of the IgG-secreting cells. This in turn could stimulate synthesis of IgM to new determinants on the surface of *T. pallidum*, with further depression of IgG synthesis. Immune complexes, composed of treponemal antigen and specific antitreponemal immunoglobulins, on the surfaces of T cells could also interfere with appropriate T- and B-cell interactions necessary for optimal IgG responses (1,2). Suppression of IgG formation could thus explain the failure of the host to produce effective opsonizing and/or treponemicidal antibodies until the time of restoration of normal T-cell function.

Immunosuppression to a Heterologous Antigen During *Treponema pallidum* Infection

In an attempt to indirectly test this hypothesis, studies were designed to assess the primary humoral response to sheep erythrocytes (SRBC), a T-dependent antigen, in syphilitic rabbits. In our initial studies (28), the number of plaque-forming cells (PFC) to SRBC in the spleens of control and IV-infected rabbits were assayed 7 days after sensitization using a Jerne plaque assay. A three- to fourfold increase in the IgM PFC (direct) responses of syphilitic rabbits was observed in the second and third week of infection, and significant increases persisted throughout the first 6 weeks (Fig. 1). The most striking finding in the syphilitic rabbits, however, was the marked reduction in the IgG PFC (indirect) response. Whereas uninfected animals usually had 500 to 1000 indirect PFC per 10^6 spleen cells, rabbits infected 1 to 2 weeks before sensitization with SRBC all had less than 200 indirect plaques per 10^6 spleen cells. By the fourth to sixth week of infection the IgG PFC responses were further diminished, often being

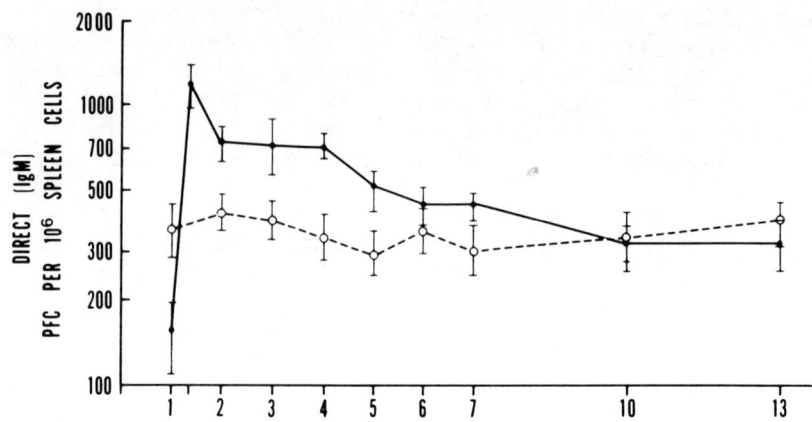
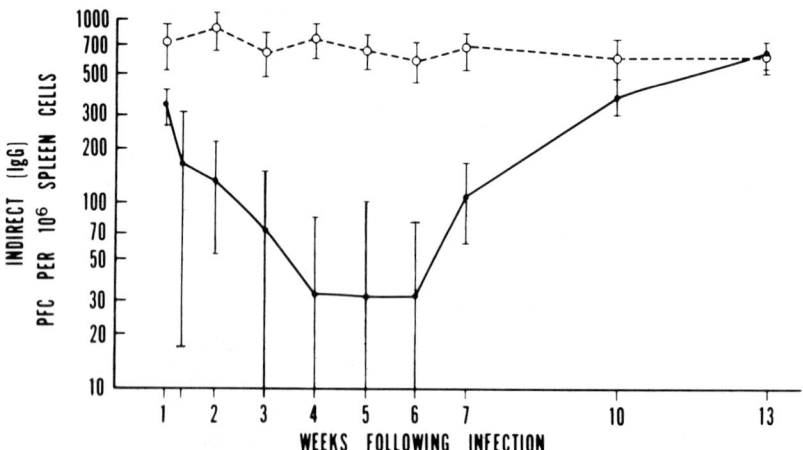

Figure 1 Altered responsiveness of rabbits to SRBC after intravenous infection with *T. pallidum*. 2×10^9 SRBC were administered intravenously 7 days before each assay. Each point in the arithmetric mean (±1 SD) of the PFC per spleen of three control (○) or three infected (●) rabbits. (*Source*: Reference 28.)

Table 1 Alterations in the Primary In Vivo and Secondary In Vitro Anti-SRBC Response[a]

Response	Uninfected		Infected	
	IgM	IgG	IgM	IgG
Primary, in vivo	282 ± 23	649 ± 43	612 ± 108[b]	26 ± 43[b]
	394 ± 37	426 ± 51	538 ± 94[c]	18 ± 33[c]
Secondary, in vitro	42,867	25,000	36,067[b]	1,866[b]
	49,485	31,000	7,520[c]	200[c]

[a]Values for primary responses indicated PFC per 10^6 cells ± SD. Those for secondary responses indicate PFC per culture.
[b]Sheep erythrocytes (2×10^9) were given intravenously 11 days after infection with *T. pallidum* and the in vivo assay performed on day 18. The control animal was sensitized and the assay performed at the same time.
[c]Sheep erythrocytes (2×10^9) were given intravenously 28 days after infection with *T. pallidum* and the in vivo assay performed on day 35. The control animal was sensitized and the assay performed at the same time.
Source: Reference 29.

equal to the background values of nonsensitized controls, indicating effective obliteration of the IgG response. Similar results were obtained irrespective of the route of treponemal challenge or when comparisons between PFC per spleen and PFC per 10^6 cells were made. We also found that infection appeared to cause quantitative changes rather than a shift in the kinetics of the response. Of even greater importance, treatment of infected animals with benzathine penicillin G resulted in a return to normal levels of responsiveness to the heterologous immunogen. Quantitative assays of humoral antibody to SRBC also showed that 2-mercaptoethanol-resistant (IgG) hemagglutinins and hemolysins were significantly depressed in infected rabbits (28).

In order to gain further insight into the nature of the suppressed IgG responses we then examined the secondary in vitro immune responses of splenic and peripheral blood lymphocytes (29). Splenic lymphocytes from uninfected rabbits which had been sensitized to SRBC showed marked increases in both IgM and IgG PFC after 4 days of culture in the presence of SRBC (Table 1). In contrast, cells obtained from rabbits early in the course of syphilis (<21 days after treponemal challenge and before the appearance of generalized lesions) appeared to mount a normal IgM response but had greatly reduced numbers of IgG PFC (Table 1). Similar results were obtained with

Table 2 Altered Secondary Responses When Two Sensitizing Doses of SRBC Were Administered at the Height of Syphilitic Infection[a]

Response	Number of spleen cells added per culture	Number of PBL cells added per culture	Ig	PFC per 10^6 cells ± SD[b]		PFC/culture			
				Uninfected	Infected	Uninfected		Infected	
						No SRBC	SRBC	No SRBC	SRBC
Secondary, in vivo			M	204 ± 27	604 ± 68				
			G	884 ± 76	68 ± 68				
Secondary, in vitro	4	0	M			765	17,600	385	6,460
			G			700	59,200	45	680
	2	0	M			660	19,400	400	5,320
			G			425	53,400	0	280
	2	2	M			670	17,400	365	5,140
			G			450	53,000	40	420
	3	1	M			680	23,400	405	5,100
			G			690	50,800	0	300
	0	2	M			425	3,300	155	1,080
			G			15	14,300	5	120

[a]Sheep erythrocytes (2 × 10^9) were injected intravenously on days 21 and 35 of *T. pallidum* infection. The uninfected control received two injections of SRBC 14 days apart. The assay was performed 7 days after the second injection of SRBC.
[b]SD, standard deviation.

cells from several other experimental rabbits sensitized with SRBC 3, 7 or 14 days after IV infection and *T. pallidum*. When PFC were calculated per spleen, the results paralleled PFC per 10^6 cells. Different results were obtained with other rabbits sensitized with SRBC at the height of the generalized syphilitic eruption (28, 35, or 42 days after IV challenge), in that decreases both in secondary IgM and IgG responses in vitro were observed; the results of a representative experiment are shown on Table 1.

Further evidence that cells from infected rabbits were incapable of a normal response was obtained in experiments in which rabbits received two doses of SRBC at 14-day intervals. Under these conditions cells from control rabbits gave predominantly IgG responses in vivo (Table 2); this response was greatly decreased with infection, and IgM PFC were increased during syphilis. As in our previous studies, differences between control and infected rabbits were shown not to be due to shifts in the kinetics of the response. Results of sensitization in vitro paralleled the in vivo observations; the IgG response predominated with cells from control rabbits and this response was greatly diminished in cell cultrues from syphilitic rabbits (Table 2).

Attempts to Delineate the Nature of the Immunologic Unresponsiveness in Experimental Syphilis

In assessing the results of these early studies, we reasoned that the nature of the unresponsiveness might be multifactoral. Among the contending factors, glycosaminoglycans (GAG) and IC appeared most worthy of future investigation. Recent studies had called attention to the fact that GAG or the acidic mucopolysaccharides (14) are capable of suppressing the blast response of normal lymphocytes to Concanavalin A. This mucoid material is also most apparent at the time when lesions are progressing (6,14,30).

In terms of possible mechanisms, we felt that amorphous material, other treponemal antigens, or the spirochetes themselves could be competing with SRBC for uncommitted macrophages. Overloading of macrophages with mucoid material and/or treponemal antigens was foreseen as possibly inhibiting their ability to process and present SRBC antigens to lymphocytes. Although this could certainly account for the in vivo unresponsiveness of infected spleen cells, it was more difficult to envision antigen carryover on the surfaces of macrophages being sufficient, after extensive washing, to produce the observed in vitro effects. Another possibility was that masking of antigenic sites on the surface of treponemes with host proteins inhibited host cell interactions. A recent study (31) has shown that a variety of avidly associated host proteins are present on the surface of washed treponemes including non-parasite-specific IgG and IgM plus complement components. Coating of the organism with host macromolecules could interfere with macrophage recognition and processing, as well as appropriate T- and B-cell interactions, and thereby result in decreased immunogenicity.

We also reasoned that immune complexes, rather than antigen alone, could be responsible for the observed immunoregulatory effects (32-42). The rabbit is known to mount early humoral responses to nontreponemal and treponemal antigens so that by the third week of infection complexes formed in vivo in antigen excess might paralyze macrophages, thereby rendering them incapable of ingesting SRBC.

In an attempt to delineate the nature of the unresponsiveness, we extended our studies to inbred rabbits so that lymphocytes from both normal and infected animals could be cocultured in vitro. Splenic or lymph node lymphocytes from the syphilitic rabbits were admixed in varying proportions with splenic lymphocytes from their uninfected SRBC-sensitized siblings and cultured in vitro in the presence of SRBC for either 5 or 6 days. Results from experiments in which rabbits were sensitized with SRBC once (28 days after infection) or twice (21 and 28 days after infection) are shown in Table 3. As observed previously using lymphocytes from outbred rabbits (28), cells from normal, uninfected rabbits yielded vigorous IgM and IgG PFC responses, whereas the PFC responses of lymphocytes from infected rabbits were substantially lower in comparison. Addition of lymph node or splenic lymphocytes from infected rabbits, even at low ratios (1 infected lymphocyte per 40 normal splenic lymphocytes), suppressed PFC responses; the most profound effects were on the IgG-secreting cells.

Experiments were then performed to determine whether suppression could be ascribed to either an adherent or nonadherent cell population. Normalized data from two experiments are presented in Table 4. Suppression of normal IgM and IgG responses were observed when adherent or nonadherent fractions of spleen or lymph node cells from syphilitic rabbits were added to cultures at a ratio of 1:20; the levels of suppression were similar to those obtained with unfractionated spleen cells from infected animals. The addition of normal cells (fractionated or unseparated) to cultures of infected cells failed to restore IgG PFC responses to normal, suggesting that an absence of helper T cells was not responsible. Depletion of adherent cells left a nonadherent population of normal cells which gave a minimal PFC response; normal responsiveness was, to a great extent, restored by adding back adherent cells at a 1:20 ratio. These findings led us to question whether immune complexes or antibody bound to the surface membranes of cells from infected rabbits might interfere with the cellular interactions required for maximal humoral responses to the heterologous antigen.

To test this hypothesis, lymph node and spleen cells from infected, inbred rabbits were treated with pronase, trypsin, or hyaluronidase,

Table 3 Suppression of the Secondary In Vitro Response of Normal Rabbit Splenic Lymphocytes Cocultured with Splenic or Lymph Node Lymphocytes from Syphilitic Rabbits[a]

Cells (×10^6) added per culture			Experiment 1				Experiment 2			
Normal spleen cells	Infected spleen cells	Infected lymph node cells	PFC per culture		Suppression (%)		PFC per culture		Suppression (%)	
			IgM	IgG	IgM	IgG	IgM	IgG	IgM	IgG
2	0	0	37,333	21,333			28,333	46,333		
0	2	0	4,627	186			8,400	400		
0	0	2	106	33			260	0		
1	1	0	6,600	320	82	98	12,400	1,600	56	96
1.5	0.5	0	9,467	399	75	98	15,600	2,400	45	95
2	0.1	0	11,333	2,267	70	89	17,200	7,600	39	84
2	0.05	0	14,267	2,933	62	86	19,600	11,200	31	76
1	0	1	1,667	0	96	100	9,600	800	66	98
1.5	0	0.5	9,067	0	76	100	8,800	2,000	69	96
2	0	0.1	12,933	1,067	65	95	11,600	4,400	59	91
2	0	0.05	18,667	1,599	50	93	16,400	9,200	42	80

[a]The infected rabbit in experiment 1 received 2 × 10^9 SRBC on day 28 of infection, whereas the infected rabbit in experiment 2 received two injections of SRBC on days 21 and 28. Control animals, which had received heat-killed *T. pallidum*, were sensitized at the same times. Cells were placed in culture together with SRBC 7 days after sensitization. Data are reported as PFC per culture on day 5.
Source: Reference 43.

Table 4 Suppression of the Secondary In Vitro Response of Normal Rabbit Splenic Lymphocytes Cocultured with Adherent and Nonadherent Splenic Lymphocytes from Syphilitic Rabbits[a]

Cells ($\times 10^6$) added per culture		PFC per culture	
Normal	Infected	IgM	IgG
2 (unseparated)	0	19,767	39,417
2 (unseparated)	0.1 (unseparated)	7,550	3,500
2 (unseparated)	0.1 (adherent)	5,650	5,950
2 (unseparated)	0.1 (nonadherent)	8,825	6,750
0	2 (unseparated)	11,200	1,550
0.1 (unseparated)	2 (unseparated)	14,350	1,860
0.1 (adherent)	2 (unseparated)	13,450	2,140
0.1 (nonadherent)	2 (unseparated)	10,700	1,250
2 (nonadherent)	0	2,125	440
2 (nonadherent) + 0.1 (adherent)	0	11,230	18,540
2 (nonadherent)	0.1 (adherent)	1,675	525
2 (nonadherent)	0.1 (nonadherent)	1,425	325

[a]Normalized data from two experiments with inbred rabbits are expressed as PFC per culture on day 5. In both experiments, SRBC were administered intravenously 21 and 28 days after infection with *T. pallidum*. Control animals in each experiment were sensitized 21 and 28 days after having received heat-killed *T. pallidum*.
Source: Reference 43.

extensively washed, and then admixed with splenic cells from normal SRBC-sensitized animals. In addition, the first-wash fluid obtained during preparation of the lymph node and spleen cells was decanted, filtered through a series of membrane filters, and added in microliter concentrations to cultures of normal cells. The normalized results of two studies in which the infected and control inbred rabbits had received one injection of SRBC are presented in Table 5. Pronase or trypsin treatment of infected spleen or lymph node cells abolished their ability to suppress Ig responses of normal lymphocytes; treatment with hyaluronidase had no effect. Enzyme treatment of infected cells, however, did not enhance their ability to respond alone in culture to SRBC. Treatment of normal lymphocytes with each of the enzymes prior to placing the cells in culture had no effect on their ability to respond. Of equal importance, the cell-free wash fluids of infected cells were capable of suppressing both the IgM and IgG responses of normal spleen cells (Table 6).

These results suggested that antigen-antibody complex interference with helper T cell function might be responsible for the observed aberrations in immune responsiveness (37-42). Helper T cells are known to exert regulatory effects on B-cell responses to most antigens by (1) controlling the differentiation of antigen-stimulated specific B cells into antibody-secreting cells, (2) influencing the switch from production of IgM to IgG antibodies, and/or (3) determining the rate of selection of specific cells by antigen in the immune response as reflected in the change of affinity of humoral antibody with time. With regard to immune complexes, there is also ample evidence to suggest that suppression occurs only when T cells are exposed to and allowed to take up AG-Ab complexes (32). Complexes formed in certain critical ratios have been shown to "freeze" membrane receptors of Ag-reactive cells (37,38) and are capable of reducing secondary responses to both heterologous and homologous antigens in vitro (35). Moreover, antigen carryover on surfaces of spleen cells is much greater with complexes than with antigen (36), and artificial complexes formed in antigen excess have been shown to suppress in vitro responses to a greater degree than complexes formed at equivalence

Table 5. Effect of Cell-Free Washings of Splenic or Lymph Node Lymphocytes on PFC Responses of Normal Lymphocytes[a]

Additions per culture	PFC per culture		Percentage of suppression	
	IgM	IgG	IgM	IgG
None	22,367	14,700	—	—
Normal spleen cell wash:				
50 µl	20,850	13,450	7	9
100 µl	19,900	14,100	11	4
Infected spleen cell wash:				
50 µl	10,234	2,450	54	83
100 µl	8,775	2,267	61	88
Infected lymph node cell wash:				
50 µl	16,467	3,550	26	76
100 µl	12,334	2,267	45	85

[a]Normalized data from two experiments with inbred rabbits are expressed as PFC per culture on day 5. In both experiments the normal lymphocytes were obtained from control animals sensitized with SRBC 21 days after having received heat-killed *T. pallidum*. Source: Reference 43.

Table 6 Pronase and Trypsin Abrogation of the Suppressive Effect of Lymph Node Cells on the PFC Response of Normal Rabbit Splenic Lymphocytes[a]

Cells ($\times 10^6$) added per culture		Infected lymph node cells					
		Untreated		Pronase treated		Trypsin treated	
Normal	Infected	IgM	IgG	IgM	IgG	IgM	IgG
0	2	140	30	190	30	170	30
1	1	940	0	21,400	16,500	20,600	13,600
1.5	0.5	1,630	90	22,200	13,800	21,700	15,000
2	0.1	1,810	250	21,400	14,800	20,200	15,900
2	0.05	3,040	290	22,800	13,700	23,200	14,200
2	0.01	4,250	390	23,100	14,200	22,000	18,400

[a]Normalized data from two experiments with inbred rabbits are expressed as PFC per culture on day 5. In both experiments, SRBC were administered intravenously 21 days after infection with *T. pallidum*. Control animals in each experiment were sensitized 21 days after having received heat-killed *T. pallidum*. PFC response of 2×10^6 normal rabbit spleen cells: IgM = 22,367; IgG = 14,700.
Source: Reference 43.

(34,35). Retention of treponemal immune complexes on the surface of T cells of infected rabbits might freeze the cell membrane, causing unresponsiveness to SRBC in vitro.

Detection of Immune Complexes in the Sera of Rabbits with Experimental Syphilis

On the basis of these findings, we then directed our attention to the possible role of IC in the observed non-antigen-specific immune suppression (43). Sera from normal and intravenously infected animals were examined for complexes by the Raji cell assay and the polyethylene glycol-complement consumption (PEG-CC) assay. As shown in Table 7, ≥83% of the sera obtained between the fourth and seventh weeks of infection were positive for IC using the Raji cell assay; these results were significantly different from those obtained with sera collected before the onset of or after the regression of lesions ($P < 0.0005$, χ^2 analysis). These data should not be misconstrued as representing a chronological study.

A total of 201 serum samples, including 138 that had been analyzed by the Raji cell assay, were evaluated for IC using the PEG-CC assay. Because this test measures complement consumption, mean values and

Table 7 Detection of Immune Complexes in the Sera of Rabbits Infected Intravenously with *T. pallidum* by the Raji Cell and PEG-CC Assays

	Raji cell assay[a]			PEG-CC assay[b]			
						Percentage of complement consumption	
Sample	Number positive/ Number tested	Percentage positive	Range of SD above mean	Number positive/ Number tested	Percentage positive	Mean	Range
Preinfection	4/30	13	2.06-2.18	0/35	0	21.3	8-30
Postinfection							
Week 1	0/20	0	—	0/14	0	21.8	14-30
Week 2	5/21	24	2.30-4.22	3/14	21	23.4	10-37
Week 3	16/41	39	2.06-5.37	16/37	43	37.8	17-91
Week 4	46/51	90	2.34-10.41	31/43	72	55.1	19-100
Week 5	25/27	93	5.37-10.25	18/22	82	60.7	17-95
Week 6	5/6	83	4.38-9.11	7/12	58	49.8	21-84
Week 7	13/15	87	5.12-8.87	4/12	33	36.0	17-73
Week 10	1/15	7	2.08	1/12	8	22.7	10-39

[a]The ranges of only the positive values obtained are expressed in terms of the number of SD above the mean for sera from normal rabbits.
[b]Those samples considered positive had values greater than 2 SD above the mean of preinfection levels; 21.6 + (2 × 4.35) = 30.3. The ranges of all values tested are presented.

Table 8 Detection of Immune Complexes in the Sera of Rabbits Infected Intradermally and Intratesticularly with T. pallidum by Raji Cell and PEG-CC Assays

Sample	Raji cell assay[a]			PEG-CC assay[b]			
	Number positive/ Number tested	Percentage positive	Range of SD above mean	Number positive/ Number tested	Percentage positive	\multicolumn{2}{c}{Percentage of complement consumption}
						Mean	Range
Post ID infection							
First 2 weeks	2/12	30	2.30-2.96	4/25	16	21.9	13-46
Weeks 3, 4 and 5	17/30	57	2.04-3.76	15/35	43	40.3	15-68
Weeks 6 and 7	7/18	42	2.28-2.87	7/20	35	35.5	12-51
Week 10	4/12	33	2.09-2.78	2/8	25	25.3	10-49
Post IT infection							
Days 9 to 14	3/15	20	2.30-2.96	2/15	13	20.9	18-41

[a]The ranges of only the positive values obtained are expressed in terms of the number of SD above the mean for sera from normal rabbits.
[b]Those samples considered positive had values greater than 2 SD above the mean of preinfection levels; $21.6 + (2 \times 4.35) = 30.3$. The ranges of all values tested are presented.

ranges for all the sera were obtained and are shown in Table 7. Once again IC were detected as early as the second week of infection; the most profound increases in IC by the PEG-CC assay were similarly noted between the third and seventh week of infection ($P < 0.0005$, χ^2 analysis), as compared with results before the development or after the resolution of lesions.

Of the 138 sera from normal and intravenously infected rabbits which were examined by both IC assays, 67 were positive using the Raji cell assay. Of these 67 sera 20 were negative when examined by the PEG-CC procedure. Of the 71 sera that had been negative in the Raji cell assay, 11 were considered positive in the PEG-CC assay. The sample proportions of positives were 0.42 for the PEG-CC assay and 0.49 for the Raji cell assay. Using McNemar's test for correlated proportions, the hypothesis was accepted that the population proportions of positives, at the 5% level, for the two procedures were equal.

Glycosaminoglycan materials were demonstrated in the sera throughout the course of infection (data not shown); however, there was no direct association between the levels observed and the presence of overt disseminated disease, as GAG was detectable both prior to the onset of lesions and after their regression.

Sera from intradermally and intratesticularly infected animals were also examined for IC and GAG. Twelve rabbits were infected intradermally at each of four sites with 10^6 organisms. Serum samples collected from these rabbits throughout a 10-week period, as well as serum samples from 15 individual rabbits with orchitises (9 to 14 days after IT infection) were evaluated using both the Raji cell and PEG-CC assays. The results of these studies are shown in Table 8. Chancres at each site of injection had developed in all intradermally infected animals by day 6; these continued to progress through a necrotic stage, followed by complete resolution and healing between the 9th and 10th weeks. Intratesticularly infected rabbits had no visible signs of infection other than their orchitis. Both the incidence and levels of IC, as shown in Table 8, were lower in these two groups of animals when these data are compared with those obtained with IV infection (Table 7). In all the sera from intratesticularly and intradermally infected animals throughout the study GAG was present. These results emphasize one difference between the IV model and the ID and IT models.

In conjunction with these studies, dose response curves were also constructed to determine the effect of syphilitic serum on the response of primed cells in the Jerne plaque technique. Rabbits were sensitized once or twice (Table 9) with SRBC. After 1 week their lymphocytes were placed in tissue culture with increasing concentrations of sera that had been studied for quantification of IC and GAG. Sera obtained from syphilitic rabbits 7 or 14 days after *T. pallidum* infection contained relatively high levels of GAG but did not inhibit PFC responses. By contrast, serum obtained 28 or 35 days into infection,

Table 9 Suppression of the Secondary In Vitro Response to SRBC by Immune Complexes in the Serum of Syphilitic Rabbits

Source of serum added to cultures	Immune complexes[a]		Glycosamino-glycan[b]	Amount added (μl)	PFC per culture[c]		Percentage of suppression	
	Raji	C1q-SPA			IgM	IgG	IgM	IgG
None Preinfection	— <2	— <2	— —	— 15 30 45	40,500 41,700 39,200 43,800	23,100 21,350 22,500 19,200	— 0 3 0	— 8 3 17
Infected Day 7	<2	<2	1.0	15 30 45	42,100 36,400 37,250	22,800 19,900 20,150	0 10 8	1 14 13
Day 14	<2	<2	0.5	15 30 45	38,700 41,200 35,640	24,100 21,500 19,600	4 0 12	0 7 15
Day 28	10.25	3.42	1.0	15 30 45	8,900 2,750 1,050	950 300 50	78 93 97	96 99 <99
Day 35	9.69	7.42	0.5	15 30 45	26,300 14,400 8,700	7,800 2,360 650	35 64 78	66 90 97
Day 35	8.87	3.48	0.5	15 30 45	12,600 4,350 1,200	1,800 600 110	69 89 97	92 97 99

[a] Immune complex data are expressed as the number of standard deviations above the mean of normal sera values.
[b] Glycosaminoglycan is expressed in milligrams per milliliter of serum.
[c] Data for the PFC are expressed per culture on day 5. Spleen cells from a normal rabbit were obtained 7 days after a single injection of SRBC.
Source: Modified from Reference 43.

Table 10 Suppression of the Secondary In Vitro Response of Normal Rabbit Splenic Lymphocytes by Artificial Complexes[a]

Additions to 1 ml cultures cultures containing 2×10^6 lymphocytes		Response to SRBC (day 5)			
		PFC per culture		Percentage of Suppression	
		IgM	IgG	IgM	IgG
None		28,600	13,200	—	—
VDRL antigen (Difco)	60 µl	29,600	12,500	0	5
FTA test antigen (Difco)	60 µl	27,600	14,400	3	0
T. pallidum immune serum	60 µl	26,800	12,800	6	3
VDRL antigen (Difco) + T. pallidum immune serum (30 min. at 37°C)	15 µl	20,350	9,600	29	27
	30 µl	18,200	4,200	36	68
	45 µl	14,700	2,150	49	84
	60 µl	10,400	1,050	64	92

[a]Sheep erythrocytes (2×10^9) were given intravenously 7 days prior to obtaining spleen cells and placing them in culture. Data are reported as PFC per culture.

which contained the same GAG concentration but also had high levels of IC, caused a striking depression of PFC responses, with the effect being more profound in the case of IgG. This effect was dose related within the range studied. In six subsequent experiments the overall correlation between the presence of CIC and the degree of immune suppression was striking ($r^2 > 0.8$), whereas no association with GAG was seen.

A second line of presumptive evidence which suggests that immune complexes may play a role in the observed suppression stems from studies using artificial complexes. These complexes were made by incubating in vitro commercial VDRL or fluorescent treponemal antibody (FTA) test antigens in antigen excess with immune complex-negative, hyperimmune serum from an animal repeatedly infected with T. pallidum. Increasing concentrations added to cultures of normal splenic lymphocytes primed with SRBC suppressed secondary PFC responses, with the effect on IgG being more pronounced (Table 10).

Conclusion

At the present time, there is considerable controversy concerning the existence of abnormal immunologic responsiveness in active syphilitic infection. Part of the problem is semantic in origin because, unfortunately, the term immunosuppression has been used to describe humoral responses. In fact, our initial studies (28) showed that IgM responses to SRBC were increased in infected rabbits, whereas IgG responses were obliterated. These changes occurred at a time when other IgG was being produced, e.g., that detected in the VDRL or FTA reactions.

The fact that antibodies of various kinds are present early in syphilitic infection by no means excludes the subsequent induction of suppressor mechanisms; suppression of IgG responsiveness could explain the failure to mount Ab that is treponemicidal in vivo. Interaction between the immune system and specific antigens in a number of parasitic infections (8,44) and granulomatous diseases (45,46) is known to produce responses in which suppressor mechanisms overwhelm the existing effector mechanisms. In addition to specific T suppressor cells and their products, immune complexes and certain bacterial products can also exert suppressive influences. An organism as complex as *T. pallidum* undoubtedly presents a variety of immunogenic determinants to the host. The nature of all treponemal antigens is as yet unknown; it is not known whether FTA-ABS, TPHA, or TPI antibodies are directed against the same or different antigenic determinants. While the importance of these antigens in the diagnosis of the disease seems clear, their role in host resistance is controversial (see also Chap. 12).

While most of our evidence is indirect, the results with the IV infection model are in accord with the hypothesis that immune complexes formed at the height of the treponemal burden act to suppress certain IgG responses, a possible explanation for the host's failure to produce an appropriate treponemicidal antibody by the end of the primary stage of syphilis. A strong association appears to exist among (1) overt clinical disease in the experimental host, (2) the treponemal burden in the involved tissues, (3) elevated levels of IC in the sera, and (4) the ability of these sera to nonspecifically suppress the in vitro Ig response of normal rabbits to a heterologous antigen. This evidence is derived from the IV model; the results obtained with the ID model, although convincing, were less sound. Overall, our findings (43) appear to be consistent with previous studies that have shown that (1) IC may be carried over on spleen cells which are placed in culture and subsequently alter immune responsiveness (35,36), and (2) IC are present in active syphilitic infection in the human (47,48).

Although our results (43) support the contention that immune complexes reflect disease activity and may exert an immunoregulatory effect in experimental syphilis, they could alternatively merely represent by-products of the infection. In favor of their potential immunosuppressive effect in syphilis is the strong correlation which we have observed between IC in the sera of infected animals and the ability of these sera to induce non-antigen-specific suppression in an in vitro system. Arguments that the immune response in experimental syphilis is "normal" and that persistence of treponemes is in no way related to an induced immunosuppressive state have been based on observations in intratesticularly infected animals (23,24). As the intensity of antigen load and circulating IC are much less stricking in the IT model, one may question the validity of generalized conclusions which ignore host responses and the progression of disease in contrasting models of infection. Direct comparisons of the above-mentioned studies with ours are further complicated by the fact that the in vivo and in vitro parameters of non-antigen-specific suppression, characteristic of both IV and ID infections, have not been demonstrated with the IT model. Other factors may also exert immunoregulatory effects in experimental syphilis and thus contribute to the pathogenesis of *T. pallidum*. As communication between inducer, regulatory, and effector cell subsets determines not only the intensity but also the type of response following antigenic insult (49), future studies in experimental syphilis must be less simplistic than those of the past few years.

Further studies are necessary to document whether antibody, either alone or complexed with treponemal antigens, exerts an adverse effect upon the course of infection, possibly via negative feedback effects on T-cell function. In terms of antibody alone, autolymphocytotoxins may be important; a recent study (50) suggests that complement-dependent lymphocytotoxins are regularly present in the sera of patients with secondary syphilis. Hopefully, studies aimed at (1) determining the state of relative antigen or antibody excess in IC, (2) characterizing the antigens in the complexes, and (3) determining the size and charge characteristics of the complexes in experimental syphilis will provide us with insights regarding their biological significance in syphilis and contribute to our basic understanding of the delicate balance between immunoregulatory and suppressive forces.

References

1. A. N. Theofilopoulos and F. J. Dixon. The biology and detection of immune complexes. *Adv. Immunol.* 28:89-200 (1979).
2. WHO Scientific Group. The role of immune complexes in diseases. *WHO Tech. Ser.* 606 (1977).
3. J. H. Schwab. Suppression of the immune response by microorganisms. *Bacteriol. Rev.* 39:121-143 (1975).

4. N. H. Bishop and J. N. Miller. Humoral immunity in experimental syphilis. II. The relationship of neutralizing factors in immune serum to acquired resistance. *J. Immunol. 177:* 197-207 (1976).
5. D. M. Musher and R. F. Schell. The immunology of syphilis. *Hosp. Pract. 1045-50* (1975).
6. T. B. Turner and D. H. Hollander. Biology of the treponematoses. *Who Monogr. Ser. 34* (1957).
7. R. A. Nelson, Jr. and M. M. Mayer. Immobilization of *Treponema pallidum* in vitro by antibody produced in syphilitic infection. *J. Exp. Med. 89*:369-393 (1949).
8. B. R. Bloom. Games parasites play: How parasites evade immune surveillance. *Nature 271*:21-26 (1979).
9. G. M. Levene and D. J. M. Wright. Cell-mediated immunity and lymphocytes transformation in syphilis. *Proc. R. Soc. Med. 64*:426-428 (1971).
10. G. M. Levene, D. J. M. Wright, J. L. Turk, and A. G. S. Brimble. Reduced lymphocyte transformation due to a plasma factor in patients with active syphilis. *Lancet 2*:246-247 (1969).
11. D. M. Musher, R. F. Schell, and J. M. Knox. In vitro lymphocyte response to *Treponema refringens* in human syphilis. *Infect. Immun. 9*:654-657 (1974).
12. D. M. Musher, R. F. Schell, R. H. Jones, and A. M. Jones. Lymphocyte transformation in syphilis: An in vitro correlate of immune suppression in vivo? *Infect. Immun. 11*:1261-1264 (1975).
13. E. From, K. Thestrup-Pedersen, and H. Thulin. Reactivity of lymphocytes from patients with syphilis towards *T. pallidum* antigen in the leucocyte migration and lymphocyte transformation tests. *Br. J. Vener. Dis. 56*:224-229 (1976).
14. R. F. Bey, R. C. Johnson, and T. J. Fitzgerald. Suppression of lymphocyte response to Concanavalin A by mucopolysaccharide material from *Treponema pallidum*-infected rabbits. *Infect. Immun.* 2664-69 (1979).
15. C. S. Pavia, J. B. Baseman, and J. D. Folds. Selective response of lymphocytes from *Treponema pallidum*-infected rabbits to mitogens and *Treponema retteri*. *Infect. Immun. 15*:417-422 (1977).
16. C. S. Pavia, J. D. Folds, and J. B. Baseman. Depression of lymphocyte response to concamavalin A in rabbits infected with *Treponema pallidum* (Nichols strain). *Infect. Immun. 14*: 320-322 (1976).
17. C. S. Pavia, J. D. Folds, and J. B. Baseman. Selective in vitro response of thymus-dependent-derived lymphocytes from *Treponema pallidum* infected rabbits. *Infect. Immun. 18*: 603-611 (1977).

18. V. Wicher and K. Wicher. In vitro cell response to *Treponema pallidum* infected rabbits. I. Lymphocyte transformation. *Clin. Exp. Immunol.* 24:480-486 (1977).
19. S. M. Maret, J. B. Baseman, and J. D. Folds. Cell-mediated immunity in *Treponema pallidum* infected rabbits: In vitro response of splenic and lymph node lymphocytes to mitogens and specific antigens. *Clin. Exp. Immunol.* 39:38-43 (1980).
20. H. C. Festenstein, C. Abrahams, and V. Bokkenheuser. Runting syndrome in neonatal rabbits infected with *Treponema pallidum*. *Clin. Exp. Immunol.* 2:311-320 (1967).
21. D. R. Turner and D. J. M. Wright. Lymphadenopathy in early syphilis. *J. Pathol.* 110:304-308 (1973).
22. V. Wicher and K. Wicher. In vitro cell response to *Treponema pallidum*-infected rabbits. III. Impairment in production of lymphocyte mitogenic factor. *Clin. Exp. Immunol.* 24:496-500 (1977).
23. S. A. Lukehart, S. A. Baker-Zander, and S. Sell. Characterization of lymphocyte responsiveness in early experimental syphilis. I. In vitro response to mitogens and *Treponema pallidum* antigens. *J. Immunol.* 124:454-460 (1980).
24. S. Baker-Zander and S. S. Sell. A histopathologic and immunologic study of the course of syphilis in the experimentally infected rabbit. *Am. J. Pathol.* 101:387-404 (1980).
25. J. L. Ware, J. D. Folds, and J. B. Baseman. Serum of rabbits infected with *Treponema pallidum* (Nichols) inhibits in vitro transformation of normal rabbit lymphocytes. *Cell. Immunol.* 42:363-372 (1979).
26. V. Wicher and K. Wicher. In vitro cell response of *Treponema pallidum*-infected rabbits. II. Inhibition of lymphocyte response to phytohaemagglutinin by serum of *T. pallidum*-infected rabbits. *Clin. Exp. Immunol.* 24:487-495 (1977).
27. K. Wicher, V. Wicher, and D. Kamanski. Effect of *Treponema pallidum*-infected testis supernatants on the cellular response of normal rabbit lymphocytes. *Infect. Immun.* 27:846-850 (1980).
28. R. E. Baughn and D. M. Musher. Altered immune responsiveness associated with experimental syphilis in the rabbit: Elevated IgM and depressed IgG responses to sheep erythrocytes. *J. Immunol.* 120:1691-1695 (1978).
29. R. E. Baughn and D. M. Musher. Aberrant secondary antibody responses to sheep erythrocytes in rabbits with experimental syphilis. *Infect. Immun.* 25:133-138 (1979).
30. T. J. Fitzgerald, R. C. Johnson, and E. T. Wolff. Mucopolysaccharide material resulting from the interaction of *Treponema pallidum* (Nichols strain) with cultured mammalian cells. *Infect. Immun.* 22:575-584 (1978).

31. J. F. Alderete and J. B. Baseman. Surface-associated host proteins on virulent *Treponema pallidum*. *Infect. Immun.* 26: 1048-1056 (1979).
32. B. A. Askonas, A. J. McMichael, and M. E. Roux. Clonal dominance and the preservation of clonal memory cells mediated by antigen-antibody. *Immunology* 31541-551 (1976).
33. E. Diener and M. Feldmann. Relationship between antigen and antibody induced suppression of immunity. *Transplant. Rev.* 8:76-103 (1972).
34. H. N. Eisen and F. Karush. Immune tolerance and an extracellular regulatory role for bivalent antibody. *Nature* 202: 667-682 (1964).
35. E. L. Morgan and C. H. Tempelis. The role of antigen-antibody complexes in mediating immunologic unresponsiveness in the chicken. *J. Immunol.* 119:1293-1298 (1977).
36. D. W. Scott and B. D. Waksman. Mechanisms of immunologic tolerance. I. Induction of tolerance to bovine gamman globulin by injection of antigen into infant organs in vitro. *J. Immunol.* 102:347-354 (1969).
37. S. Kotiainen. Blocking antigen-antibody complexes on the T-lymphocyte surface identified with defined protein antigens. II. Lymphocyte activation during the in vitro response. *Immunology* 28:535-542 (1974).
38. S. Kotiainen and N. A. Mitchinson. Blocking antigen-antigen complexes on the T-lymphocyte surface identified with defined protein antigens. I. Lymphocyte activation during in vitro incubation before adoptive transfer. *Immunology* 28:523-533 (1975).
39. M. Rabinovitch, R. E. Manejias, and U. Nussenzweig. Selective phagocytic paralysis induced by immobilized immune complexes. *J. Exp. Med.* 142:827-838 (1975).
40. J. L. Ryan, R. D. Arbeit, H. B. Dickler, and P. A. Henkart. Inhibition of lymphocyte mitogenesis by immobilized antigen-antibody complexes. *J. Exp. Med.* 142:814-826 (1975).
41. C. L. Sidman and E. R. Unanue. Control of B-lymphocyte function. I. Inactivation of mitogenesis by interaction with surface immunoglobulin and Fc-receptor molecules. *J. Exp. Med.* 144:882-896 (1976).
42. J. M. Mansfield and J. A. Wallace. Suppression of cell-mediated immunity in experimental African trypanosomiasis. *Infect. Immun.* 10335-339 (1974).
43. R. E. Baughn, K. S. K. Tung, and D. M. Musher. Detection of circulating immune complexes in the sera of rabbits with experimental syphilis: Possible role in immunoregulation. *Infect. Immun.* 29:575-582 (1980).

44. A. N. Jayawardena and B. H. Waksman. Suppressor cells in experimental trypanosomiasis. *Nature* 265:539-541 (1977).
45. J. M. Dwyer, R. J. Mangi, B. Gee, and F. S. Kantor. Comparison of the anergy of sarcoidosis with experimentally induced anergy in guinea pigs. *Ann. N.Y. Acad. Sci.* 278:29-35 (1976).
46. S. M. Hillinger and G. P. Herzig. Impaired cell-mediated immunity in Hodgkin's disease mediated by suppressor lymphocytes and monocytes. *J. Clin. Invest.* 59:1620-1627 (1977).
47. J. Sølling, K. Sølling, K. U. Jacobsen, and E. From. Circulating immune complexes in syphilis. *Acta Derm. Venereol.* 58:263-267 (1978).
48. S. Engel and W. Diezel. Persistent serum immune complexes in syphilis. *Br. J. Vener. Dis.* 56:221-222 (1980).
49. H. Cantor and R. K. Gershon. Immunological circuits: Cellular composition. *Fed. Proc. Fed. Am. Soc. Exp. Biol.* 38:2058-2064 (1976).
50. N. H. L. DeJong, J. A. M. Koehorst, J. J. Van der Sluis, and A. M. Boer. Autolymphocytotoxins in syphilis. *Br. J. Vener. Dis.* 56:297-301 (1980).

15
Histopathology and Immunopathology of Experimental Syphilis

STEWART SELL
University of Texas
Health Science Center at Houston
Houston, Texas

Phases of Experimental Syphilis   298
Systemic Manifestations   298
Local Manifestations   300
Effect of Cortisone on Experimental Lesions   308
Latency and Tertiary Lesions   308
Summary   309
References   310

Infection with *Treponema pallidum* is limited to a narrow host range. The only natural host of pathogenic treponemes is man. Experimental infection may be induced in certain species of higher apes and the rabbit, and manifestations of tissue lesions have only been demonstrated in man and the rabbit (1). Chimpanzees infected with *T. pallidum* develop circulating antibody to *T. pallidum*, but lesions do not occur (2). The rabbit therefore provides the major experimental model for study of the host-parasite relationship in syphilis. Hamsters (3), guinea pigs (4), and irradiated mice (5) have also been utilized for certain special experimental studies, but the reaction to infection is different from that in humans and rabbits.

In the rabbit the injection of T. *pallidum* into the shaved skin produces raised firm dermal lesions similar to those that occur upon natural infection of humans, i.e., the primary chancre (6,7). Intratesticular inoculation results in development of an acute orchitis (Fig. 1) that provides another model for primary syphilis (6,8-14). In addition, intravascular inoculation of large numbers of organisms may result in disseminated skin lesions in shaved areas (15). This model has some similarities to secondary syphilis in humans (16). In this chapter recent histologic and immunologic studies in our laboratory on the primary response to experimental T. *pallidum* infection in the rabbit will be described.

Phases of Experimental Syphilis

The response of rabbits to experimental intradermal or intratesticular inoculation of T. *pallidum* may be divided into three phases: inductive, reactive, and latent (6,17,18). The *inductive* phase features a rapid increase in T. *pallidum* in connective tissue. The end of the inductive phase is signaled by an increasing lymphocytic infiltrate. The *reactive* phase is characterized by a rapid drop in the numbers of T. *pallidum* that coincides with the infiltration of the infected tissue with large numbers of macrophages. The *latent* phase is distinguished by resolution and focal scarring at the site of infection, the continued presence of small numbers of organisms, and the return to a clinically normal state. The duration of each phase is dependent on the number of organisms injected. At the dose used for most of our experiments (10^7 to 10^8 viable T. *pallidum* per site) the following times are usually observed, with considerable variation among individual rabbits: induction phase, days 0-11; reactive phase, days 12-21; latent phase, after day 21 (11-14). Experimental results described in this chapter will show that the inflammatory response to T. *pallidum* infection is largely responsible for the lesions observed and that clearance of organisms from sites of infection is the result of phagocytosis and destruction by macrophages as a component of a delayed hypersensitivity reaction initiated by specifically sensitized T cells.

Systemic Manifestations

Experimental infection with T. *pallidum* is associated with marked local swelling and inflammation (see Fig. 1, Chap. 13), as well as hyperplasia of draining lymph nodes and spleen (Fig. 1). Within a few hours of infection dissemination of organisms occurs. The spleen and lymph nodes increase in size within 1 week. Marked hyperplasia of

15. Histopathology and Immunology of Experimental Syphilis 299

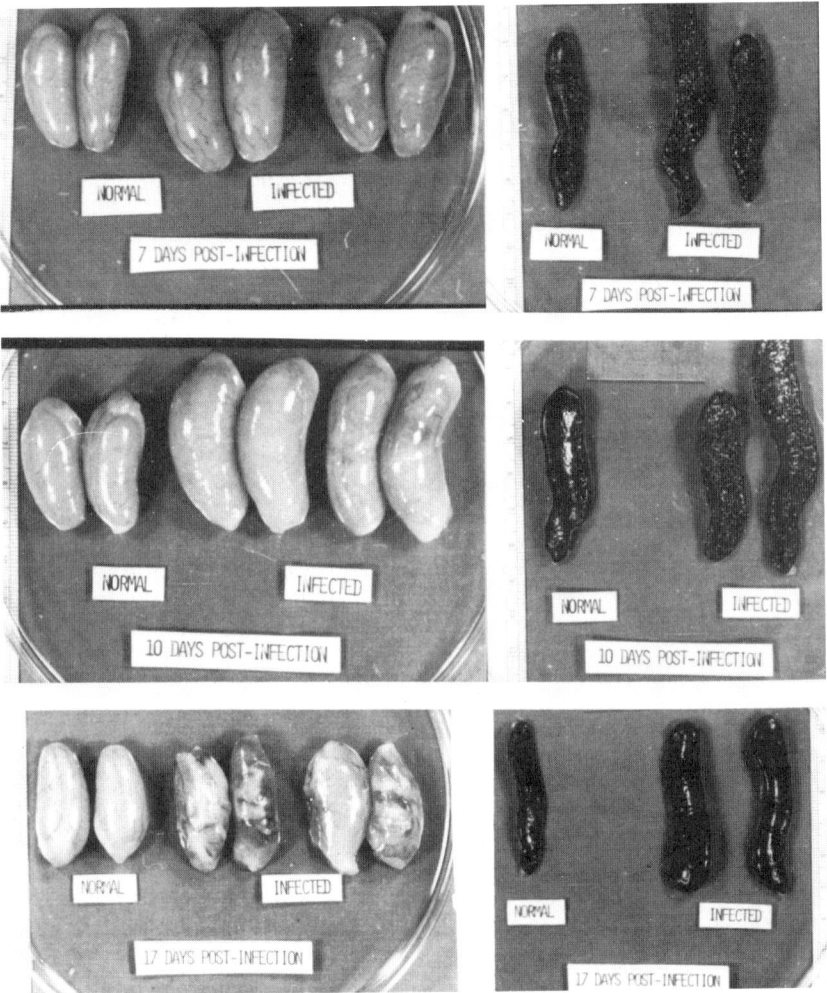

Figure 1 Gross appearance of testicles (lest) and spleens (right) following intratesticular inoculation of 2 to 10×10^7 viable organisms. There is marked swelling and enlargement of the testicles on day 10. Although there is less swelling on day 17, there are focal areas of hemorrhage and exudation. Note the dullness and granular appearance of infected spleens as compared to normal ones. (*Source*: Modified from Ref. 14.)

the diffuse cortex of the lymph nodes and periarterial (T cells) zones of the spleen is seen early (Fig. 2), followed by striking hyperplasia of germinal centers (13,14). A decrease in the percentage of T cells in the spleen and nodes on day 10 is interpreted as being due to the dissemination of large numbers of these cells to the sites of infection (14). A month after infection the lymph node and spleen have returned to about normal size. There is no evidence of hypoplasia at any time after infection (13,14).

Specific increases in the responsiveness of spleen and lymph node lymphocytes to T. pallidum antigens in the form of sonicates occur within 3 days of infection and remain elevated for at least 2 years after infection (Fig. 3) (11). The blast transformation response is eliminated by treatment of reactive cell populations with anti-T-cell serum, but is retained in T-cell-enriched cell populations (11). Thus the proliferative response to specific T. pallidum antigens is a property of the T-cell population. We have not found blast transformation response to nonspecific stimulation, such as Concanavalin A (ConA) or anti-Ig, to be depressed at any phase of the infection (11,14, see Chap. 16). Circulating humoral antibody as measured by VDRL or fluorescent treponemal antibody absorption (FTA-ABS) appears about day 10. Fluorescent treponemal antibody absorption titers remain elevated for the lifetime of the untreated infected animal but VDRL titers decline after resolution of lesions. (14).

Sera from approximately 40% of infected animals will cause a lowering of the specific T. pallidum response of sensitized lymphocytes, as compared to the response in normal rabbit serum. The response to ConA is not affected. This "suppressive" effect is not significantly associated with the presence of antibodies to T. pallidum nor with the presence of immune complexes per se (19). Similar specific suppression of sheep red blood cell (SRBC)-induced responses of lymphocytes from rabbits immunized with SRBC is observed using sera from SRBC-immunized rabbits; sera from T. pallidum-infected rabbits do not suppress the SRBC response. The significance of this phenomenon in the course of the host response to T. pallidum remains unclear. There is no apparent difference in the overall course of infection in rabbits which demonstrate such a serum effect as compared to those who do not (19). We have postulated that the presence of such serum factors may be a manifestation of the normal mechanism(s) that serve to shut off or limit specific immune responses (7,13,19).

Local Manifestations

Following inoculation of approximately 10^7 viable T. pallidum, Nichols strain, into the shaved skin or testicle there is little or no noticeable change for several days. However, by immunofluorescence increasing numbers of organisms may be identified in the dermis of the skin (7)

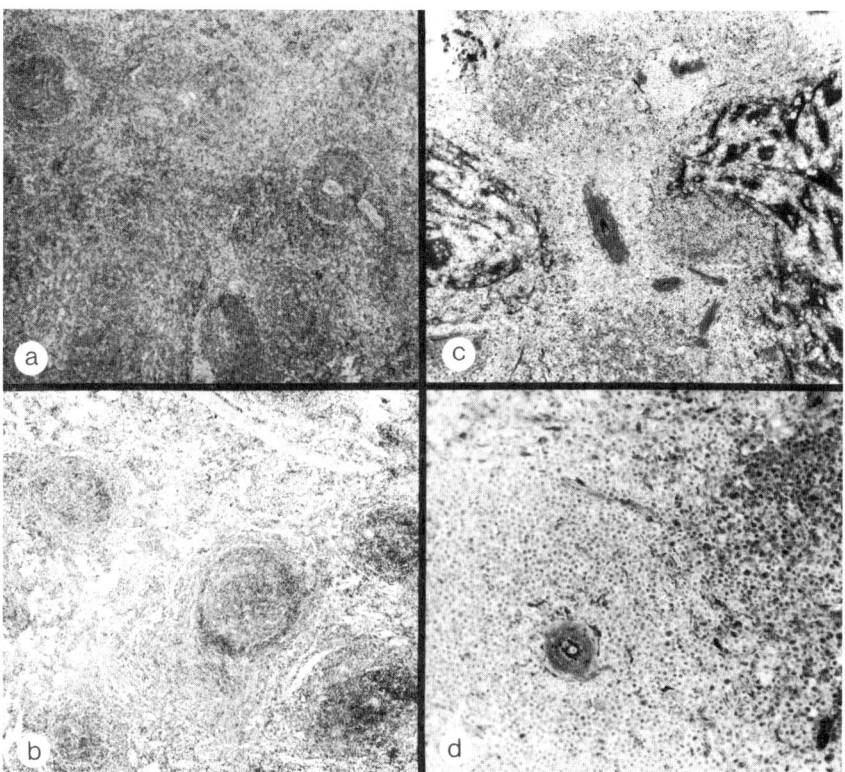

Figure 2 Histologic changes in spleen after intratesticular infection with *T. pallidum*: (a) normal spleen, hematoxylin and eosin; (b) spleen 10 days after infection (hematoxylin and eosin); (c) spleen 10 days after infection, stained for T cells; and (d) spleen 10 days after infection, stained for T cells, higher magnification. The follicles and periarticular (T-cell) zones, which label for T cells, are markedly enlarged after *T. pallidum* infection. (*Source*: Modified from Ref. 13.)

or the interstitial tissues of the testes (Fig. 4). By days 3-6 atrophy of the testicular tubules begins and an increasing mononuclear infiltrate is observed (Fig. 5); some polymorphonuclear cells are also seen. The number of organisms visualized reaches a maximum at days 10-11 (12). Cellular infiltration, initially mostly T cells (Fig. 6), gradually shows a predominance of macrophages with an increasing but minor component of plasma cells (11,14). The number of identifiable organisms now falls dramatically so that by day 17 and later only rare organisms are identifiable (Fig. 7). The lesions then slowly resolve, with focal areas of scarring (Fig. 6). After 2 months the testicular tubules have regenerated (14).

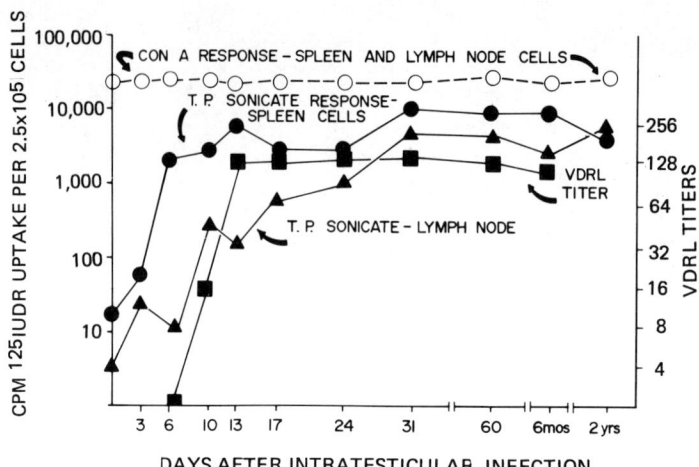

Figure 3 Lymphocyte blast transformation and Veneral Disease Research Laboratories (VDRL) antibody titers in experimental syphilis. An increased lymphocyte response to sonicate of $T.\ pallidum$ is observed within 3 days after infection; VDRL titers become elevated by day 10. These responses remain elevated for up to 2 years after infection. The non-antigen-specific response to Concanavalin A remains constant with no evidence of "suppression." (*Source*: Data from Refs. 11 and 14.)

During the reactive stage, when the number of organisms is declining rapidly, fragments of fluorescent material are seen in foci of macrophage infiltration; these fragments stain specifically with reagents for $T.\ pallidum$ (14). By electron microscopy typical treponemes are located almost exclusively extracellularly on day 10 (Fig. 7). However, upon entering the reactive stage many $T.\ pallidum$ structures are seen within membrane-delineated vacuoles in macrophages. In many instances swollen and disarticulated organisms are visualized, as well as unidentifiable phagocytic debris (20). Some identifiable fragments of $T.\ pallidum$ are seen in lipid-containing digestive vacuoles. From these observations we conclude that the major mechanism of clearance of organisms from infected sites is by phagocytosis and digestion by macrophages, following initiation of an inflammatory response by specifically sensitized T lymphocytes (20).

The possible role of immunoglobulin antibody in this process remains unclear (Chap. 13). The onset of the reactive phase, and the rapid clearance of organisms from infected sites, correlates closely with the appearance of circulating antibody (14, 21). Antibody has been shown to be required for phagocytosis of $T.\ pallidum$ by macrophages in vitro

(22); immunoglobulin antibody neutralizes *T. pallidum* in vitro (23); passively transferred immune serum protects nonimmune rabbits against intradermal infection (23-27); and passive transfer is induced by the IgG fraction of immune serum (28). However, passive transfer of specific immunity by serum is not completely effective in preventing disease and a prominent coating of organisms by immunoglobin in vivo is not apparent by immunofluorescence (7,12,14). In addition, infiltration of infected sites by polymorphonuclear cells would be expected if antibody activation of complement was a major component of the inflammatory reaction, i.e., an Arthus reaction (29), and this is not the case (12,14). Thus it seems unlikely that humoral antibody plays a major role in the initial clearing of organisms during the reactive stage. On the other hand, a role for antibody cannot be ruled out (Chap. 13). Components of antibody and complement could be involved in the alteration and activation of macrophages. In addition, long-term resistance

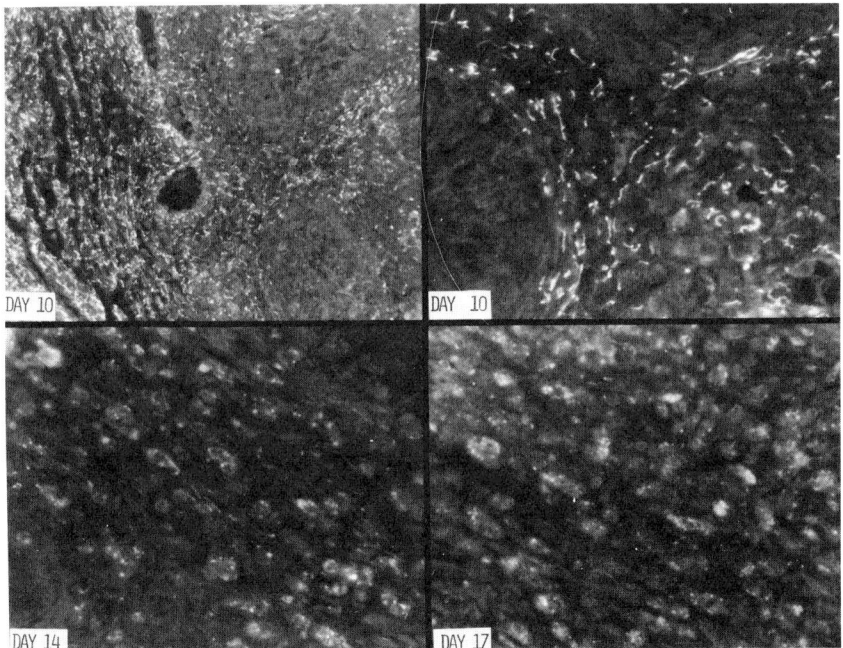

Figure 4 Immunofluorescent identification of *T. pallidum* in infected rabbit testes. During the inductive stage, day 10, increasing numbers of typical spiroform structures are present in the interstitial tissue and tubular basement membrane. During the reactive stage, days 14 and 17, fewer organisms are seen and labeled fragments may be seen in association with foci macrophages. (*Source*: Data from Refs. 12 and 14.)

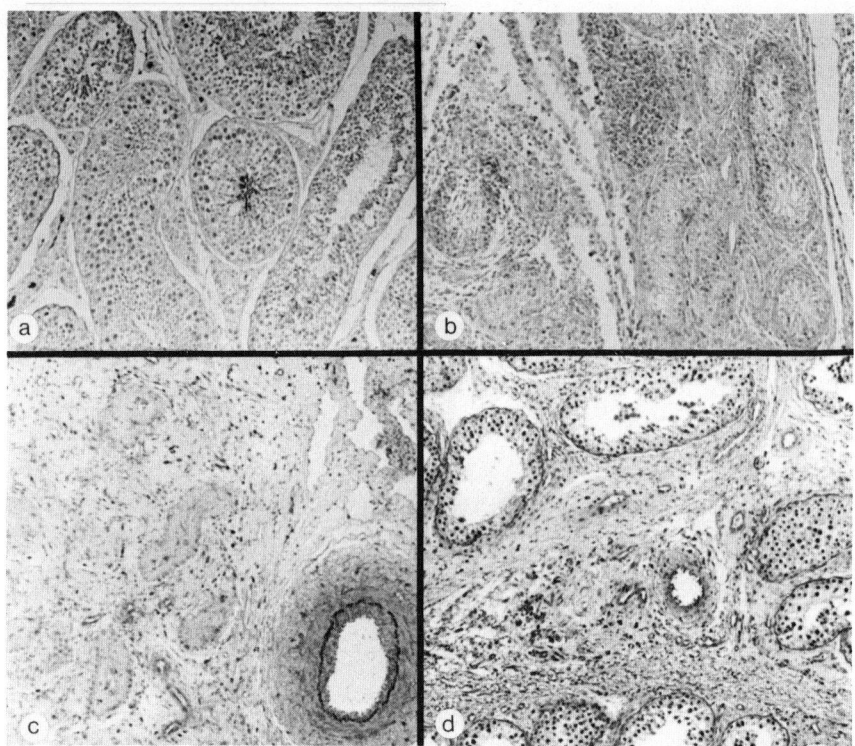

Figure 5 Light-microscopic pictures of testicles during syphilis infection. (a) Normal. (b) Day 11. (c) After 3 months. (d) After 6 months. During the inductive and reactive stage there is infiltration of the interstitial tissue with mononuclear cells, edema, and atrophy of the testicular tubules. (c) illustrates an area of scarring with atrophic tubules. (d) illustrates a focus of scarring surrounded by regenerating tubules.

to reinfection could depend upon antibody to *T. pallidum* (14,30). Reinoculation of infectious organisms into previously infected immune animals results in disappearance of organisms at the site of inoculation, with evidence of a slight delayed hypersensitivity reaction as well as mild acute inflammation (S. Sell and Nauro, unpublished observations). This effect could be explained by a direct toxic effect of antibody or antibody and complement on infecting organisms. Experiments testing the ability of immune cells to provide passive protection against *T. pallidum* have given inconsistent and conflicting results (31,32).

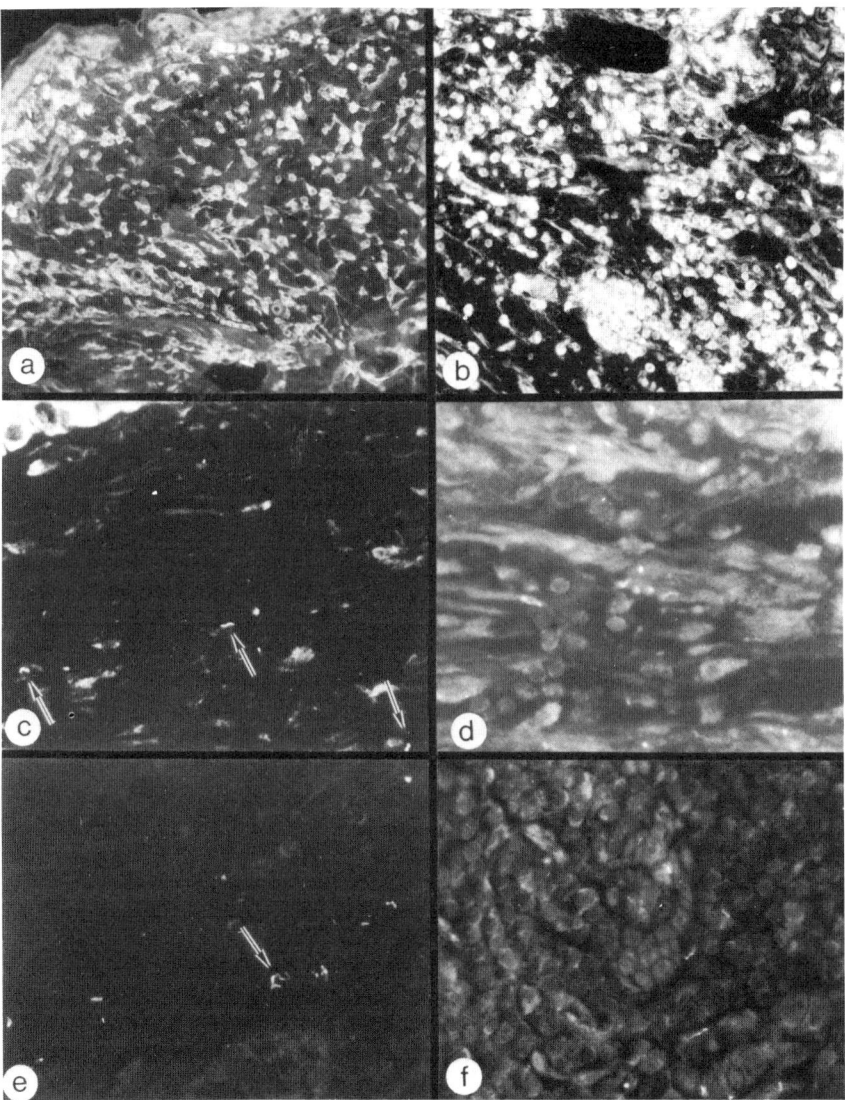

Figure 6 Immunofluorescent localization of T cells and *T. pallidum* in infected skin and testicles. (a) T cells in skin, day 14. (b) T cells in testis 10 days after intratesticular inoculation. (c) *T. pallidum* and fragments in subepidermal granulomatous zone 6 weeks following intradermal inoculation. (d) Granulomatous area in testis containing a few *T. pallidum* 20 days after intratesticular infection. (e) *T. pallidum* in testicle 6 weeks after intradermal inoculation. (f) Spleen containing identifiable *T. pallidum* 13 days after intratesticular inoculation. (*Source*: Modified from Ref. 7.)

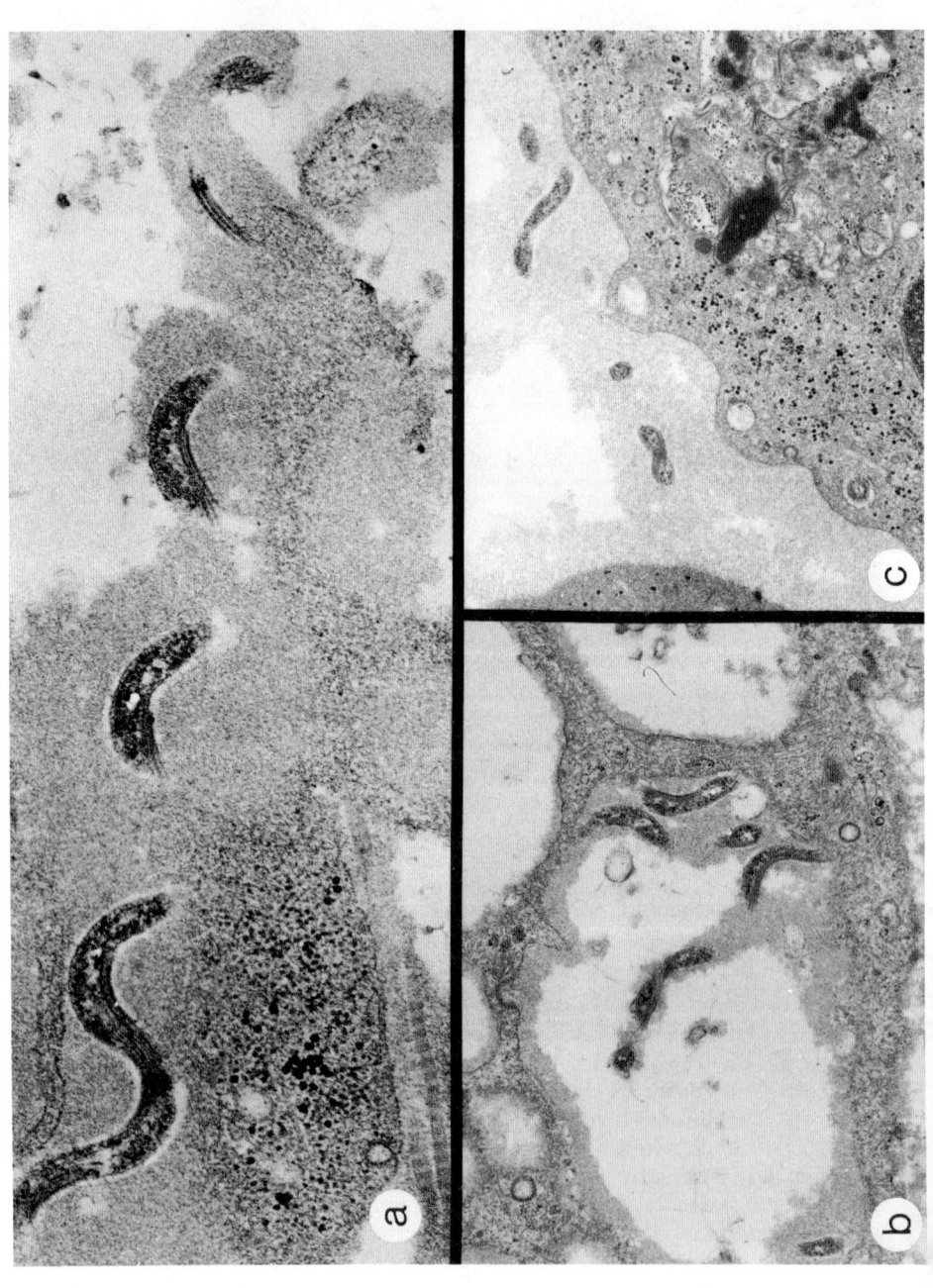

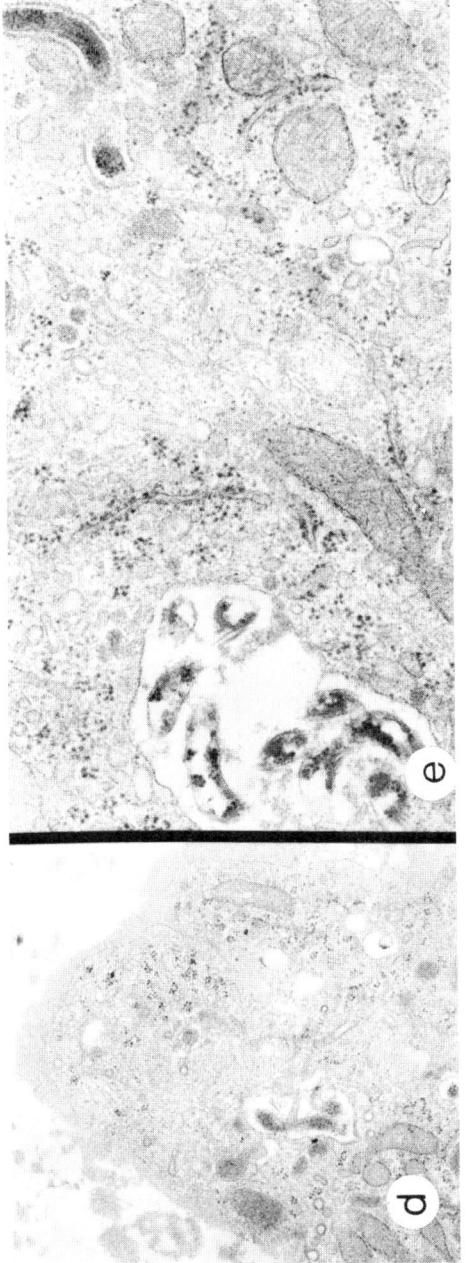

Figure 7 Electron-microscopic identification of *T. pallidum* in infected testicular lesions. (a) Typical extracellular *T. pallidum* illustrating spiroform structures with characeristic axial filaments. Note coating of organisms, adjacent cell fragment, and collagen fibers with amorphous material. (b) Macrophage with numerous large endocytotic vesicles. The surface of the macrophage (bottom of picture), the internal surface of the vesicles, and organisms within the vesicles are coated with amorphous material. (c) Extracellular organisms and macrophage containing a large phagocytic vesicle with unidentifiable debris. (d) Macrophage containing vesicle with disarticulated *T. pallidum*. (e) Higher magnification of macrophage shows a vesicle with swollen disentegrating *T. pallidum* (lower left) as well as intact organism in another vesicle (upper right). Note the good preservation of the cellular organelles. (*Source*: Modified from Ref. 20.)

Effects of Cortisone on Experimental Lesions

The well-known enhancing effect of cortisone on *T. pallidum* infection (6) has been reexamined (33). Cortisone administration essentially inhibits the development of a measurable immune response and increases the duration of the initiation stage of the experimental disease. Cortisone administration delays the development of reactive lymphocytes in spleen and lymph node, postpones production of humoral antibody, permits a greater increase in the number of organisms at the site of infection, inhibits the local mononuclear cell infiltration, and greatly increases the amount of amorphous extracellular "ground substance" at the site of infection. However, when cortisone treatment is stopped, there is a rapid development of a T-cell response to treponemal antigen; together with the prompt appearance of circulating antibody, a rapid and massive infiltration of the infected sites by T cells and macrophages, and expeditious clearance of organisms by phagocytosis. Electron microscopy demonstrates that both in untreated and cortisone-treated syphilitic rabbits the presence of large amounts of amorphous "ground substance" does not inhibit the ability of macrophages to ingest and destroy organisms (20). Macrophages, lymphocytes, and organisms in the lesions of untreated rabbits are coated with this material and it is markedly increased in cortisone-treated rabbits. Many intracytoplasmic vesicles in macrophages, some containing *T. pallidum* and *T. pallidum* fragments, are lined by the same material.

Latency and Tertiary Lesions

The period of latency implies the continued presence of organisms in the absence of clinical disease or tissue lesions. The presence of organisms during latency has been demonstrated by the ability of extracts of tissue, particularly lymphoid tissue, to transfer the disease to previously uninfected rabbits (6,17). *Treponema pallidum* has been tentatively identified in human gummas (tertiary lesions) by transfer to rabbits (34,35) and by immunofluorescence (36,37). Latency represents a state of concomitant immunity, since rabbits in latency resist rechallenge with viable organisms (6,14,17). Specific antibodies to *T. pallidum* may be responsible for maintenance of latency.

There is little or no convincing evidence that establishment of latency depends upon an abnormality of the immune response to *T. pallidum*. During the early latent phase of experimental syphilis, at a time of resolution of the inflammatory lesions, rare organisms may be visualized in tissues by immunofluorescence. These appear to be located extracellularly in zones of scarring. It is postulated that these organisms have found an extracellular niche that shields them from immune attack (11-14,38). In this niche the organisms may remain dormant but viable for a long time. The lack of demonstrable lesions in systemic sites, where it is known that organisms are located, implies that a certain minimum number of organisms may be necessary to provide a stimulus for initiation of an immune-mediated inflammatory reaction. Following intradermal reinoculation a small number of organisms may be visualized in the testes (Fig. 7), but little or no inflammatory reaction is observed, even when the dermal reaction is greatest (7). On the other hand, primary inoculation into the testes results in a prompt and vigorous cellular inflammatory response (12). The observation that T. pallidum may be found within host cells (39,40), even within the nucleus (41), has led to the conclusion that intracellular location may be important in protection against immune attack and latency (39-41). However, we have not been able to demonstrate intracellular *persistence* of organisms (20). It is possible that intracellular location of T. pallidum results in destruction, even in cells other than macrophages.

Although tertiary lesions have not been observed in the rabbit, gummatous inflammatory reactions seen in humans (Chap. 6) may represent a response to T. pallidum that temporarily escape dormancy and begin to proliferate, perhaps related to a decline in immune responsiveness. Such foci restimulate immune reactivity, resulting in the chronic inflammation seen, as in gummas or meningovascular syphilis. It is postulated that small numbers of nonproliferating T. pallidum may remain viable but dormant for long periods of time in isolated avascular areas. If proliferation occurs, sufficient numbers of organisms would be generated to incite a chronic inflammatory response leading to the characteristic lesions of tertiary disease.

Summary

Experimental intradermal or intratesticular infection of rabbits with T. pallidum initiates a prompt systemic hyperphasia of lymphoid organs, the appearance of T lymphocytes responsive to T. pallidum antigens, the extensive local cellular inflammatory reaction. During the local cellular immune response the early infiltrates consist mainly of T cells. Later, organisms are cleared from infected sites by phagocytosis and digestion by macrophages. The evolution of the inflammatory response is essentially that of a delayed hypersensitivity reaction. The presence of extracellular amorphous "ground substance" coating T. pallidum as well as inflammatory cells does not prevent phagocytosis and digestion of organisms.

Although humoral antibody does not appear to be necessary for the inflammatory reaction observed, it could play a role in resistance to reinfection by other immune mechanisms. Although some sera from infected rabbits will decrease the specific lymphocyte transformation response in vitro when compared to sera from normal rabbits, we have found no effect on non-antigen-specific transformation and there is no evidence for an immunosuppressive effect in vivo.

We conclude that macrophage destruction of *T. pallidum*, as a component of a delayed hypersensitive reaction, is the major mechanism for removing organisms from sites of infection during the primary response to syphilitic infection. Latency is most likely the result of the localization of organisms in "protective niches" that are inaccessable to products of the immune response. Tertiary lesions may result when dormant but viable organisms begin to proliferate and stimulate a chronic inflammatory response.

Acknowledgments

This work was supported by USPHS Grant No. AI-14262 from the National Institute of Allergy and Infectious Disease. Most of the experiments described in this chapter were carried out directly by Sheila Lukehart, Ph.D., and Sharon Baker-Zander. The electron-microscopic studies were done in collaboration with Henry Powell, M.D., and Mike Costello. Determination of immune complexes was done by A. Theofilopolous, M.D. I am most grateful to them for their major contribution to these studies and to James N. Miller for his continued stimulation and advice.

References

1. World Health Organization. *Treponematosis research. WHO Tech. Rep.* 455 (1970).
2. W. J. Brown, U. S. G. Kuhn III, E. A. Tolliver, and L. C. Norins. Experimental syphilis in the chimpanzee. Immunoglobulin class of early antibodies reactive with *Treponema pallidum*. *Br. J. Vener. Dis.* 46:198-200 (1970).
3. R. F. Schell, J. L. LeFrock, J. K. Chan, and O. Bagasra. LSH hamster model of syphilitic infection. *Infect. Immun.* 28:909-193 (1980).
4. K. Wicher, V. Wicher, and M. C. Wang. Cellular and humoral immune response of guinea pig infected with *Treponema pallidum*. *Int. Arch. Allergy Appl. Immun.* 51:284-297 (1976).
5. J. R. Klein, A. A. Monjan, P. H. Hardy, Jr., and G. A. Cole. Abrogation of genetically controlled resistance of mice. *Nature* 283:572-574 (1980).
6. T. B. Turner and D. H. Hollander. Biology of the treponematoses. *WHO Monogr. Ser.* 35, 1-278 (1957).
7. S. Sell, D. Gamboa, S. A. Baker-Zander, S. A. Lukehart, and J. N. Miller. Host response to *Treponema pallidum* in intradermally-infected rabbits: Evidence for persistence of infection at local and distant sites. *J. Invest. Dermatol.* 75:470-475 (1980).

8. W. H. Brown and L. Pearce. Experimental syphilis in the rabbit: 1. Primary infection in the testicle. *J. Exp. Med.* 31:475-498 (1920).
9. W. H. Brown and L. Pearce. Experimental syphilis in the rabbit: 2. Primary infection in scrotum. Part 1. Reaction to infection. *J. Exp. Med.* 31:709-727 (1920).
10. W. H. Brown and L. Pearce. Experimental syphilis in the rabbit. 2. Primary infection in scrotum: Part 2. Scrotal lesions and the character of the scrotal reaction. *J. Exp. Med.* 31:729-748 (1920).
11. S. A. Lukehart, S. A. Baker-Zander, S. Sell. Characterization of lymphocyte responsiveness in early experimental syphilis. I. In vitro response to mitogens and *Treponema pallidum* antigens. *J. Immunol.* 124:454-460 (1980).
12. S. A. Lukehart, S. A. Baker-Zander, R. M. C. Lloyd. Characterization of lymphocyte responsiveness in early experimental syphilis. II. Nature of cellular infiltration and *Treponema pallidum* distribution in testicular lesions. *J. Immunol.* 124:461-467 (1980).
13. S. Sell, S. A. Baker-Zander, and R. M. C. Lloyd. T-cell hyperplasia of lymphoid tissue of rabbits infected with *T. pallidum*: Evidence for a vigorous immune response. *Sex. Transmit. Dis.* 7:74-84 (1980).
14. S. Baker-Zander and S. Sell. A histopathologic and immunologic study of the course of syphilis in the experimentally infected rabbit. *Am. J. Pathol.* 101:387-403 (1980).
15. D. M. Musher and R. F. Schell. The immunology of syphilis. *Hosp. Prac.* 10:45-50 (1975).
16. *Public Health Service.* Syphilis. *U. S. Publ.* 1660:1 (1968).
17. A. M. Chesney. Immunity in syphilis. *Medicine* 5:463 (1926).
18. P. Collart, P. Fraceschini, D. Durel. Experimental rabbit syphilis. *Br. J. Vener. Dis.* 47:389-400 (1971).
19. S. A. Baker-Zander, S. Sell, and S. A. Lukehart. Serum regulation of in vitro lymphocyte responses in early experimental syphilis. *Infect. Immun.* 37:568-578 (1982).
20. S. Sell, S. A. Baker-Zander, and H. C. Powell. Experimental syphilitic activities in rabbits: Ultrastructural appearance of *T. pallidum* during phagocytosis and dissolution by macrophages in vivo. *Lab. Investig.* 46:355-364 (1982).
21. N. H. Bishop and J. N. Miller. Humoral immunity in experimental syphilis. II. The relationship of neutralizing factors in immune serum to acquired resistance. *J. Immunol.* 117:197-207 (1976).
22. S. A. Lukehart and J. N. Miller. Demonstration of the in vitro phagocytosis of *Treponema pallidum* by rabbit peritoneal macrophages. *J. Immunol.* 121:2014-2024 (1978).

23. N. H. Bishop and J. N. Miller. Humoral immunity in experimental syphilis. I. The demonstration of resistance conferred by passive immunization. *J. Immunol.* 117:191-196 (1976).
24. P. L. Perine, R. S. Weiser, and S. J. Klebanoff. Immunity to syphilis. I. Passive transfer in rabbits with hyperimmune serum. *Infect. Immun.* 8:787-790 (1973).
25. T. B. Turner, P. H. Hardy, Jr., B. Newman, and E. E. Nell. Effects of passive immunization on experimental syphilis in the rabbit. *Johns Hopkins Med. J.* 133:241-251 (1973).
26. N. H. Bishop and J. N. Miller. Humoral immunity in experimental syphilis. I. The demonstration of resistance conferred by passive immunization. *J. Immunol.* 117:191-196 (1976).
27. R. S. Weiser, D. Erickson, P. L. Perine, and N. N. Pearsall. Immunity to Syphilis: Passive transfer in rabbits using serial doses of immune serum. *Infect. Immun.* 13:1502-1407 (1976).
28. R. G. Titus and R. S. Weiser. Experimental syphilis in the rabbit: Passive transfer of immunity with immunoglobulin G from immune serum. *J. Infect. Dis.* 140:904-913 (1979).
29. S. Sell. *Immunology, Immunopathology and Immunity*, 3rd ed. Harper and Row, Hagerstown, Maryland (1980).
30. J. S. Pepose, N. H. Bishop, S. Feigenbaum, J. N. Miller, and P. M. Zeltzer. The humoral immune response in rabbits infected with *Treponema pallidum*: Comparison of antibody levels measured by the staphylococcal protein A-IgG (SPA-TP) microassay with VDRL, FTA-Abs, and TPI antibody responses during the development of acquired resistance to challenge. *Sex. Transmit. Dis.* 7:125-129 (1980).
31. M. Metzger and W. Smogor. Passive transfer of immunity to experimental syphilis in rabbits by immune lymphocytes. *Arch. Immunol. Ther. Exp.* 23:625-630 (1975).
32. R. E. Baughn, D. M. Musher, C. B. Simmons. Inability of spleen cells from chancre-immune rabbits to confer immunity to challenge with *Treponema pallidum*. *Infect. Immun.* 17:535-540 (1977).
33. S. A. Lukehart, S. A. Baker-Zander, R. M. C. Lloyd; and S. Sell. Effect of cortisone on host parasite relationships in early experimental syphilis. *J. Immunol.* 127:1361-1368 (1981).
34. C. H. Browning and I. Mackenzie. Recent methods. In *Diagnosis and Treatment of Syphilis*. Constable, London, 1924.
35. R. H. Kampmeier. The late manifestations of syphilis: skeletal, visceral and cardiovascular. *Med. Clin. North. Am.* 48:667-697 (1964).
36. A. R. Yobs, J. W. Clark, S. E. Mothershed, J. C. Bullard, and C. W. Artley. Further observations on the persistence of *Treponema pallidum* after treatment in rabbits and humans. *Br. J. Vener. Dis.* 44:116-130 (1968).

37. H. H. Handsfield, S. A. Lukehart, S. Sell, and K. K. Holmes. Demonstration of *Treponema pallidum* in a cutaneous gumma by indirect immunofluorescence. *Arch. Derm.* In press.
38. M. A. Medici. The immunoprotective niche—A new pathogenic mechanism for syphilis, the systemic mycoses and other infectious diseases. *J. Theor. Biol.* 36:617–625 (1972).
39. H. A. Azar, T. D. Pham, and A. K. Kurban. An electron microscopic study of a syphilitic chancre. *Arch. Pathol.* 90:143–150 (1970).
40. J. A. Sykes and J. N. Miller. Intracellular location of *Treponema pallidum*, Nichols strain, in the rabbit testis. *Infect. Immun.* 4:307–314 (1971).
41. J. A. Sykes, J. N. Miller, and A. J. Kalan. *Treponema pallidum* within cells of a primary chancre from a human female. *Br. J. Vener. Dis.* 50:40–44 (1974).

16
Cell-Mediated Immunity

JAMES D. FOLDS
School of Medicine
University of North Carolina
Chapel Hill, North Carolina

Cell-Mediated Immunity in Human Syphilis   316
Studies on *Treponema pallidum*-Infected Rabbits   321
References   326

The venereal disease syphilis has become the focus of considerable interest, especially concerning the role of the body's defense mechanisms in eradicating its causative agent, *Treponema pallidum*. Progress in the study of the host's immune mechanisms against this agent has been hampered by the inability to grow *T. pallidum* in large quantities and also the failure to produce pure *T. pallidum*. Research and study have also been slowed by the lack of a useful animal model with which to do these investigations on syphilis. Still some significant observations have been made. *Treponema pallidum* is susceptible to antibiotic therapy, but due to several factors, patients are not always treated promptly. If left untreated, syphilis can become a progressive disease. Ample evidence indicates that humoral responses against treponemal and nontreponemal antigens probably play a role in the host's defense mechanisms. These antibodies are not, however, totally effective in removing treponemes or arresting the disease (1). Considerable controversy exists concerning the possible role of cell-mediated immunity (CMI) in host defense against treponemes. In this chapter, observations on indirect measures of CMI in syphilis will be reviewed.

Cell-Mediated Immunity in Human Syphilis

Early in the research of syphilis the use of skin-testing procedures to measure delayed-type hypersensitivity, often associated with CMI, yielded observations about the immune mechanisms against syphilis. Noguchi (2) and Michelson (3) noted that skin tests were negative in primary syphilis and early secondary syphilis, but reactive in late secondary and latent syphilis. Similar observations were made in an extensive study by Thivolet et al. (3a) using a relatively pure preparation of *Treponema pallidum*.

The current interest concerning cell-mediated immunity (CMI) during *T. pallidum* infection in man began in 1969 with a report of Levene, Turk, Wright, and Grimble (4). Their brief preliminary study suggested that lymphocytes in the peripheral blood of patients with primary and secondary syphilis did not respond in vitro to the mitogen phytohemagglutinin (PHA). Furthermore, the plasma of secondary syphilitics reduced the responsiveness of lymphocytes to PHA in vitro to levels below that of normal persons. These researchers also suggested that this impaired responsiveness may be related to a depression of CMI, which could be at least partially responsible for the manifestations of secondary syphilis. Plasma from early primary or latent syphilitics did not exhibit the inhibitory factor found in plasma from secondary syphilitics; lymphocytes from patients with latent syphilis responded well in vitro to PHA.

A subsequent study by Levene, Wright, and Turk (5) disclosed histologic evidence that certain populations of lymphocytes in the spleen and lymph nodes of patients with either congenital or secondary syphilis were depleted. Depletion of lymphocytes in the paracortical areas of the lymph nodes and of the area surrounding the central arteriole of the spleen has been associated with defective CMI. Evidence presented in their report indicates that children with congenital syphilis showed abnormalities similar to those seen in neonatal rabbits infected with *T. pallidum*, i.e., depletion of lymphocytes near the central arteriole of the spleen (6). Furthermore, Levene et al. (5) found that in untreated secondary syphilitics there was a depletion of lymphocytes in the paracortical areas of the lymph nodes. The authors related these studies to earlier reports by Noguchi (2) and Michelson (3), which demonstrated negative skin tests in primary and early secondary syphilis but reactive skin tests in late secondary and latent syphilis, and suggested that impaired CMI in early syphilis might permit progression of the disease.

Fulford and Brostoff (7) applied another parameter to the study of patients at various stages of syphilis: They used the inhibition of leukocyte migration in vitro as an index of CMI (8). They observed that the peripheral blood lymphocytes from patients with primary stage syphilis migrated in the presence of the Reiter protein. This indicated a failure of CMI. Lymphocytes from patients with secondary syphilis

16. Cell-Mediated Immunity

were neither stimulated to migrate nor inhibited from migration by the Reiter protein; lymphocytes from patients with late active syphilis demonstrated strong inhibition of migration. These data indicate that early in infection certain in vitro parameters of CMI are not active, whereas in later stages of the disease CMI is apparently active.

Musher, Schell, and Knox (9) studied the in vitro response of lymphocytes from humans with primary or secondary syphilis. In their study they used PHA, pokeweed mitogen (PWM), streptolysin O (SLO), and treponemes (*Treponema refringens*) as stimulating agents. Lymphocytes from patients with primary and secondary syphilis responded normally to PHA and PWM, but showed a depressed response to SLO and treponemes. In contrast to the work of Levene et al. (4), serum from syphilitic patients in this study did not depress the ability of normal lymphocytes to respond to mitogens. Furthermore, culturing syphilitic lymphocytes in normal serum did not restore their responsiveness to SLO or treponemes. Their study also reported that normal lymphocytes were stimulated in vitro by treponemes and a dose response curve was demonstrated. Antibiotic therapy of primary or secondary syphilitics resulted in the lymphocyte response in vitro returning to a level equal to the response of normal lymphocytes to treponemes. A subsequent study by Musher et al. (10) suggested a more generalized depression of lymphocyte responsiveness in vitro. While lymphocytes from primary or secondary syphilitics responded well to mitogens such as PHA or PWM, they failed to respond in vitro to *T. refringens, Treponema reiter, T. pallidum, Monilia,* or trichophytins. The authors suggested that human infection with *T. pallidum* resulted in a complex immune response in which CMI was depressed while humoral immunity remained intact. They also suggested that the depressed lymphocyte responsiveness was more generalized than originally thought.

From, Thestrup-Pedersen, and Thulin (11) studied three parameters of cell-mediated immunity in humans: skin reactivity, leukocyte migration, and lymphocyte transformation. They found reduced skin test reactivity during the early stages of syphilis. Lymphocyte reactivity in both the leukocyte migration test and lymphocyte transformation studies was reduced initially but was stimulated after the patients were treated. The authors suggested that the decrease in skin reactivity and in vitro lymphocyte response in syphilitics may be due to high antigen loads before treatment. They also suggested that plasma contains specific inhibitors of lymphocyte reactivity which might be responsible; however, they were unable to demonstrate the presence of plasma inhibitors if the plasma was frozen and thawed before study.

Friedman and Turk (12,13) reported on studies of syphilitic patients in England (1975) and Ethiopia (1978). The lymphocyte transformation test was used for both studies. Stimulating agents included *T. pallidum* sonicates, PHA, and purified protein derivative (PPD). In their studies using English patients, the researchers found that individuals with early primary seronegative syphilis and secondary syphilis with macular rash appeared to have diminished lymphocyte responses to both T. *pallidum* sonicates and PPD, whereas patients with seropositive primary syphilis and secondary syphilis with a papular rash appeared to have an enhanced response to T. *pallidum* in vitro. In their studies of syphilitic patients from Ethiopia, lymphocytes from patients with cardiovascular syphilis responded significantly to T. *pallidum* in vitro. Antibiotic therapy resulted in enhanced lymphocyte responsiveness to T. *pallidum* in vitro in about half the patients.

Friedman and Turk (13) attributed the difference between the disease in England and in Ethiopia to the fact that delayed hypersensitivity does not develop as frequently in Ethiopia as in Europe, as well as to possible differences in immunological responsiveness. They further suggested that many of the late complications of syphilis may be due to the tissue-damaging effects of delayed hypersensitivity reactions. Other factors which may explain the differences in the disease on the two continents may include (1) a concomitant infection with other organisms and (2) the effects of dietary factors related to foods and herbal medications taken by the Ethiopians.

Recent data from my laboratory using lymphoblastic transformation confirms data published earlier by others. Procedures for my research essentially follow those already published (14). In brief, lymphocytes were isolated from human peripheral blood by Ficoll Hypaque gradients. These were then cultured in the presence of mitogens or T. *pallidum* extracts for 5 days. Tritiated thymidine was added for the last 18 hr of culture. Lymphocytes were cultured either in the patient's serum (autologous serum) or in the serum from the normal control individual. Table 1 gives lymphocyte transformation data on three secondary syphilitic patients with Venereal Disease Research Laboratories (VDRL) tests. Data are expressed in terms of tritiated thymidine incorporation into DNA. Lymphocytes from patient 1 responded poorly to Concanavalin A (ConA) in autologous serum; however, their response to ConA in normal human serum was significant. These lymphocytes also responded poorly to T. *pallidum* extracts in vitro in autologous syphilitic serum or normal human serum. Patient 2 showed a similar pattern of diminished responsiveness to ConA in syphilitic serum, but a good response when cultures were established in normal human serum. Lymphocytes of patient 3 demonstrated depressed blast transformation responses to both ConA and T. *pallidum* extract when cultured in either syphilitic or normal serum. Lymphocytes taken from control individuals of the same age and cultured under the same conditions as syphilitic patients have good responses in normal human serum to ConA, but decreased responses when cultured in syphilitic serum. These normal lymphocytes failed to respond to T. *pallidum* extracts when cultured in either syphilitic or normal serum.

Table 2 gives blast transformation data from one patient with secondary syphilis studied just before antibiotic therapy and 2 weeks after

16. Cell-Mediated Immunity

Table 1 Effect of Concanavalin A and *T. pallidum* Extract on Blastic Transformation of Lymphocytes from Syphilitic and Normal Persons

	Syphilitic serum (cpm)[a]	Normal human serum (cpm)
Patient 1 (VDRL titer = 1:128) (untreated[b])		
ConA[c]	1,175	14,059
T. pallidum[d] control	4,454	388
	2,314	311
Patient 2 (VDRL titer = 1:164)		
ConA	4,171	25,860
T. pallidum control	1,427	372
	1,127	468
Patient 3 (VDRL titer = 1:128)		
ConA	420	1,693
T. pallidum control	115	80
	173	188
Control 1 (VDRL = NR)		
Con A	5,990	19,906
T. pallidum control	3,241	353
	5,887	397
Control 2 (VDRL = NR)		
ConA	13,709	58,157
T. pallidum control	1,188	588
	3,253	409
Control 3 (VDRL = NR)		
ConA	9,669	22,293
T. pallidum control	104	137
	334	252

[a] Counts per minute of tritiated thymidine.
[b] Patient blood drawn just prior to treatment.
[c] Concanavalin A concentration (10 μg) giving maximum stimulation.
[d] *Treponema pallidum* concentration (15 μg) giving maximum stimulation.

Table 2 Effect of Treatment on Blastic Transformation of Syphilitic and Normal Lymphocytes

Patient	Autologous (syphilitic) serum (cpm)[a]	Normal human serum (cpm)
Untreated		
ConA[b]	245	279
T. pallidum control[c]	252	133
	238	154
Normal control		
ConA	43,263	48,817
T. pallidum control	167	119
	206	162
Lymphocytes collected 2 weeks after treatment		
Treated		
ConA	53,650	71,454
T. pallidum control	20,854	8,939
	628	915
Normal control		
ConA	13,709	58,157
T. pallidum control	1,188	778
	2,837	409

[a]Counts per minute of tritiated thymidine.
[b]Concanavalin A concentration (10 µg) giving maximum stimulation.
[c]T. pallidum concentration (15 µg) giving maximum stimulation.

therapy. Before therapy, the patient's lymphocytes failed to respond to ConA or T. pallidum extracts in either syphilitic serum or normal serum. However, 2 weeks after treatment, a vigorous response was observed to both ConA and T. pallidum extracts. These data indicate that after treatment the patient's lymphocytes are capable of recognizing T. pallidum antigens and responding to these antigens in vitro. Also, syphilitic serum does not decrease lymphocyte responsiveness to T. pallidum extracts or the ability of ConA to stimulate lymphocytes in vitro.

These data, derived from a small number of patients with syphilis, appear to confirm earlier observations. It appears that early in syphilis, peripheral blood lymphocytes respond poorly to ConA and T. pallidum extracts and that the serum of syphilitic patients appears less effective in supporting responses of normal lymphocytes to ConA.

16. Cell-Mediated Immunity

After treatment, lymphocytes from syphilitics respond to both ConA and *T. pallidum* extracts and serum from syphilitic patients was capable of supporting normal lymphocytes responses to ConA.

Studies on *Treponema pallidum*-Infected Rabbits

Rabbits frequently serve as experimental models for the study of *T. pallidum* infection (15). Rabbits injected intratesticularly with viable *T. pallidum* (Nichols) develop a characteristic course of infection, beginning with an acute orchitis at 8-13 days (16,17). Most of the animals will show no lesions 30-35 days after injection of treponemes (16). In a few rabbits lesions will recur at some later date, but these occurrences are inconsistent and random. *Treponema pallidum*-infected rabbits develop both VDRL and fluorescent treponemal antibody absorption (FTA-ABS) antibodies which can be detected as early as 10 days after infection (17).

Several parameters of CMI have been studied in rabbits infected with *T. pallidum* (Nichols). These include histological studies, delayed hypersensitivity in the skin, macrophage migration inhibition, leukocyte migration, and lymphocyte transformation in vitro to both mitogens and specific antigens. There is considerable controversy concerning CMI in infected rabbits. Several investigations (15-19) have suggested that CMI may be impaired early in infection. Other studies (20-22) indicate intact CMI. Most of these studies were carried out using outbred rabbits and different culture conditions and preparations of antigen; therefore comparisons are difficult. In this section the work of several investigators will be discussed, with points of difference indicated.

Festenstein et al. (6) reported that infection of rabbits with *T. pallidum* prior to the second week of life resulted in a runting syndrome which ultimately brought on the premature death of the rabbits. Infected rabbits also had an increased number of histiocyte-like cells in the spleen while still having normal thymus glands. Depletion of lymphocytes in the white pulp areas of the spleens of these rabbits was also observed. It has been suggested that these data are consistent with depletion of lymphocytes in areas of the spleen thought to be thymus dependent (23,14).

Lymphocyte transformation in vitro is frequently used as an indicator of intact CMI in a variety of diseases (24-27). Pavia, Folds, and Baseman (16) reported that peripheral blood lymphocytes from rabbits bits infected with *T. pallidum* failed to respond to ConA in vitro. This observation was followed by other studies with phytohemagglutinin (PHA), pokeweed mitogen (PWM), and *Treponema phagedenis* biotype Reiter, in which lymphocyte responses were depressed (18). The depression of lymphocyte transformation was greatest during the first 34 days of infection. Although culturing lymphocytes in autologous serum (taken from an infected rabbit on the day lymphocytes were cultured) most effectively depressed mitogen responses, a lesser degree of depression was observed when cultures were established in either fetal calf serum or pooled normal serum. After 4 weeks of infection, normal levels of blastogenesis were usually observed.

Wicher and Wicher (17) reported similar findings in their study of the effects of PHA on PBL. They established cultures in 15% normal inactivated autologous rabbit serum. They found that the response to PHA was significantly suppressed only in lymphocytes from infected rabbits and that the maximal suppression was at about 30 days after infection. The authors (17) also discovered a significant increase in lymphocyte transformation in the presence of cardiolipin reagent 20 days after infection. This correlated well with the appearance of a maximum titer of Wassermann antibodies. The same workers also reported the production of a mitogenic factor in cultures of lymph node and spleen cells from infected rabbits that had been incubated in serum-free medium containing the Reiter protein. This factor found in supernatant cultures mentioned above was capable of stimulating blastogenesis in peripheral blood lymphocytes from normal rabbits.

Several investigators have also indicated the presence of a factor or factors in serum which block in vitro lymphocyte proliferation (16,18, 28,29). This factor is present in the greatest concentration during the height of orchitis (29) and disappears when the lesion subsides in most cases. It may, however, persist for as long as 6 months (28). In another experiment Wicher and Wicher (28) indicated that this factor was present in normal rabbit serum. According to Ware, Folds, and Baseman (29), it was present only in syphilitic serum and its effect was negated by greatly increasing the mitogen concentration. It was also possible to store serum at $-70\,°C$ and recover activity.

Recent results by Lukehart, Baker-Zander, and Sell (21) have failed to confirm the findings of studies on depressed lymphocyte transformation. These workers found that lymphoid cells from the spleen and lymph nodes from infected rabbits responded to both ConA and *T. pallidum*. All cultures were established in the presence of a pool of normal rabbit serum. These results partially correlate with data published by Maret, Baseman, and Folds (30) in their study of spleen and lymph node cells from *T. pallidum*-infected rabbits. In this study, cultures were established in both autologous serum and normal rabbit serum. In normal serum, both spleen and lymph node cells responded to ConA, PHA, and *T. pallidum*; however, in autologous serum responsiveness to *T. pallidum* antigens was depressed, while good responses to both PHA and ConA were observed. Hardy et al. (22) also reported that lymph node and spleen cells from infected rabbits responded to *T. pallidum* antigens and mitogens in vitro. Their cultures were performed in the presense of fetal calf serum. Lukehart et al. (21) offered several possible explanations for these differences in data. They suggested that peripheral blood lymphocytes may not be the preferred cells for a study of responsiveness, because T and B cells are not easily separated as in spleen and lymph nodes; i.e., T and B cells of peripheral blood share many of the same surface characteristics (31). Also, the later appearance of sensitized lymphocytes in peripheral blood may reflect the sequestering of these cells at the site of infection and in regional lymph nodes (32). It is also important to consider the source of serum used in establishing the lymphocyte culture. Autologous serum has a profound effect on the responsiveness of lymphocytes to either mitogens or specific *T. pallidum* antigens. Normal rabbit serum in many instances enhances responsiveness of lymphocytes, whereas fetal calf serum may stimulate lymphocyte transformation (33).

Schell and Musher presented evidence for the stimulation of cell-mediated immunity in syphilis (34). They gave indirect evidence for the presence of CMI by demonstrating that infecting rabbits with *T. pallidum* renders them resistant to challenge with *Listeria monocytogenes*. This indirect demonstration of acquired cellular resistance was first reported by Blanden and co-workers (35). This enhanced ability to kill an unrelated organisms, presumably due to activation of macrophages, was demonstrated between 3 and 5 weeks after infection with *T. pallidum*. The researchers suggested that activation of macrophages and CMI may be associated with latency. Schell and Musher (36) further demonstrated that acquired cellular resistance (ACR) could be transferred using spleen cells from *T. pallidum*-infected rabbits. They further showed that treatment of spleen cells from *T. pallidum*-infected rabbits with antithymus serum could abolish the listeriocidal effects (37). This was further evidence that infection with *T. pallidum* stimulated CMI.

Other studies by Baughn et al. (38), Graves and Johnson (39), and Graves (40) demonstrated that activation of macrophages by *Mycobacterium bovis*, bacille Calmette-Guérin (BCG), or *Propionibacterium acnes* failed to kill *T. pallidum* but was sufficient to prevent the growth of *Listeria*. These authors concluded that macrophages probably do not participate in host resistance to *T. pallidum* infection. More recently, however, Hardy et al. (41) presented evidence that prior sensitization of rabbits to BCG followed by simultaneous injection of BCG and *T. pallidum* modified the course of treponemal infection. These findings suggested that local macrophage activation modified the experimental infection and also suggested a similar role for CMI. In vitro studies by Lukehart (Chap. 18), which showed treponeme-like structures in macrophages following in vitro incubation, may provide support for this concept.

Inhibition of leukocyte migration in the presence of specific antigen has been reported to be an in vitro measure of CMI (25). In this test migration inhibition is measured using either peripheral blood leukocytes or sensitized lymphocytes and guinea pig peritoneal exudate macrophages. The lymphocytes are placed in capillary tubes or soft agarose along with specific antigen and incubated for 24-48 hr. At the end of incubation, the migration of cells out of the capillary tube is measured in both cultures containing antigen and control cultures without antigen. Inhibition of migration in the presence of antigen characterizes intact cell-mediated immunity. Wicher and Wicher (19) studied leukocyte migration inhibition in rabbits experimentally infected with *T. pallidum* antigen. They reported that in early stages of infection, low concentrations of Reiter protein, *T. pallidum* antigen, and VDRL antigen stimulate migration. In later stages, after the fourth week, inhibition of migration was observed. Metzger et al. (42) demonstrated similar results using macrophage migration inhibition. They observed an inhibition of migration in the presence of *T. pallidum* antigen 1 month after infection and up to 4 to 6 months. Pavia et al. (43) also demonstrated stimulation of macrophage migration early after *T. pallidum* infection; however, they observed an inhibition between 3 and 15 weeks after infection. The antigen used for these studies was *T. phagedenis* biotype Reiter at concentrations of 3 to 25 mg protein.

Results from these leukocyte migration inhibition studies suggest that CMI may be delayed in developing during the early stages of experimental *T. pallidum* infection in rabbits. These results are consistent with findings using delayed hypersensitivity skin testing and in vitro lymphocyte transformation studies.

The immune response to a *T. pallidum* infection is complex and may be different from responses to other microbes. As previously discussed, humoral antibodies are produced early after infection, but activation of effective CMI seems to be delayed. Perhaps CMI is related to the development of latent syphilis, but the exact mechanisms are not understood. Several possible explanations may be given for the delay.

1. It is possible that delayed activation of T-cell responses may occur. This may prevent adequate early host responses to the antigens of *T. pallidum* which would permit establishment of the organism in the host. The data obtained from studies that showed differences in reactivity to mitogens and antigens from animals infected by different routes of infection may explain this. Results from experiments using peripheral blood demonstrate reactivities to mitogens and antigens different from those seen with spleen or lymph node cells.

2. Virulent treponemes may possess a slime layer (44) which helps protect the treponemes from host defenses or prevent activation of certain populations or subpopulations of lymphocytes. Fitzgerald and Johnson (45) recently reported on the nature of surface mucopolysaccharides of *T. pallidum* and suggested that the complex at the surface may interfere with antitreponemal antibodies. Alderete and Baseman (46) demonstrated surface-associated host proteins on *T. pallidum* which were acquired immediately after infection. It was suggested that these proteins may serve to protect the treponeme against host defenses by masking treponemal antigens. This type of surface coat

may serve to protect the treponeme against phagocytosis and other defense mechanisms and may also be associated with survival of the organisms through the primary and secondary phases of the disease. Alderete and Baseman (46) have also suggested that the presence of host treponemal proteins may induce autoimmune phenomena by coating the treponeme with IgG or IgM and eliciting responses against the host's own immunoglobulins. Rheumatoid factors and cryoglobulins have been detected in syphilitic serum (47,48). Furthermore, Bey et al. (49) showed that the testicular fluid and serum from rabbits infected intratesticularly with *T. pallidum* inhibited the mitogenic response of normal rabbit peripheral blood lymphocytes to Concanavalin A. They suggested that this was due to the presence of the mucopolysaccharide material present in the testicular fluid. It was also suggested that mucopolysaccharide material present in *T. pallidum*-infected rabbits may be the inhibitory factor responsible for suppression of mitogen stimulation of rabbit peripheral blood lymphocytes in vitro (49). It is possible that treponemal mucopolysaccharides and/or host protein on the surface of the treponeme may give rise to a transient suppression of lymphocyte responses during the early stages of infection. It is conceivable that these types of mechanisms protect the treponeme, allowing it to become established in the host.

3. Immune complexes may prevent early activation of T lymphocytes and cell-mediated immunity. Baughn and Musher (50) suggested that immune complexes may be involved in delaying immune responses to *T. pallidum*. They also showed that humoral immunity to T-dependent antigen (sheep erythrocytes) was depressed if rabbits were injected with *T. pallidum* and sheep erythrocytes simultaneously. Baughn and Musher (51) suggested several possibilities to explain this lack of responsiveness, such as immune complex formation, interference of mucoid material with phagocytosis by macrophages, and/or the overloading of macrophages. Sølling et al. (52) demonstrated the presence of immune complexes in a case of syphilitic nephropathy and suggested that immune complexes may be involved in immunopathogenesis of syphilitic nephropathy. Furthermore, Baughn, Musher, and Tung (53) presented evidence that artificial immune complexes were capable of suppressing immune responsiveness in vitro.

4. Several investigators have reported the presence of plasma factors which may influence CMI. Plasma factors have been reported which will suppress transformation of normal or syphilitic lymphocytes by PHA (4,28) or ConA (16,29). One such factor is present only during primary or secondary syphilis and is lost upon storage at 4 or 20 °C (29). This serum factor, which is sensitive to trypsin, is distinct from the one which blocks ConA responsiveness described by Bey et al. (49).

5. It is also conceivable that *T. pallidum* infection stimulates the formation of suppressor T lymphocytes, as suggested by Pavia, Folds, and Baseman (14), and perhaps localization of treponemes is related to

an inhibition of suppressor T lymphocytes. There is no proof for this hypothesis at the present time.

6. Since *T. pallidum* persist in patients and experimentally infected animals in the presence of humoral antibodies, it is possible that blocking antibodies may exist during *T. pallidum* infection (54). These antibodies may block the early CMI responses and prevent cell-mediated immune mechanisms from removing the infecting agent. At the present time a clear understanding of immune mechanisms does not exist. Much of the existing data from human experiments and rabbit models is in conflict and more definition of the immune response is necessary.

In conclusion, despite a great deal of recent effort, it is apparent that the exact mechanisms of host-parasite interactions in syphilitic infection have eluded our understanding. The recent exciting observation of Klein et al. (55) on the growth of *T. pallidum* in mice provides a new model for study. The inbred mouse has many advantages, most notably, a well-defined immunological response, and should give opportunity to study immunity under carefully defined conditions.

Acknowledgments

The author wishes to acknowledge the collaboration of Dr. Joel Baseman, Dr. Charles Pavia, Dr. Melissa Maret, and Dr. Joy Ware. The technical assistance of Ms. Ann Rauchbach and the secretarial assistance of Ms. Sue McFarland and Ms. Susan Moore is also greatfully acknowledged. The editorial assistance of Mr. Alvin Hall is appreciated. This work was supported in part by the North Carolina Program Project on Sexually Transmitted Diseases.

The literature search for this chapter was completed in March 1980.

References

1. D. M. Musher and R. F. Schell. The Immunology of syphilis. *Int. J. Dermatology* 15:566 (1976).
2. H. Noguchi. A cutaneous reaction in syphilis. *J. Exp. Med.* 14:577 (1911).
3. H. E. Michelson. The superficial lymph glands in early syphilis. *Arch. Dermatol. Syphilol.* 25:457 (1932).
3A. J. Thivolet, A. Simeray, M. Rolland, and F. Challut. Etude de l'intradermoréaction aux suspensions de tréponèmes formolées (souche Nichols pathogène) chez les syphilitiques et les sujets normaux. *Ann. Inst. Pasteur Lille* 85:23 (1953).
4. G. M. Levene, J. L. Turk, D. J. M. Wright, and A. G. S. Grimble. Reduced lymphocyte transformation due to a plasma factor in patients with active syphilis. *Lancet* 3:246 (1969).

5. G. M. Levene, D. J. M. Wright, and J. L. Turk. Cell-mediated immunity and lymphocyte transformation in syphilis. *Proc. R. Soc. Med.* 64:426 (1971).
6. H. Festenstein, C. Abrahams, and V. Bokkenhauser. Runting syndrome in neonatal rabbits infected with *Treponema pallidum*. *Clin. Exp. Immunol.* 2:311 (1967).
7. K. W. M. Fulford and J. Brostoff. Leukocyte migration and cell-mediated immunity. *Br. J. Vener. Dis.* 48:483 (1972).
8. M. Soborg. *In vitro* detection of cellular hypersensitivity in man. Specific migration inhibition of white blood cells from brucella positive persons. *Acta Med. Scand.* 182:167 (1967).
9. D. M. Musher, R. F. Schell, and J. M. Knox. *In vitro* lymphocyte response to *Treponema refringens* in human syphilis. *Infect. Immun.* 9:654 (1974).
10. D. M. Musher, R. F. Schell, R. H. Jones, and A. M. Jones. Lymphocyte transformation in syphilis: An *in vitro* correlate of immune suppression *in vivo*? *Infect. Immun.* 11:1261 (1975).
11. E. From, K. Thestrup-Pedersen, and H. Thulin. Reactivity of lymphocytes from patients with syphilis towards *T. pallidum* antigen in the leukocytes migration and lymphocyte transformation tests. *Br. J. Vener. Dis.* 52:224 (1976).
12. P. S. Friedman and J. L. Turk. A spectrum of lymphocyte responsiveness in human syphilis. *Clin. Exp. Immunol.* 21:59 (1975).
13. P. S. Friedman and J. L. Turk. The role of cell-mediated immune mechanisms in syphilis in Ethiopia. *Clin. Exp. Immunol.* 31:59 (1978).
14. C. S. Pavia, J. D. Folds, and J. B. Baseman. Cell-mediated immunity during syphilis: A review. *Br. J. Vener. Dis.* 54:144 (1978).
15. A. M. Payne. Treponematoses research. *WHO Tech. Rep.* 445:5 (1970).
16. C. S. Pavia, J. D. Folds, and J. B. Baseman. Depression of lymphocyte response to concanavalin A in rabbits infected with *Treponema pallidum* (Nichols). *Infect. Immun.* 14:320 (1976).
17. V. Wicher and K. Wicher. *In vitro* cell response of *Treponema pallidum*-infected rabbits. I. Lymphocyte transformation. *Clin. Exp. Immunol.* 24:480 (1977).
18. C. S. Pavia, J. B. Baseman, and J. D. Folds. Selective response of lymphocytes from *Treponema pallidum*-infected rabbits to mitogens and *Treponema reiteri*. *Infect. Immun.* 15:417 (1977).
19. V. Wicher and K. Wicher. Cell response in rabbits infected with *T. pallidum* as measured by the leukocyte migration inhibition test. *Br. J. Vener. Dis.* 51:241 (1975).
20. S. Sell. The rabbit immune system: Characterization of cell surface markers and functional properties of rabbit lymphocytes. *Mol. Immunol.* 16:1045 (1979).

21. S. A. Lukehart, S. A. Baker-Zander, and S. Sell. Characterization of lymphocyte responsiveness in early experimental syphilis. I. In vitro response to mitogens and T. pallidum antigens. J. Immunol. 124:454 (1980).
22. P. H. Hardy, E. E. Nell, J. R. Klein, and R. A. Dredergast. Specific stimulation of cells from various lymphoid tissues of rabbits with early syphilitic infection. 18th Interscience Conference on Antimicrobial Agents and Chemotherapy, Abstract No. 197 (1978).
23. D. M. V. Parrott, M. A. de Sousa, and J. East. Thymus-dependent areas in the lymphoid organs of neonatally thymectomized mice. J. Exp. Med. 123:191 (1966).
24. F. S. Kantor. Infection, anergy and cell-mediated immunity. N. Engl. J. Med. 292:629 (1975).
25. R. Rocklin. Mediators of cellular immunity, In Basic and Clinical Immunology, 2nd ed. (H. Fudenberg, D. Stites, J. Caldwell, J. Wells, Eds.). Lange Medical Publications, Los Altos, California, 1978, p. 128.
26. A. Fleer, M. Van Der Hart, B. J. T. Blok-Schut, and P. T. A. Schellekens. Correlation of PPD and BCG-induced leukocyte migration inhibition, delayed cutaneous hypersensitivity, lymphocyte transformation in vitro and humoral antibodies to PPD in man. Eur. J. Immunol. 6:163 (1976).
27. M. G. Whitaker and C. G. Clark. Depressed lymphocyte function in carcinoma of the breast. Br. J. Surg. 58:717 (1971).
28. V. Wicher and K. Wicher. In vitro cell response of Treponema pallidum infected rabbits. II. Inhibition of lymphocyte response to phytohemagglutinin by serum of T. pallidum-infected rabbits. Clin. Exp. Immunol. 29:487 (1977).
29. J. L. Ware, J. D. Folds, and J. B. Baseman. Serum of rabbits infected with Treponema pallidum (Nichols) inhibits in vitro transformation of normal lymphocytes. Cell. Immunol. 42:363 (1979).
30. S. M. Maret, J. B. Baseman, and J. D. Folds. Cell-mediated immunity in Treponema pallidum infected rabbits: In vitro response of splenic and lymph node lymphocytes to mitogens and specific antigens. Clin. Exp. Immunol. 39:38 (1980).
31. H. W. Sheppard, D. Redelman, and S. Sell. In vitro studies of the rabbit immune system. II. Differential mitogen responses of isolate T and B cells. Cell. Immunol. 24:34 (1976).
32. S. A. Lukehart, S. A. Baker-Zander, R. M. Cheri Lloyd, and S. Sell. Characterization of lymphocyte responsiveness in early experimental syphilis. II. Nature of cellular infiltration and Treponema pallidum distribution in testicular lesions. J. Immunol. 124:461 (1980).
33. A. Coutinho and G. Moller. Thymus-independent B-cell induction and paralysis. Adv. Immunol. 21:113 (1975).
34. R. F. Schell and D. M. Musher. Detection of non-specific resistance to Listeria monocytogenes in rabbits infected with Treponema pallidum. Infect. Immun. 9:658 (1974).

35. R. V. Blanden, M. J. Lefford, and G. B. Mackaness. The host response to Calmette-Guérin Bacillus in mice. *J. Exp. Med. 129*: 1079 (1969).
36. R. F. Schell and D. M. Musher. Transfer of non-specific resistance to *Listeria monocytogenes* using spleen cells from syphilitic rabbits. *Proc. Soc. Exp. Biol. Med. 148*:516 (1975).
37. R. F. Schell, D. M. Musher, K. Jacobson, and P. Schwethelm. Induction of acquired cellular resistance following transfer of thymus-dependent lymphocytes from syphilitic rabbits. *J. Immunol. 114*:550 (1975).
38. R. E. Baughn, D. M. Musher, and J. M. Knox. Effect of sensitization with *Propionibacterium acnes* on the growth of *Listeria monocytogenes* and *Treponema pallidum* in rabbits. *J. Immunol. 118*:109 (1977).
39. S. R. Graves and R. C. Johnson. Effect of pretreatment with *Mycobacterium bovis* (strain BCG) and immune syphilitic serum on rabbit resistance to *Treponema pallidum*. *Infect. Immun. 12*:1029 (1975).
40. S. Graves. Susceptibility of rabbits to *Treponema pallidum* after infection with *Mycobacterium bovis*. *Br. J. Vener. Dis. 55*:394 (1979).
41. P. Hardy, D. Graham, E. Nell, and A. Dannenberg. Macrophages in immunity to syphilis: Suppressive effect of concurrent infection with *Mycobacterium bovis* BCG on the development of syphilitic lesions and growth of *Treponema pallidum* in tuberculin-positive rabbits. *Infect. Immun. 26*:751 (1979).
42. M. Metzger, J. Podiwinska, and W. Smogor. Cell-mediated immunity in experimental syphilis in rabbits. *Arch. Immunol. Ther. Exp. Engl. Transl. 25*:25 (1977).
43. C. S. Pavia, J. D. Folds, and J. B. Baseman. Development of macrophage migration inhibition in rabbits infected with virulent *Treponema pallidum*. *Infect. Immun. 17*:651 (1977).
44. J. A. Zeigler, A. M. Jones, R. H. Jones, and K. M. Kubica. Demonstration of extracellular material at the surface of pathogenic *T. pallidum* cells. *Br. J. Vener. Dis. 52*:1 (1976).
45. T. J. Fitzgerald and R. C. Johnson. Surface mucopolysaccharides of *Treponema pallidum*. *Infect. Immun. 24*:244 (1979).
46. J. F. Alderete and J. B. Baseman. Surface-associated host proteins of virulent *Treponema pallidum*. *Infect. Immun. 26*:1048 (1979).
47. K. K. Mustakallio, A. Lassus, and O. Wager. Autoimmune phenomena in syphilitic infection: Rheumatoid factor and cryoglobulins in different stages of syphilis. *Int. Arch. Allergy 31*:417 (1967).
48. A. Peltier and C. L. Christian. The presence of the "rheumatoid factor" in sera from patients with syphilis arthritis and rheumatism. *Arthritis Rheum. 11*:1 (1959).

49. R. F. Bey, R. C. Johnson, and T. J. Fitzgerald. Suppression of lymphocyte response to concanavalin A by mucopolysaccharide material from *Treponema pallidum*-infected rabbits. *Infect. Immun.* 26:64 (1979).
50. R. E. Baughn and D. M. Musher. Altered immune responsiveness associated with experimental syphilis in the rabbit: Elevated IgM and depressed IgG responses to sheep erythrocytes. *J. Immunol.* 120:1691 (1978).
51. R. E. Baughn and D. M. Musher. Aberrant secondary antibody responses to sheep erythrocytes in rabbits with experimental syphilis. *Infect. Immun.* 25:133 (1979).
52. J. Sølling, K. Sølling, K. U. Jacobsen, S. Olsen, and E. From. Circulating immune complexes in syphilitic nephropathy. *Br. J. Vener. Dis.* 54:53 (1978).
53. R. E. Baughn, K. S. K. Tung, and D. M. Musher. Detection of circulating immune complexes in the sera of rabbits with experimental syphilis: possible role in immunoregulation. *Infect. Immun.* 29:575 (1980).
54. I. Hellstrom and K. E. Hellstrom. Immunological enhancement as studied by cell culture techniques. *Annu. Rev. Microbiol.* 24:373 (1970).
55. J. R. Klein, A. A. Monjan, P. H. Hardy, and G. A. Cole. Abrogation of genetically controlled resistance of mice to *Treponema pallidum* by irradiation. *Nature* 238:572 (1980).

17
T-Cell-Mediated Resistance

RONALD F. SCHELL,
JOHN K. CHAN,* and
JACK L. LEFROCK
Division of Infectious Diseases and Clinical Microbiology
Hahnemann University School of Medicine
Philadelphia, Pennsylvania

Indirect Evidence for T-Cell Involvement 332
Direct Evidence for T-Cell Involvement 333
Summary 343
References 343

The course of treponemal infection and its eventual resolution are associated with the development of both humoral and cell-mediated responses. However, the precise roles these defense mechanisms play in eliminating virulent treponemes from the host's tissue are not clearly understood. The humoral immune response appears to afford only modest protection. Injection of large quantities of immune serum, or daily injections of purified immunogloblin G from convalescent rabbits, delayed the appearance or diminished the severity of lesions in newly infected animals (1-7), but immune serum did not prevent the establishment of infection, even though serum was administered before treponemal challenge (1-8). This finding suggests that humoral responses do not decide the outcome of treponemal infection.

Present affiliation: Memorial Hospital Medical Center of Long Beach, Long Beach, California

Indirect Evidence for T-Cell Involvement

The importance of cell-mediated (T-cell-dependent) immunity in control of treponemal infection has been inferred from several clinical and experimental observations:

1. Skin testing of patients with latent or tertiary syphilis elicited delayed-type hypersensitivity responses to treponemal antigens (9-11). Delayed-type hypersensitivity is used frequently to assess the development of cell-mediated immunity.
2. The gumma, a chronic lesion of late syphilis, is characterized by massive infiltration of lymphocytes and macrophages (12), similar to cell-mediated infections such as tuberculosis (13) and brucellosis (14).
3. Lymphocytes are depleted in the thymus-derived areas of the spleen in congenital syphilis in man and in the lymph nodes of patients with late primary, secondary, and early latent syphilis (15). Similar observations have been made in neonatal rabbits infected with *Treponema pallidum* (16).
4. Dysfunction of T cells in syphilitic animals has been shown by the inability of infected rabbits to respond normally to stimulation with sheep erythrocytes, a T-dependent antigen (17,18). Syphilitic rabbits were resistant, however, to challenge with *Listeria monocytogenes*, an organism commonly used to monitor the development of acquired cellular resistance (19). This nonspecific resistance to *Listeria* could be conferred on recipient rabbits and abrogated by treating cells with antirabbit thymocyte serum and complement (20,21).
5. Rabbits have been successfully vaccinated with viable, irradiated treponemes against challenge with *T. pallidum* (22). Classically, live vaccines have been more efficacious in inducing resistance against organisms that are associated with cell-mediated immunity (23,24).

Several in vitro methods for assessing lymphocyte responsiveness have also provided evidence for a role of cell-mediated immunity in syphilis. Patients with primary and secondary syphilis responded poorly to T-cell mitogens, treponemal antigens, and such nontreponemal antigens as *Candida*, *Trichophyton*, and tuberculin (25-30). Lymphocytes from syphilitic rabbits were less reactive to specific T-cell mitogens, while responses to classical B-cell mitogens remained normal (31-33). Inhibition of macrophage migration, an in vitro correlate of cell-mediated immunity, has also been reported to occur in tissues from patients with late or congenital syphilis (29,34) and from treponemal rabbits (35-37).

These approaches, however, have fallen short of proving that cell-mediated responses are involved in protection against treponemal infection. A significant effort was made by Metzger et al. (38) to correlate the appearance and extent of inhibition of macrophage migration with the ability of immunized rabbits to resist challenge to *T. pallidum*. No correlation was found: Immune or partially immune rabbits resisted challenge to *T. pallidum*, but their lymphocytes exerted only an equivocal effect on macrophage migration. Metzger also attempted to define the protective role of cell-mediated immunity in syphilis by using the immunosuppressive agent cyclophosphamide (39). Treatment of rabbits with cyclophosphamide prior to challenge with *T. pallidum* completely abolished their cell-mediated response (inhibition of macrophage migration), yet the production of nonspecific and specific treponemal antibodies was not affected. The severity of the lesions in the treated rabbits was given as additional support for a protective role of cell-mediated responses in syphilis.

Direct Evidence for T-Cell Involvement

The most direct method to determine the role of cell-mediated immunity in resistance would be to confer resistance on normal recipients with immune cells from animals resistant to treponemal infection. Metzger and Smogor (40) have demonstrated that such protection can be conferred. Normal outbred rabbits infused with syphilitic immune lymph node cells were partially protected from a subsequent intradermal challenge with *T. pallidum*. Adoptively immunized rabbits had fewer lesions and a significant delay in their appearance, compared to rabbits that received normal lymphocytes or no cells. Although these studies were performed with outbred rabbits, the authors concluded that protection was due to cell-mediated immunity. By contrast, Baughn et al. (41) observed that immunity against chancres could not be transferred to inbred rabbits with spleen cells from syngeneic rabbits resistant to rechallenge with *T. pallidum*. Recipients of immune cells developed syphilitic lesions indistinguishable from those in controls. The inbredness of these rabbits was verified by mixed-leukocyte reactions, and the transferability of cell-mediated responses was proven by parallel experiments with tuberculin. The authors concluded that cell-mediated mechanisms do not play a central role in immunity to syphilis.

The differing ability of lymph node and spleen cells to confer immunity may account in part for the contradictory results obtained by these investigators. A higher proportion of either T or B cells may be found in lymph nodes than in spleen cells obtained from rabbits infected with *T. pallidum*. The proportion of T and B cells in the population of cells transferred was not determined by either set of investigators. Another explanation may be the so-called allogenic effect: the protection observed by Metzger and Smogor (40) may have resulted from cooperation between the transferred syphilitic immune cells and the recipients' immunologically competent system.

Attempts to elucidate the mechanisms by which animals respond to treponemal infection have been hindered by the unavailability of suitable inbred animals. Treponemal disease cannot be regularly induced in guinea pigs (42) or mice (43-47), although some success has been achieved with inbred strains (42,48). Inbred rabbits can regularly develop clinical manifestations of syphilis (41), but commercially inbred rabbits are difficult to obtain. This unavailability of suitable inbred strains of animals compromises immunologic studies involving the transfer of acquired resistance to treponemal infection. Survival of treponemal immune cells cannot be guaranteed in recipient outbred animals due to allogenic differences.

Inbred hamsters, however, are readily available. They become infected with *T. pallidum* Bosnia A or *Treponema pertenue*, the causative agents of endemic syphilis and frambesia (yaws) respectively (49,50), and develop cutaneous lesions which persist for 6 to 9 months (Chap. 7). For example, LSH hamsters infected with 4×10^5 *T. pallidum* Bosnia A developed an erythematous reaction at the inoculation site 3 weeks after infection. Within 24 to 48 hr the skin ulcerated and became a large crusted lesion or an open lesion, while the periphery of the lesions continued to expand. The timing of the appearance and resolution of these lesions varied with the size of the inoculum. The infected hamsters' lymph nodes also increased significantly in weight and contained sizable numbers of treponemes for several weeks. Similar responses were observed in CB hamsters infected with *T. pertenue* (49). In addition, CB and LSH hamsters infected with either *T. pallidum* Bosnia A or *T. pertunue* for 10 to 16 weeks were resistant to reinfection with homologous or heterologous virulent treponemes (49,50).

The ability to acquire resistance to reinfection and produce pathologic changes which are amenable to quantitation makes the hamster an ideal model to define the mechanism of resistance to treponemal infection. The following studies—all performed with inbred hamsters—were designed to determine the ability of immune cells from convalescent donors to confer protection against treponemal infection upon syngeneic recipients. Leukocytes were administered whole or as purified populations enriched for B or T lymphocytes to define the contributions of these cell types in the modulation of resistance to treponemal infection. The protocols for these studies have been described in detail elsewhere (51-55).

A large group of hamsters was infected intradermally in the inguinal region with 10^5 *T. pallidum* Bosnia A. Cutaneous lesions characteristic of syphilitic infection developed in all animals 24 to 30 days after infection. A total of 4 months after infection the hamsters were treated with 4000 units of penicillin to terminate syphilitic infection. After another 2 weeks five hamsters were reinfected intradermally with *T. pallidum* Bosnia A and were shown to be resistant to the development of further syphilitic lesions. Immune spleen cells were obtained from 30 of these hamsters 16 days after treatment with penicillin. Concomitantly, normal cells were obtained from 30 age-matched hamsters treated with penicillin.

Normal hamsters were then injected intravenously with pooled normal or immune cells (10^8 per animal) and challenged intradermally with 10^4 T. pallidum Bosnia A. No syphilitic lesions were detected in hamsters that had received immune cells, and their lymph node weights were significantly lower ($P < 0.001$) than those of recipients of normal cells (Table 1). The number of treponemes in their lymph nodes, although sizable (1.2×10^5), was significantly lower ($P < .001$) than for recipients of normal cells.

Similarly Guerraz et al. (56) presented preliminary evidence that resistance to *Treponema fribourg blanc* can be conferred on inbred hamsters with cells from immune donors. Normal or immune lymphoid (spleen and lymph node) cells were transferred intraperitoneally to isogenic recipients, which were infected with *T. fribourg blanc* 8 days later by inguinal scarification. Within 40 ± 3 days all animals developed cutaneous lesions. Spontaneous remission of lesions occurred in 60% of animals that had received immune cells, compared to 16% of animal infusion with normal cells.

These results clearly demonstrate that immune cells can confer resistance to treponemal infection on recipient hamsters.

Table 1 Influence of Transferred Immune Spleen Cells on Pathology of Recipient Hamsters 48 days After Challenge with *Treponema pallidum* Bosnia A

		Lymph nodes	
Experimental group (N = 4 per group)	Number of hamsters developing lesions	Weight (mg)[a]	Mean number of treponemes per node ($\times 10^4$)
Recipients of			
Immune cells	0	15 ± 4	12
Normal cells	4	52 ± 6	101
Donors of			
Immune cells	0	18 ± 1	0
Normal cells	4	72 ± 4	153

[a]Mean $\pm$ SD.
Source: Reference 52.

Further evidence of the importance of cell-mediated immunity in treponemal infection is the inability of syphilitic immune cells to transfer resistance when preincubated with a specific anti-hamster-thymocyte serum and complement (Table 2). No significant differences were found in the time of development of syphilitic lesions by recipients of immune spleen cells or normal spleen cells, each treated with antithymocyte serum. As a corollary the lymph node weights and the number of treponemes detected there were not significantly different for these groups. Similar results were obtained after treatment of frambesial immune cells with antithymocyte serum and complement (53). All recipients of immune cells treated with antithymocyte serum had cutaneous lesions 21 days after frambesial infection, in contrast to recipients of immune cells treated with normal rabbit serum (Table 3). However, their lymph node weights and numbers of treponemes were significantly ($P < 0.001$) lower than in hamsters infused with normal cells treated with either antithymocyte serum or normal rabbit serum. These results show that cells susceptible to antithymocyte serum are involved in resistance to treponemal infection.

Successful transfer of resistance with immune cells and inhibition of this ability by treatment with antithymocyte serum does not mean that resistance is dependent upon T cells. These results cannot exclude a role for B cells. The transferred immune cells might include a population of antibody-producing cells which have a treponemicidal or treponemistatic effect. Likewise, treatment of immune cells with antithymocyte serum would bring into play its cytolytic activity against helper T cells and might thus inhibit the development of protective antibodies in recipients. Such influence of T cells on the development of antibody is well documented (57).

We therefore sought more direct evidence for T-cell involvement in treponemal infection. Various populations of lymphocytes were separated without killing the T cells. These preparations were enriched for T cells by passage through glass and nylon-wool columns, a fractionation procedure which has been shown to remove T cells and macrophages from cell preparations in hamsters (58) and mice (59).

In a double-blind study 35 hamsters were infected intradermally in the inguinal region with 10^6 T. pertenue. After 16 weeks the animals were treated with penicillin (4000 units) to terminate infection. Immune spleen and lymph node cells were obtained from 30 of these hamsters 16 days after treatment with penicillin. No treponemes were observed in the suspensions of immune cells. The remaining hamsters were reinfected with T. pertenue and did not develop cutaneous lesions.

Suspensions of pooled immune or normal lymphoid cells, unfractionated or B-cell depleted, were transferred intravenously (7×10^7 viable cells per hamster). Although inbred hamsters were used, all recipients were preirradiated as an additional measure to preclude cooperation between transferred cells and the recipients' immune system. Hamsters

Table 2 Effect of Antithymocyte Serum on the Ability of Immune Spleen Cells to Confer Resistance to T. pallidum Bosnia A

Experimental group[a] (N = 4 per group)	Lesions		Lymph nodes	
	Number of hamsters developing lesions	Development time (days)[b]	Weight (mg)[c]	Mean number of treponemes per node ($\times 10^4$)
Recipients of				
Immune cells, untreated	0	0	15 ± 4	12
Immune cells, ATS treated	4	24 ± 3	80 ± 5	318
Normal cells, untreated	4	30 ± 5	52 ± 6	101
Normal cells, ATS treated	4	25 ± 2	67 ± 3	224
Donors of				
Immune cells	0	0	18 ± 1	0
Normal cells	4	28 ± 4	72 ± 4	153

[a] ATS = antithymocyte serum plus complement.
[b] Mean ± SE.
[c] Mean ± SD; the SE for each mean was 0.011.
Source: Reference 52.

Table 3 Effect of Antithymocyte Serum on the Ability of Immune Cells to Confer Resistance to *T. pertenue*[a]

Experimental group[b] (N = 6 per group)	Number of hamsters developing lesions	Lymph nodes	
		Weight (mg)[c]	Number of treponemes per node ($\times 10^4$)
Recipients of:			
Immune cells, NRS treated	0	7 ± 1	2 ± 1
Immune cells, ATS treated	6	43 ± 4	19 ± 4
Normal cells, NRS treated	6	64 ± 7	98 ± 9
Normal cells, ATS treated	6	71 ± 4	84 ± 4
Donors of			
Immune cells	0	34 ± 3	2 ± 2
Normal cells	6	85 ± 5	462 ± 9

[a]At 21 days after infection.
[b]NRS = normal rabbit serum, ATS = antithymocyte serum plus complement.
[c]Mean ± SD.
Source: Reference 53.

were reconstituted with 6×10^7 bone marrow cells from a normal hamster. The recipient hamsters were subsequently infected intradermally with 10^6 *T. pertenue*.

To determine whether suspensions of frambesial immune cells depleted of B cells could confer resistance, four groups of hamsters were experimentally infected with *T. pertenue*. Within 8 days all these animals developed cutaneous lesions. The lesions gradually enlarged and became necrotic. In animals that had received suspensions of immune cells, either fractionated or depleted of B cells; the lesions regressed and were completely healed by 21 days after infection (Table 4). At that time all recipients were sacrificed. The lymph nodes of hamsters that had received B-cell-depleted or unfractionated immune cells weighed less and contained significantly fewer treponemes than those in animals that had received normal cells. These results show that B-cell-depleted immune cell suspensions are capable of conferring resistance to challenge with *T. pertenue*.

17. T-Cell-Mediated Resistance

A similar experiment yielded direct evidence for involvement of T cells in host defense against syphilitic infection. Irradiated, bone marrow-reconstituted hamsters received suspensions of B-cell-depleted or unfractionated cells from normal hamsters or from hamsters immune to infection with *T. pallidum* Bosnia A. A fifth group received only bone marrow cells. In the two groups that had received immune cells, B-cell-depleted or unfractionated, no lesions were detected 24 days after infection (Table 5). In the other three groups all animals had lesions. Similarly, the lymph nodes of animals that had received immune cells, B-cell-depleted or unfractionated, had significantly lower weights and fewer treponemes than those of animals that had received normal lymphoid cells or bone marrow cells. Thus immune cell suspensions depleted of B cells closely resembled the unfractionated suspensions in their ability to confer resistance to syphilitic infection. These results confirmed that T cells can confer protection on hamsters against treponemal infection.

To verify that our suspensions of fractionated lymphocytes were highly enriched in T cells, we incubated them—as well as suspensions of the unfractionated immune cells—with antithymocyte serum in the presence of complement, antihamster immunoglobulin, or classical T- or B-cell mitogens. For cells treated with both rabbit antihamster immunoglobulin and fluorescein-labeled goat antirabbit immunoglobulin,

Table 4 Ability of B-Cell-Depleted Suspensions of Immune Spleen Cells to Confer Resistance to *T. pertenue* in X-Irradiated, Bone Marrow-Reconstituted Hamsters[a]

		Lymph nodes	
Recipients of (N = 6 per group)	Number of hamsters developing lesions	Weight (mg)[b]	Number of treponemes per node ($\times 10^4$)[b]
Normal cells			
Unfractionated	6	72 ± 9	109 ± 29
B cell depleted	6	47 ± 4	118 ± 18
Immune cells			
Unfractionated	0	16 ± 1	5 ± 1
B cell depleted	0	13 ± 1	10 ± 5

[a]21 days after infection.
[b]Mean ± SD.
Source: Reference 54.

Table 5 Ability of B-Cell-Depleted Suspensions of Immune Spleen Cells to Confer Resistance to *T. pallidum* Bosnia A in X-Irradiated, Bone Marrow-Reconstituted Hamsters[a]

Recipients of (N = 3 or 4 per group)	Lesions/sites[b]	Lymph nodes Weight (mg)[c]	Mean number of treponemes per node ($\times 10^3$)
Normal cells			
Unfractionated	8/8	29 ± 3	174
B cell depleted	6/6	44 ± 7	146
Immune cells			
Unfractionated	0/8	17 ± 4	4
B cell depleted	1/8	15 ± 5	33
Bone marrow cells (control)	6/6	42 ± 10	123

[a]At 21 days after infection with 7×10^5 *T. pallidum*.
[b]Each hamster was inoculated at two sites.
[c]Mean ± SD.

fractionation reduced the proportion of cells bearing immunoglobulins by 94%, from a mean ± standard error (SE) of 36 ± 2% to only 2 ± 1%. No fluorescent cells were detected after treatment with either immunoglobulin alone. In contrast, the proportion of cells susceptible to antithymocyte serum plus complement increased by 135%, from (37 ± 9)% to (87 ± 4)% (mean ± SE). The response of lymphocyte to four classic T- or B-cell mitogens (Concanavalin A, phytohemagglutinin, lipopolysaccharide, and dextran sulfate) was significantly decreased by fractionation (Table 6). However, the least decrease was seen with the T-cell mitogen Concanavalin A. These results show that the fractionated cells were stimulated preferentially by concanavalin A.

As an additional measure of the proportion of B cells in the fractionated cells, immune hamsters were inoculated with sheep erythrocytes, and after 5 days the number of direct and indirect plaque-forming cells was determined. Fractionation reduced the number by 90% (Table 7). Thus the protective activity of transferred immune cells resides largely within a population of cells that are sensitive to treatment with antithymocyte serum, perferentially stimulated by Concanavalin A, and devoid of surface immunoglobulins—in short, a population of T cells.

An especially interesting finding was that resistance to frambesial infection can be transferred with enriched T cells in the apparent absence of an anamnestic antibody response to specific treponemal antigens. No significant differences in protection were detected between recipients of B-cell-depleted and unfractionated immune cells, except that the latter group had a fourfold higher antibody response to treponemal challenge. The lower antibody titer in recipients of suspensions of B-cell-depleted immune cells might be due to the depletion of immune cells capable of producing treponemal antibodies. This hypothesis is supported by the significant decrease (90%) in the number of direct and indirect plaques produced by fractionated, sheep erythrocyte-sensitized immune cells.

These results comprise the first direct evidence that resistance to infection with *T. pallidum* Bosnia A or *T. pertunue* is primarily a T-cell-dependent phenomenon. Since earlier attempts to transfer resistance with immune serum had only limited success, these results suggest that cell-mediated immunity plays the dominant role in the destruction and elimination of treponemes. The mechanism by which these T cells confer protection is not yet clearly understood, but at least three modes may be suggested:

1. Although direct cellular cytotoxicity against treponemes has not been reported, T-cell-mediated direct cytotoxicity is well known in

Table 6 Effect of Column Fractionation on the Response to B- and T-Cell Mitogens of Lymphocytes from Syphilitic Hamsters

Mitogen (per 0.2 ml)	[^{3}H]Thymidine incorporated (counts per minute)	
	Before fractionation	After fractionation
Concanavalin A		
1 µg	265,765 ± 3,951	123,835 ± 3,274
5 µg	219,826 ± 6,514	120,409 ± 7,589
Phytohemagglutinin		
10 µg	71,911 ± 6,012	2,510 ± 96
20 µg	65,400 ± 4,946	2,794 ± 143
Lipopolysaccharide		
25 µg	29,320 ± 1,769	5,208 ± 144
50 µg	32,189 ± 1,455	6,498 ± 327
Dextran sulfate		
10 µg	28,496 ± 6,738	2,142 ± 216
15 µg	23,251 ± 7,195	1,978 ± 180
None	6,915 ± 1,072	1,142 ± 69

[a]Geometric mean ± SE of quadruplicate cultures.
Source: Reference 55.

Table 7 Effect of Column Fractionation on the Number of Plaque-Forming Cells Recovered from Syphilitic Hamsters Sensitized with Sheep Erythrocytes

Assay	Number of PFC[a]		Reduction (%)
	Before fractionation	After fractionation	
Direct	3340 ± 10	254 ± 25	92.4
Indirect	2646 ± 215	313 ± 17	88.2

[a]Geometric mean ± SE per 10^6 viable cells.
No PFC were detected before or after fractionation in cultures treated only with antiserum to hamster IgG or RPMI 1640 medium.
Source: Reference 55.

other systems, including virus-infected cells (60) and some tumor systems (61). These T cells may act directly or indirectly against cells that contain or are sensitized to treponemal antigen and may contribute to the pathogenesis and chronicity of treponemal disease by the destruction of effector or regulatory cells.

2. Since the production of specific antibodies for many antigens requires collaboration between T and B lymphocytes (62), the immune response to treponemes could be manifested in helper T-cell activity. The fact that syphilitic and frambesial immune serum can confer partial protection indicates that specific immunoglobulin is involved in host defense. Baughn and Musher (17,18) have presented evidence that the in vivo immunoglobulin G response to sheep erythrocytes, a T-helper-dependent response, is significantly suppressed in syphilitic rabbits. The quality of the helper T-cell responses may influence the production of a treponemicidal antibody.

3. Finally, T cells may mediate destruction of virulent treponemes by macrophage activation. When interacting with sensitized lymphocytes stimulated by antigen, macrophages undergo a number of metabolic and functional changes, generally referred to as activation. One distinct feature of activated macrophages is their enhanced ability to retard the growth of or destroy ingested microorganisms (63). It seems reasonable that competent T cells would interact with treponemal antigen and induce the release of soluble mediators, which would alter the function of the macrophages to reduce the number of treponemes in tissue.

The enhanced ability of immune cells from syphilitic rabbits to suppress the growth of *L. monocytogenes* has provided evidence that activation of macrophages occurs during syphilitic infection (19,21). Harris and Thoen (64) and Hardy et al. (65), using this finding, have shown that nonspecific activation of macrophages by inoculation of rabbits with the potent activator BCG inhibits the development of syphilitic skin lesions. In contrast, several investigators (66-69) have failed to demonstrate that BCG or another potent activator, *Corynebacterium acnes*, modifies the development of syphilitic lesions, even when immune serum is present. It may be necessary for macrophages to become activated in a specific sequence or concomitantly with other effector mechanisms to kill treponemes. The question of whether macrophages are ultimately responsible for the destruction of treponemes remains unsolved.

The chronicity of treponemal infection in the hamster suggests that treponemes are protected, at least partially, from acquired immunity. One mechanism by which treponemes could evade the immune response would be to acquire host antigens on their surface. Evidence to support this hypothesis was recently provided by Aldarete and Baseman (70) and Baseman and Hayes (71). The presence of receptors for host proteins on the surface of treponemes and the consequent coating of treponemes with host protein would prevent macrophages from recognizing, processing, and presenting treponemal antigen to competent T cells. The protein coat would also prevent antibody from aiding in opsonization.

Summary

It has been shown that T-cell-dependent immunity mediates resistance to treponemal infection. The precise mode utilized by these cells to regulate the development of effective resistance needs to be defined. Studies are in progress to determine whether T cells can influence the presentation, processing, and destruction of treponemes in tandem with macrophages or immune serum.

References

1. N. H. Bishop and J. N. Miller. Humoral immunity in experimental syphilis. I. The demonstration of resistance conferred by passive immunization. *J. Immunol.* 117:191-196 (1976).
2. P. L. Perine, R. S. Weiser, and S. J. Klebanoff. Immunity to syphilis. I. Passive transfer in rabbits with hyperimmune serum. *Infect. Immun.* 8:787-790 (1973).
3. M. Sepetjian, D. Salussola, and J. Thivolet. Attempt to protect rabbits against experimental syphilis by passive immunization. *Br. J. Vener. Dis.* 49:335-337 (1973).
4. T. B. Turner, P. H. Hardy, B. Newman, and E. E. Nell. Effects of passive immunization on experimental syphilis in the rabbit. *John Hopkins Med. J.* 133:241-251 (1973).

5. R. S. Weiser, D. Erickson, P. L. Perine, and N. N. Pearsall. Immunity in syphilis: Passive transfer in rabbits using serial doses of immune serum. *Infect. Immun.* 13:1402-1407 (1976).
6. S. Graves and J. Alden. Limited protection of rabbits against infection with *Treponema pallidum* by immune sera. *Br. J. Vener. Dis.* 55:399-403 (1979).
7. R. G. Titus and R. S. Weiser. Experimental syphilis in the rabbit: Passive transfer of immunity with immunoglobulin G from immune serum. *J. Infect. Dis.* 140:904-913 (1979).
8. T. B. Turner. Protective antibodies in the serum of syphilitic rabbits. *J. Exp. Med.* 69:867-890 (1939).
9. L. C. Marshak and S. Rothman. Skin testing with a purified suspension of *Treponema pallidum*. *Am. J. Syph. Gonorrhea and Vener. Dis.* 35:35-41 (1951).
10. G. W. Csonka. "Luotest": A preliminary evaluation in the diagnosis of late syphilis. *Med. Biol. Illus.* 4:389-391 (1950).
11. H. J. Magnuson, E. W. Thomas, S. Olansky, B. I. Kaplan, L. DeMello, and J. C. Culter. Inoculation syphilis in human volunteers. *Medicine* 35:33-82 (1953).
12. T. B. Turner. Syphilis and the treponematoses. In *Infectious Agents and Host Reactions* (S. Mudd, Ed.). W. B. Saunders, Philadelphia, 1970, pp. 346-390.
13. G. P. Youmans. *Tuberculosis*. W. B. Saunders, Philadelphia, 1979, pp. 209-244.
14. S. S. Elberg. Immunity to Brucella infections. *Medicine* 52: 339-356 (1973).
15. D. R. Turner and D. J. M. Wright. Lymphadenopathy in early syphilis. *J. Pathol.* 110:305-308 (1973).
16. H. Festenstein, C. Abrahams, and V. Bokkenheuser. Runting syndrome in neonatal rabbits infected with *Treponema pallidum*. *Clin. Exp. Immunol.* 71:311-320 (1967).
17. R. E. Baughn and D. M. Musher. Altered immune responsiveness associated with experimental syphilis in the rabbit: Elevated IgM and depressed IgG responses to sheep erythrocytes. *J. Immunol.* 120:1691-1695 (1978).
18. R. E. Baughn and D. M. Musher. Aberrant secondary antibody responses to sheep erythrocytes in rabbits with experimental syphilis. *Infect. Immun.* 25:133-138 (1979).
19. R. F. Schell and D. M. Musher. Detection of nonspecific resistance to *Listeria monocytogenes* in rabbits infected with *Treponema pallidum*. *Infect. Immun.* 9:658-662 (1974).
20. R. Schell, D. Musher, K. Jacobson, and P. Schwethelm. Induction of acquired cellular resistance following transfer of thymus-dependent lymphocytes from syphilitic rabbits. *J. Immunol.* 114: 550-553 (1975).

21. R. F. Schell and D. M. Musher. Transfer of nonspecific resistance to *Listeria monocytogenes* using spleen cells from syphilitic rabbits. *Proc. Soc. Exp. Biol. Med. 148*:516-518 (1975).
22. J. N. Miller. Immunity in experimental syphilis. VI. Successful vaccination of rabbits with *Treponema pallidum*, Nichols strain, attenuated by γ-irradiation. *J. Immunol. 110*:1206-1215 (1973).
23. D. W. Smith, A. A. Grover, and E. Weigeshaus. Nonliving immunogenic substances of mycobacteria. *Adv. Tuber. Res. 16*: 191-227 (1968).
24. W. R. Barclay. In *Immunization in Tuberculosis* (E. C. Chamberlayne, Ed.). Fogarty International Center Proceedings No. 14., Washington, D. C., 1972, pp. 245-247.
25. D. M. Musher, R. F. Schell, and J. M. Knox. 1974. In vitro lymphocytes response to *Treponema refringens* in human syphilis. *Infect. Immun. 9*:654-657 (1974).
26. D. M. Musher, R. F. Schell, R. H. Jones, and A. M. Jones. Lymphocyte transformation in syphilis: An in vitro correlate of immune suppression in vivo? *Infect. Immun. 11*:1261-1264 (1975).
27. G. M. Levene, J. L. Turk, D. J. M. Wright, and A. G. S. Grimble. Reduced lymphocyte transformation due to a plasma factor in patients with active syphilis. *Lancet 2*:246-247 (1969).
28. F. S. Kantor. Infection, anergy and cell-mediated immunity. *N. Engl. J. Med. 292*:629-634 (1975).
29. E. From, K. Thestrup-Pedersen, and H. Thulin. Reactivity of lymphocytes from patients with syphilis towards *T. pallidum* antigen in the leukocyte migration and lymphocyte transformation test. *Br. J. Vener. Dis. 52*:224-229 (1976).
30. R. F. Bey, R. C. Johnson, and T. J. Fitzgerald. Suppression of lymphocyte response to concanavalin A by mucopolysaccharide material from *Treponema pallidum*-infected rabbits. *Infect. Immun. 26*:64-69 (1979).
31. C. S. Pavia, J. B. Baseman, and J. D. Folds. Selective response of lymphocytes from *Treponema pallidum* infected rabbits to mitogens and *Treponema reiteri*. *Infect. Immun. 15*:417-422 (1977).
32. C. S. Pavia, J. D. Folds, and J. B. Baseman. Depression of lymphocyte response to concanavalin A in rabbits infected with *Treponema pallidum* (Nichols strain) *Infect. Immun. 14*:320-322 (1976).
33. C. S. Pavia, J. D. Folds, and J. B. Baseman. Selective in vitro response of thymus-derived lymphocytes from *Treponema pallidum*-infected rabbits. *Infect. Immun. 18*:603-611 (1977).
34. K. W. M. Fulford and J. Brostoff. Leucocyte migration and cell-mediated immunity in syphilis. *Br. J. Vener. Dis. 48*:483-488 (1972).

35. V. Wicher and K. Wicher. In-vitro cell response of *Treponema pallidum* infected rabbits. I. Lymphocyte transformation. *Clin. Exp. Immunol.* 29:480-486 (1977).
36. V. Wicher and K. Wicher. Cell response in rabbits infected with *Treponema pallidum* as measured by the leucocyte migration inhibition test. *Br. J. Vener. Dis.* 51:240-245 (1975).
37. C. S. Pavia, J. B. Baseman, and J. D. Folds. Development of macrophage migration inhibition in rabbits infected with virulent *Treponema pallidum*. *Infect. Immun.* 17:651-654 (1977).
38. M. Metzger, J. Podiwinska, and W. Smogor. Cell-mediated immunity in experimental syphilis in rabbits *Arch. Immunol. Ther. Exp.* 25:25-34 (1977).
39. M. Metzger. Theme 2: Recent advances in the immunology of syphilis. Role of humoral versus cellular mechanisms of resistance in the pathogenesis of syphilis. *Br. J. Vener. Dis.* 55:94-98 (1979).
40. M. Metzger and W. Smogor. Passive transfer of immunity to experimental syphilis in rabbits by immune lymphocytes. *Arch. Immunol. Ther. Exp.* 23:625-630 (1975).
41. R. E. Baughn, D. M. Musher, and C. B. Simmons. Inability of spleen cells from chancre-immune rabbits to confer immunity to challenge with *Treponema pallidum*. *Infect. Immun.* 17:535-540 (1977).
42. K. Wicher and A. Jakubowski. Effect of cortisone on the course of experimental syphilis in the guinea pig. I. Effect of previously-administered cortisone on guinea pigs infected with *Treponema pallidum* intradermally, intratesticularly, and intravenously. *Br. J. Vener. Dis.* 40:213-216 (1964).
43. A. Bessemans and A. DeMoor. Réceptivité des petits animaux de laboratoire à la syphilis et à la pallidoidose. *Ann. Inst. Pasteur* 63:569-591 (1939).
44. A. Vaisman. *La Syphilis Inapparente Expérimentale chez la Souris.* Tancrede, Paris, 1936, p. 67.
45. B. Gueft and P. D. Rosahn. Experimental mouse syphilis, a critical review of the literature. *Am. J. Syph.* 32:59-88 (1948).
46. Y. Ohta. *Treponema pallidum* antibodies in syphilitic mice as determined by immunofluorescence and passive hemagglutination techniques. *J. Immunol.* 108:921-926 (1972).
47. R. F. Schell, D. M. Musher, K. Jacobson, and P. Schwethelm. New evidence for the noninfectivity of *Treponema pallidum* for mice. *Br. J. Vener. Dis.* 51:19-21 (1975).
48. J. R. Klein, A. A. Monjan, P. H. Hardy, and G. A. Cole. Abrogation of genetically controlled resistance of mice to *Treponema pallidum* by irradiation. *Nature* 283:572-574 (1980).
49. R. F. Schell, J. L. LeFrock, J. P. Babu, and J. K. Chan. Use of CB hamsters in the study of *Treponema pertenue*. *Br. J. Vener. Dis.* 55:316-319 (1979).

50. R. F. Schell, J. L. LeFrock, J. K. Chan, and O. Bagasra. LSH hamster model of syphilitic infection. Infect. Immun. 28:909-913 (1980).
51. R. F. Schell, J. L. LeFrock, and J. P. Babu. Passive transfer of resistance to frambesial infection in hamsters. Infect. Immun. 21:430-435 (1978).
52. R. F. Schell, J. K. Chan, and J. L. LeFrock. Endemic syphilis: Passive transfer of resistance with serum and cells in hamsters. J. Infect. Dis. 140:378-383 (1979).
53. J. K. Chan, R. F. Schell, and J. L. LeFrock. Inability of immune cells treated with anti-thymocyte serum to confer on hamsters resistance to cutaneous infection with Treponema pertenue. Infect. Immun. 25:208-212 (1979).
54. J. K. Chan, R. F. Schell, and J. L. LeFrock. Ability of enriched immune T cells to confer resistance in hamsters to infection with Treponema pertenue. Infect. Immun. 26:448-452 (1979).
55. R. F. Schell, J. K. Chan, J. L. LeFrock, and O. Bagasra. Endemic syphilis: Transfer of resistance to Treponema pallidum strain Bosnia A in hamsters with a cell suspension enriched in thymus-derived cells. J. Infect. Dis. 141:752-758 (1980).
56. F. T. Guerraz, M. Sepetjian, J. C. Monier, and D. Salussola. Changes in the susceptibility of the golden hamster to cutaneous treponemal infection after transfer of lymphoid cells from infected donors. Br. J. Vener. Dis. 53:146-147 (1977).
57. M. K. Hoffman. Macrophage and T cells control distinct phases of B cell differentiation in the humoral immune response in vitro. J. Immunol. 125:2076-2081 (1980).
58. J. W. Blasecki and K. J. Houston. Identification, functional characterization and partial purification of thymus-derived lymphocytes in inbred hamsters. Immunology 35:1-11 (1978).
59. M. H. Julius, E. Simpson, and L. A. Herzenberg. A rapid method for the isolation of functional thymus-derived murine lymphocytes. Eur. J. Immunol. 3:645-649 (1973).
60. M. Rola-Pleszczynski, R. C. Hurtado, J. N. Woody, K. W. Sell, M. M. Vincent, S. A. Hensen, and J. A. Bellanti. Identification of the cell population involved in viral-specific cell-mediated cytotoxicity in man: Evidence for T cell specificity. J. Immunol. 115:239-242 (1975).
61. P. M. Sondel, C. O'Brien, L. Porter, S. F. Schlossman, and L. Chess. Cell-mediated destruction of human leukemic cells by MHC identical lymphocytes: Requirement for a proliferative trigger in vitro. J. Immunol. 117:2197-2203 (1976).
62. R. K. Gershon. T cell control of antibody production. In Contemporary Topics in Immunobiology, Vol. 3. (M. D. Cooper and N. L. Warner, Eds.). Plenum, New York and London, 1974, pp. 1-9.

63. G. Mackaness. Resistance to intracellular infection. *J. Infect. Dis.* 123:439-445 (1971).
64. D. L. Harris and C. O. Thoen. Inhibition of skin lesions due to *Treponema pallidum* in BCG-infected rabbits. *Abstr. Annu. Meet. Am. Soc. Microbiol.* E 32:86 (1977).
65. P. H. Hardy, D. J. Graham, E. E. Nell, and A. M. Dannenberg. Macrophages in immunity to syphilis: Suppressive effect of concurrent infection with *Mycobacterium bovis* (BCG) on the development of syphilitic lesions and growth of *Treponema pallidum* in tuberculin-positive rabbits. *Infect. Immun.* 26:751-763 (1979).
66. R. Schell, D. Musher, K. Jacobson, P. Schwethelm, and C. Simmons. Effect of macrophage activation on infection with *Treponema pallidum*. *Infect. Immun.* 12:505-511 (1975).
67. R. E. Baughn, D. M. Musher, and J. M. Knox. Effect of sensitization with *Propionibacterium acnes* on the growth of *Listeria monocytogenes* and *Treponema pallidum* in rabbits. *J. Immunol.* 118:109-113 (1977).
68. S. R. Graves and R. C. Johnson. Effect of pretreatment with *Mycobacterium bovis* (strain BCG) and immune syphilitic serum on rabbit resistance to *Treponema pallidum*. *Infect. Immun.* 12:1029-1036 (1975).
69. S. Graves. Rate of clearance of virulent *Treponema pallidum* (Nichols) from the blood stream of normal, *Mycobacterium bovis* BCG-treated, and syphilitic rabbits. *Infect. Immun.* 27:264-267 (1980).
70. J. F. Alderete and J. B. Baseman. Surface-associated host proteins on virulent *Treponema pallidum*. *Infect. Immun.* 26:1048-1056 (1979).
71. J. B. Baseman and E. C. Hayes. Molecular characterization of receptor binding proteins and immunogens of virulent *Treponema pallidum*. *J. Exp. Med.* 151:573-586 (1980).

18
Macrophages and Host Resistance

SHEILA A. LUKEHART
University of Washington
School of Medicine
Seattle, Washington

Histologic Evidence for Macrophage Function 350
The Role of Activated Macrophages in Resistance to
   Treponema pallidum 351
Summary 360
References 360

Primary syphilitic infection is manifest in humans and intradermally infected rabbits as a raised erythematous lesion or chancre. At the site of infection, multiplication of *Treponema pallidum* occurs, with resultant infiltration by mononuclear cells and formation of the gross lesion. The bacteria, which are abundant in early chancres, are then virtually cleared from the local site, and the lesion heals without antibiotic therapy. The mechanism by which the host is able to destroy the bacteria and clear them from the local site is not known. It has been proposed by early investigators (1) and, more recently, by Lukehart and co-workers (2-4), Baker-Zander and Sell (5), Sell et al. (6), and Hardy et al. (7) that macrophages may be the ultimate effector cell which is responsible for the destruction and clearance of *T. pallidum* in tissue. Evidence for and against this hypothesis will be presented and discussed.

Histologic Evidence for Macrophage Function

Monocytosis has long been recognized as a characteristic of active syphilitic infection in humans (8-10) and experimentally infected rabbits (11,12). Cytologic examination of blood from infected humans and rabbits revealed a significant increase in the number of circulating monocytes, accompanied by a decrease in the proportion of peripheral blood lymphocytes. These hematologic changes parallel the degree of activity at the primary site of infection.

Histologic examination of tissue from cutaneous and testicular lesions supports a role for macrophages in treponemal clearance. Several investigators (1,13-15) have reported an increase in the number, size, and apparent phagocytic activity of large mononuclear cells in these tissues. Pearce and Rosahn (1) commented that "the monocyte appears as an important and perhaps one of the most essential participants in the cellular reaction to *T. pallidum.*"

Electron-microscopic evidence exists for the intracellular location of *T. pallidum* in phagocytic and nonphagocytic cells. Azar et al. (16) reported *T. pallidum* within neutrophils, macrophages, and plasma cells in a primary human chancre. Sykes et al. (17) confirmed the presence of organisms within these cells as well as fibroblasts and epithelial and endothelial cells. Lauderdale and Goldman (18) examined tissue from an experimental rabbit orchitis and reported the presence of treponemes in Leydig cells, fibroblasts, macrophages, and polymorphonuclear leukocytes. Significantly, treponemes in various stages of degradation were observed only within known phagocytic cells. Ovcinnikov and Delektorskij (19) conducted a detailed electron-microscopic examination of treponeme-phagocyte interactions in early and resolving rabbit dermal lesions; treponemes were found within typical phagocytic vacuoles in association with lysosomal structures.

Although these studies suggest that the macrophages may be able to engulf and digest *T. pallidum*, they do not show a clear temporal correlation between macrophage activity and the disappearance of organisms from the infected site. Lukehart et al. (4) performed a careful time-course study of primary testicular infection in the rabbit. Tissues were harvested from rabbits on days 3, 6, 10, 13, 17, 21, and 28 post-infection and were examined following routine hematoxylin and eosin staining as well as immunofluorescent staining for *T. pallidum*, T lymphocytes, and immunoglobulin (including B lymphocytes). Treponemes were observed in low numbers perivascularly as early as day 3, and they increased in number until days 10-13, when organisms virtually filled the interstitial spaces. Lymphocytic infiltration began by day 7 and reached a peak at days 10-13. These lymphocytes were shown by immunofluorescence to be predominantly T cells; very few B cells were observed. During the height of the orchitis, however, immunoglobulin (presumably derived from serum) could be seen diffusely covering tissue structures. Macrophages became apparent on day 10

18. Macrophages and Host Resistance

and reached maximal numbers on day 13. Between days 13 and 17, a dramatic decrease in the numbers of demonstrable bacteria in the testes occurred. After day 13, treponemes could be demonstrated only after prolonged search. These observations suggest that bacterial clearance is the direct result of the functions of the infiltrating cells. The testes were virtually cleared of organisms within days following maximal T lymphocyte and macrophage infiltration, and treponemal fragments (demonstrable following immunofluorescent staining) can be seen within the cytoplasm of macrophages of healing lesions (5,19a). In an electron-microscopic study of tissues derived from intratesticularly infected rabbits, Sell et al. (20) demonstrated the presence of treponemes in phagocytic vacuoles in tissues from resolving testicular infection in rabbits. Again, evidence for bacterial degradation within vacuoles was provided.

The Role of Activated Macrophages in Resistance to *Treponema pallidum*

The central role of the macrophage in immunity to other infectious diseases such as listeriosis (21,22), toxoplasmosis (23), and tuberculosis (24) is well described. In these infections, destruction of the infectious organism is mediated by macrophages which have been activated by soluble products of specifically sensitized T lymphocytes. The initial sensitization of the lymphocyte and the subsequent release of macrophage-activating factors (MAF) are triggered by specific antigen. Once macrophage activation is accomplished, however, phagocytosis and destruction of unrelated organisms can occur; the effector mechanism is thus nonspecific. If such a mechanism were operative during syphilis, several factors would be required: (1) presence of specifically sensitized lymphocytes, (2) release (by lymphocytes) of factors which attract and concentrate macrophages at the local site (MIF), (3) release (by lymphocytes) of macrophage-activating factors (MAF), (4) presence of activated macrophages in vivo, (5) phagocytosis, and (6) destruction of the ingested organism. Numerous investigators have provided evidence which relates to the existence, during syphilitic infection, of the immunologic functions required by this hypothesis. The events which occur in vivo following infection with *T. pallidum* support a role for activated macrophages during early syphilis infection.

Presence of Specifically Sensitized Lymphocytes

The presence of specifically sensitized lymphocytes may be demonstrated in vitro by proliferative or blast transformation assays. Pavia et al. examined peripheral blood lymphocytes from rabbits following intratesticular infection with *T. pallidum*. Lymphocytes which were responsive to antigens obtained from *T. pallidum* (25) and *Treponema phagedenis*, biotype Reiter (26), were first demonstrable 3 weeks postinfection. Hardy et al. (27), Lukehart et al. (3), and Maret et al. (28) described *T. pallidum*-reactive lymphocytes in the spleen and lymph nodes of infected rabbits as early as the first week of infection. The responsive cells were demonstrated by Lukehart et al. to be T lymphocytes. The appearance of specifically sensitized lymphocytes during the first week of infection correlated temporally with the first apparent infiltration of the infected testes by T cells (4).

Specifically reactive lymphocytes have also been described in syphilitic humans. The earliest human study, by Chieregato and Faldarini (29), indicates that specific responsiveness to a lysate preparation of *T. pallidum*, Nichols strain, appears late in primary infection, reaches a peak during secondary disease, and persists throughout latency. Treatment and *Treponema pallidum* immobilization (TPI) seroreversal results in the loss of lymphocyte responsiveness. Lymphocytes from normal subjects do not proliferate in vitro in response to the treponemal preparation. The results of Badanoiu et al. (30), Mezzadra et al. (31), Janot et al. (32), From et al. (33), and Friedman and Turk (34,35) were very similar. Lymphocytes from patients with all stages of syphilis infection were able to respond to *T. pallidum* antigens, with the weakest response apparent during the early primary stage.

In contrast to the studies described above, Musher et al. (36,37) reported that lymphocytes from normal individuals do proliferate in response to preparations of *T. pallidum*, *Treponema refringens*, and "*Treponema reiter*" antigens. Furthermore, patients with primary and secondary syphilis demonstrate a decreased ability to respond to these antigens; "normal" responsiveness returns following treatment. The authors interpreted these results to indicate a depression of specific cellular immune function during acute syphilitic infection. A more complete discussion of a possible suppression of immunologic responses during syphilis may be found in Chap. 14 and 16.

Macrophage Accumulation at Local Sites:
Migration Inhibition Factor Production

The functional capacity of lymphocytes from syphilitic humans and rabbits to release macrophage migration inhibition factors (MIF) in response to antigen exposure has also been examined. Fulford and Brostoff (38) measured the migration inhibition of peripheral blood leukocytes from 49 syphilitic patients as well as from an equal number of age- and sex-matched control subjects in the presence or absence of protein antigen from *T. phagedenis*, biotype Reiter. The results were somewhat puzzling. Leukocytes from patients with primary syphilis demonstrated enhanced migration compared to control values, while cells from secondary and latent syphilitics showed neither significant stimulation nor inhibition of cell migration. Leukocytes from a series of six patients with late active syphilis, on the other hand, were inhibited in their migration in the presence of Reiter antigen. The authors suggested that the stimulation of migration in primary syphilis and inhibition in late active syphilis represented weak and strong delayed hypersensitivity, respectively. The absence of a notable effect on migration in secondary syphilitics was suggested to indicate a suppression of cell-mediated immunity during secondary syphilis. From et al. (33) were unable to detect any specific inhibition of leukocyte migration in a series of 20 patients with various histories of syphilitic infection. The authors did, however, note an increase in spontaneous leukocyte migration (in the absence of antigen) following treatment in nine patients with early syphilis. Bowszyc and Bowszyc (39) demonstrated macrophage migration inhibition in 87% of patients with primary syphilis and all patients with late syphilis.

Wicher and Wicher (40) examined leukocyte migration responses in a group of 48 rabbits which had been infected for periods of 1 week to 16 months. In the presence of Reiter and cardiolipin–Venereal Disease Research Laboratory (VDRL)–antigens and low concentrations of sonicated T. pallidum, a biphasic response was observed in which stimulation of migration was observed early after infection, followed by migration inhibition in later stages of the disease. The presence of higher concentrations of sonicated T. pallidum resulted in significant migration inhibition, as early as 2 weeks postinfection; inhibition was still demonstrable after 16 months of infection.

Metzger et al. (41) demonstrated the ability of rabbit lymphocytes to inhibit macrophage migration in the presence of T. pallidum antigen as early as 1 month after infection. Between the fourth and sixth month a decrease in this ability occurred, followed again by a rise in macrophage migration inhibition (MMI) capacity which persisted until the end of the 2-year observation period. Animals which were treated with penicillin 5 months postinfection demonstrated a gradual decline in MMI activity following treatment. In another group of rabbits, MMI response appeared shortly after the initiation of an artificial immunization procedure. Although the studies of Metzger indicate that lymphocytes from syphilitic animals have the ability to inhibit macrophage migration in vitro, this ability could not be strictly correlated with the immune status of the lymphocyte donor. Furthermore, guinea pigs were used as the macrophage source for these studies; thus, the in vivo relevance of this demonstration is unclear.

Pavia et al. (42), using peritoneal exudate cells from syphilitic rabbits, confirmed Metzger's observation of macrophage migration inhibition in the presence of Reiter protein 3 weeks after initial infection. This activity persisted for the course of the 15-week observation period. No inhibition was demonstrable earlier than 3 weeks postinfection.

The MIF test described above is purported to be the in vitro equivalent of delayed hypersensitivity in vivo. Delayed hypersensitivity testing, which involves the intradermal injection of a small amount of treponemal antigen, has been performed in syphilitic humans and rabbits. The presence of specifically sensitized lymphocytes and local macrophage accumulation is indicated by erythema and induration at the site of injection 24-48 hr following challenge. In 1911, Noguchi (43) performed a series of skin tests on 400 persons, of whom 146 were nonsyphilitic controls. The antigen used in these studies was a heat-killed preparation of "cultured" *T. pallidum*, which, in fact, was probably a related nonpathogenic treponeme. None of the 146 nonsyphilitic subjects and only 1 of 5 primary syphilitics gave a positive skin test. Of 50 patients with secondary syphilis, 29 were mildly reactive; the most intense responses were seen in those secondary syphilitics who had received salvarsan treatment. Consistently positive results were found in patients with tertiary (57 out of 59) and congenital (23 out of 23) syphilis, while variable results were seen in subjects with latent infection (24 out of 30) or neurologic symptoms (48 out of 77).

A similar pattern of reactivity was demonstrated more recently by Marshak and Rothman (44), Thivolet et al. (45), and Csonka (46). The antigens employed in these studies were prepared from a suspension of *T. pallidum* which had been extracted from infected rabbit testes and purified by differential centrifugation and filtration. Negative skin test results were found for nonsyphilitic control subjects, as well as for patients with primary and secondary infection. Patients with congenital or active tertiary syphilis were uniformly reactive, and subjects with latent or neurosyphilis displayed variable reactivity. In another report, Laird and Thorburn (47) demonstrated two-thirds reactivity (upon secondary challenge) in a group of 40 patients with clinical evidence of late acquired or congenital syphilis.

The results of delayed hypersensitivity studies in rabbits are inconclusive. Noguchi (43) demonstrated that while uninfected rabbits elicited no delayed skin response, all rabbits that had been injected repeatedly with living or heat-killed *T. pallidum* gave positive skin responses to the injected treponemal preparation. Rabbits with acute syphilitic orchitis and animals which had been treated with salvarsan elicited no skin response. Rich et al. (48) demonstrated that rabbits with no detectable skin response were, nevertheless, resistant to symptomatic reinfection. They concluded that "allergy" or skin reactivity was not necessary for resistance. Marshak and Rothman (44) and Thivolet et al. (45) demonstrated delayed skin reactivity in 12 out of 20 and 4 out of 14 rabbits, respectively, that had been infected for various periods of time up to 10 months. There was no correlation between skin reactivity and duration of infection. Wicher and Wicher (40) were unable to demonstrate delayed or immediate skin responsiveness to heat-killed *T. pallidum* in a group of rabbits which had been infected for 3 to 16 months.

Production of Macrophage Activating Factors

Lukehart (48a) has recently demonstrated the production of macrophage activating factors (MAF) by lymphocytes from rabbits which had been infected with T. pallidum for 2 to 12 weeks. Lymphocytes were placed in culture for 4 days with sonicated T. pallidum. The cell suspensions were then centrifuged and/or filtered to remove intact cells and the cell-free supernatants were incubated with freshly harvested peritoneal macrophages for 36 hr. The macrophage monolayers were washed carefully and infected with log phase Listeria monocytogenes. Activation of the macrophages by lymphocyte supernatants was measured by the ability of the macrophages to resist intracellular multiplication and subsequent lysis by the bacteria. The results of these experiments are shown in Table 1. Unstimulated lymphocytes from infected rabbits and "T. pallidum-stimulated" lymphocytes from normal rabbits were unable to resist intracellular multiplication of Listeria. Specifically stimulated lymphocytes from infected rabbits and mitogen-stimulated lymphocytes from all rabbits demonstrated a clear ability to limit the intracellular growth of Listeria. Antigen or mitogen alone was unable to activate the macrophages; the presence of lymphocyte products was required. These results indicate that, in the presence of specific antigen, T. pallidum-sensitized lymphocytes release MAF.

Presence of Activated Macrophages In Vivo During Syphilitic Infection

In a series of classic studies, Mackaness demonstrated activated macrophages to be the effector cells in acquired cellular resistance to infection with Listeria monocytogenes (22). Schell and Musher (49) have provided evidence that macrophages are activated in vivo following syphilitic infection by their demonstration that syphilitic rabbits show increased resistance to challenge with L. monocytogenes. This increased resistance may be prolonged by repeated stimulation of the rabbit with treponemal antigens. Furthermore, this resistance is transferable to normal recipients with spleen cells from syphilitic rabbits (50). Prior treatment of the transferred spleen cells with antithymocytic serum abrogated the effect.

Although active infection with T. pallidum appears to induce a nonspecific resistance, attempts to protect rabbits against treponemal challenge by this same mechanism have yielded conflicting results. Schell et al. (51) infected a group of rabbits with two injections of Mycobacterium bovis [strain bacille Calmette Guérin (BCG)] and challenged them intravenously with 10^7 T. pallidum. Although this BCG schedule conferred significant resistance against intravenous challenge with Listeria monocytogenes, it had no protective effect against treponemal infection. Preincubation of the challenge treponemes in immune serum, as a source of opsonin, did not alter the results. Similarly,

Table 1 Effect of Lymphocyte Products on Macrophage Activation

Lymphocyte source	Antigenic stimulus	Percentage of macrophages surviving 12 hr postchallenge[a]	Activation[b]
Syphilitic rabbit (N = 5)	None	35.7 ± 11.0	- (n.s.)[d]
	T. pallidum	74.6 ± 34.8	+ (p < 0.05)
	ConA[c]	89.5 ± 15.7	+ (p < 0.001)
Normal rabbit (N = 3)	None	21.0 ± 17.8	- (n.s.)
	T. pallidum	18.0 ± 11.1	- (n.s.)
	ConA	83.0 ± 4.24	+ (p < 0.05)
No lymphocytes (N = 2)	None	9.0 ± 1.4	- (n.s.)
	T. pallidum	8.0 ± 5.7	- (n.s.)
	ConA	10.0 ± 2.8	- (n.s.)

[a]Following challenge with viable *Listeria monocytogenes*.
[b]Activation is defined as the significant ability to resist intracellular multiplication of *L. monocytogenes* and thus survive infection. Statistical analysis of the percentage of surviving infected cells versus the percentage surviving uninfected cells was performed using Student's t test.
[c]Concanavalin A.
[d]n.s. = not significant.

Graves and Johnson (52) infected a group of rabbits with BCG prior to intravenous and intradermal challenge with *T. pallidum*. Immune syphilitic serum, a source of opsonin, was administered intravenously. In spite of increased phagocytic activity in the BCG-treated animals (measured by carbon clearance tests), no increased resistance to *T. pallidum* infection was observed. The effect of sensitization with BCG on the course of dermal lesions was also unaffected (53). Baughn et al. (54) were likewise unable to demonstrate protection against intradermal or intravenous challenge with *T. pallidum* in rabbits which had been treated with multiple injections of heat-killed *Propionibacterium acnes*. This *P. acnes* regimen was effective in conferring significant protection against challenge with *L. monocytogenes*. Furthermore, the intradermal injection of heat-killed *P. acnes* mixed with the treponemal challenge organisms failed to alter the course of treponemal infection in *P. acnes*-sensitized recipients.

In an early study, Harris et al. (55) stated that the nonspecific in vivo activation of macrophages by lecithin or trypan blue causes the early resolution of progressing testicular lesions. Similarly, Hardy et al. (7) described rapid enlargement and early onset of healing of primary lesions following inoculation of mixed BCG and *T. pallidum* in

18. Macrophages and Host Resistance

BCG-sensitized rabbits. This healing corresponded to the peak infiltration of macrophages to the site. Treponemes were identified by silver stain in phagocytic vacuoles of macrophages in those healing lesions. Similarly, Harris and Thoen (56) demonstrated that the intradermal injection of BCG close to a site of *T. pallidum* challenge inhibited the development of treponemal lesions.

Phagocytosis of Treponema pallidum by Macrophages

Several investigators have suggested that *T. pallidum* may be resistant to phagocytosis (51,52). Commonly quoted evidence for this conclusion is the report by Brause and Roberts (57), who were unable to observe phagocytosis of *T. pallidum* by human peripheral blood monocytes by means of phase-contrast and electron microscopy. In this experiment, the addition of normal human or rabbit serum plus complement did not result in detectable phagocytosis. The visualization by phase-contrast microscopy of *T. pallidum* within a phagocytic vacuole would, however, be extremely difficult. An ingested treponeme would be rounded up (2,7) and may lack detectable characteristic morphology. Furthermore, the possible opsonic role of specific antibody was not explored by these investigators.

Microscopic evidence of phagocytosis in vivo has already been presented in this chapter. In addition, other evidence exists for the phagocytosis of *T. pallidum* in vitro. Metzger and Michalska (58) reported the development of an opsonophagocytic test in which the association of ^{51}chromium-labeled *T. pallidum* with guinea pig polymorphonuclear leukocytes was measured; immune serum and complement were demonstrated to enhance this interaction. Although this evidence is suggestive of phagocytosis, Metzger and Michalska have criticized the ability of their opsonophagocytic test to differentiate true phagocytosis from adherence.

Wicher and her co-workers (59) provided evidence that leukocytes from syphilitic rabbits have higher levels of phagocytic activity than cells from normal rabbits. They examined the reduction of nitroblue tetrazolium (NBT) by peripheral blood leukocytes of rabbits injected with *T. pallidum* or control testicular extracts. A significant increase in NBT reduction was seen only in infected rabbits.

Lukehart and Miller (2) have provided definitive evidence for the phagocytosis of living and heat-killed *T. pallidum* by stimulant-induced rabbit peritoneal macrophages. Ingested treponemes were detected by indirect immunofluorescent staining (Fig. 1) and electron microscopy (Fig. 2). Treatment of macrophages with cytochalasin B, a known inhibitor of phagocytosis, blocked intracellular appearance of the organisms without affecting treponemal motility, thus eliminating the possibility that intracellular location results from active cell penetration by the treponeme. Heat-killed organisms were ingested as readily as

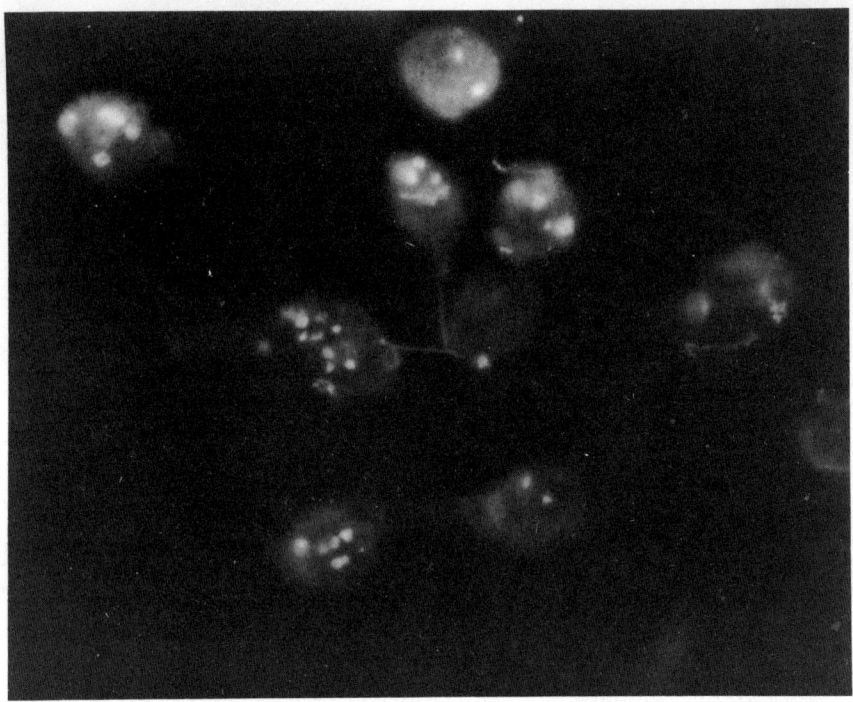

Figure 1 Immunofluorescent staining of treponemal antigens after interaction of rabbit peritoneal macrophages with *T. pallidum* in the presence of 20% heated immune rabbit serum. Note the morphologically distinct extracellular treponemes and the round cytoplasmic structures containing treponemal antigens. (× 1300)

motile *T. pallidum*. Only very low levels of phagocytosis were observed in the presence of normal rabbit serum; significantly enhanced phagocytosis occurred in the presence of immune rabbit serum. An effect of complement on phagocytosis was not demonstrated. Doe and Miller (unpublished) have confirmed these findings.

Destruction of Ingested Treponemes by
Activated Macrophages

Although activated macrophages have been demonstrated to kill and digest other ingested organisms, the direct killing of *T. pallidum* by such macrophages has not yet been described. Experiments designed to examine this possibility are currently in progress. Evidence for the

18. Macrophages and Host Resistance

destruction of *T. pallidum* within phagocytic vacuoles has been provided by electron-microscopic studies; these results have been described in more detail in Chap. 15. Even though treponemes in various stages of degradation may be seen within phagocytes, it is not yet clear whether these organisms were actually killed by the macrophages or whether the phagocytes function simply as scavenger cells which ingest organisms that have been killed by another mechanism.

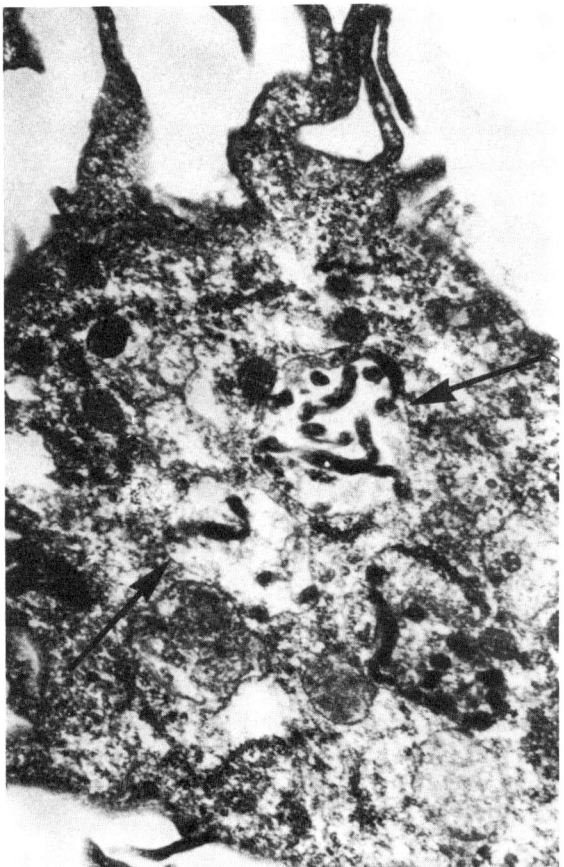

Figure 2 Electron-microscopic examination of rabbit peritoneal macrophages after interaction with *T. pallidum* in the presence of 20% heated immune rabbit serum. Note the presence of treponemes within membrane-bound vacuoles (arrows). (× 15,000) (*Source*: Reference 2.)

Summary

Activated macrophages appear to play an important role in resistance to syphilis infection. Specifically sensitized T lymphocytes, which arise early in infection, have been demonstrated to produce MIF as well as MAF. The in vivo presence of activated macrophages in syphilitic rabbits has been described. Local activation of macrophages by injection of BCG may protect animals from infection with *T. pallidum* or may accelerate the healing of existing lesions. It is now apparent that living *T. pallidum* can be phagocytized by macrophages in vitro in the presence of specific antibody. A careful histologic examination of the interactions of *T. pallidum* with host cells during the development and resolution of primary syphiliitc lesions suggests a major role for macrophages in the clearance of organisms from the local site of infection. Immunofluorescent staining and electron-microscopic studies reveal the presence of *T. pallidum* within macrophages in healing lesions. Although degradation of ingested organisms within phagocytic vacuoles has been described, the direct killing of *T. pallidum* by macrophages has not yet been demonstrated.

References

1. L. Pearce and P. D. Rosahn. The cellular reaction of experimental syphilis. Supravital and fixed material. *Proc. Soc. Exp. Biol. Med.* 28:654-656 (1931).
2. S. A. Lukehart and J. N. Miller. Demonstration of the *in vitro* phagocytosis of *Treponema pallidum* by rabbit peritoneal macrophages. *J. Immunol.* 121:2014-2023 (1978).
3. S. A. Lukehart, S. A. Baker-Zander, and S. Sell. Characterization of lymphocyte responsiveness in early experimental syphilis. I. *In vitro* response to mitogens and *Treponema pallidum* antigens. *J. Immunol.* 124:454-460 (1980).
4. S. A. Lukehart, S. Baker-Zander, R. M. C. Lloyd, and S. Sell. Characterization of lymphocyte responsiveness in early experimental syphilis. II. Nature of cellular infiltration and *Treponema pallidum* distribution in testicular lesions. *J. Immunol.* 124:461-467 (1980).
5. S. Baker-Zander and S. Sell. A histopathologic and immunologic study of the course of syphilis in the experimentally infected rabbit. *Am. J. Pathol.* 101:387-414 (1980).
6. S. Sell, D. Gamboa, S. A. Baker-Zander, S. A. Lukehart, and J. N. Miller. Host response to *Treponema pallidum* in intradermally-infected rabbits: Evidence for persistence of infection at local and distant sites. *J. Invest. Dermatol.* 75:450-475 (1980).

7. P. H. Hardy, Jr., D. J. Graham, E. E. Nell, and A. M. Dannenberg, Jr. Macrophages in immunity to syphilis: Suppressive effect of concurrent infection with Mycobacterium bovis BCG on the development of syphilitic lesions and growth of Treponema pallidum in tuberculin-positive rabbits. Infect. Immun. 26:751-763 (1979).
8. S. T. Mercer. Preliminary observation on human blood in early syphilis by the supravital method. Proc. Soc. Exp. Biol. Med. 28:1033-1035 (1931).
9. P. D. Rosahn and L. Pearce. The blood cytology in untreated and treated syphilis. Am. J. Med. Sci. 187:88-100 (1934).
10. G. Karayalain, A. Khanijov, K. Kimm, A. J. Aballi, and P. Lanzkowsky. Monocytosis in congenital syphilis. Am. J. Dis. Child, 131:782-783 (1977).
11. L. Lowenstein. The leukocytes in early acute experimental syphilis in rabbits. Am. J. Syph. Neurol. 19:39-47 (1935).
12. U. J. Wile, R. Isaacs, and C. W. Knerler. The blood cells in early syphilis. Am. J. Syph. Gonnorhea Vener. Dis. 25:133-141 (1941).
13. H. J. Morgan. A contribution to the cellular pathology of experimental syphilis. Trans. Assoc. Am. Physicians 45:67-70 (1930).
14. R. S. Cunningham, H. J. Morgan, E. Tompkins, and S. Harris. The cellular pathology of experimental syphilis as studied by the supravital method. Am. J. Syph. 17:515-521 (1933).
15. T. B. Turner and D. H. Hollander. Studies on the mechanism of action of cortisone in experimental syphilis. Am. J. Syph. Gonnorhea Vener. Dis. 38:371-387 (1954).
16. H. A. Azar, T. D. Pham, and A. K. Kurban. An electron microscopic study of a syphilitic chancre. Arch. Pathol. 90:143-150 (1970).
17. J. A. Sykes, J. N. Miller, and A. J. Kalan. Treponema pallidum within cells of a primary chancre from a human female. Br. J. Vener. Dis. 50:40-44 (1974).
18. V. Lauderdale and J. N. Goldman. Serial ultrathin sectioning demonstrating the intracellularity of T. pallidum. Br. J. Vener. Dis. 48:87-96 (1972).
19. N. M. Ovcinnikov and V. V Delektorskij. Electron microscopy of phagocytosis in syphilis and yaws. Br. J. Vener. Dis. 48:224-248 (1972).
19a. S. A. Lukehart, S. A. Baker-Zander, R. M. C. Lloyd, and S. Sell. Effect of cortisone administration on host-parasite relationships in early experimental syphilis. J. Immunol. 127:1361-1368 (1981).
20. S. Sell, S. A. Baker-Zander, H. C. Powell, and M. Costello. Digestion of Treponema pallidum by macrophages in testicular lesions of experimental syphilis. Abstracts of the Annual Meeting of the American Society for Microbiology, 1981. Abst. E66, p. 66 (1981).

21. F. C. Lane and E. R. Unanue. Requirement of thymus (T) lymphocytes for resistance to listeriosis. *J. Exp. Med.* 135:1104-1112 (1972).
22. G. B. Mackaness. The influence of immunologically committed lymphoid cells on macrophage activity in vivo. *J. Exp. Med.* 129:973-992 (1969).
23. J. L. Krahenbuhl and J. S. Remington. In vitro induction of nonspecific resistance in macrophages by specifically sensitized lymphocytes. *Infect. Immun.* 4:337-343 (1971).
24. R. J. Patterson and G. P. Youmans. Demonstration in tissue culture of lymphocyte-mediated immunity to tuberculosis. *Infect. Immun.* 1:600-603 (1970).
25. C. S. Pavia, J. D. Folds, and J. B. Baseman. Selective in vitro response of thymus-derived lymphocytes from *Treponema pallidum*-infected rabbits. *Infect. Immun.* 18:603-611 (1977).
26. C. S. Pavia, J. B. Baseman, and J. D. Folds. Selective response of lymphocytes from *Treponema pallidum*-infected rabbits to mitogens and *Treponema reiteri*. *Infect. Immun.* 15:417-422 (1977).
27. P. H. Hardy, E. E. Nell, J. R. Klein, and R. A Prendergast. Specific stimulation of cells from various lymphoid tissues of rabbits with early syphilitic infection. 18th Interscience Conference on Antimicrobial Agents and Chemotheraphy. Abst. 197 (1978).
28. S. M. Maret, J. B. Baseman, and J. D. Folds. Cell-mediated immunity in *Treponema pallidum*-infected rabbits: In vitro response of splenic and lymph node lymphocytes to mitogens and specific antigens. *Clin. Exp. Immunol.* 39:38-43 (1980).
29. G. Chieregato and G. Faldarini. La stimolazione pluriantienica in vitro dei linfociti di soggetti luetici nei vari stadi della malaffia. *Minerva Dermatol.* 43:264-269 (1968).
30. A. L. Badanoiu, M. Gavrilesco, G. Nicolau, and T. Circiumaresco. Lymphoblastogènese immunoallergique et antigène tréponèmique in vitro dans la syphilis. *Arch. Roum. Pathol. Exp. Microbiol.* 28:419-427 (1969).
31. G. Mezzadra, A. Sapuppo, C. Lazzaro, and A. Buzzoni. The-IN VITRO-lymphocyte blast transformation and syphilis. *Arch. Belg. Dermatol. Syphiligr.* 25:385-388 (1969).
32. G. Janot, M. Grandidier, P. Pupil, T. L. Thomas, J. Beurey, and E. de Lavergne, Le test de transformation lymphoblastique au cours de la syphilis. *Presse Med.* 79:1901-1904 (1971).
33. E. From, K. Thestrup-Pedersen, and H. Thulin. Reactivity of lymphocytes from patients with syphilis towards *T. pallidum* antigen in the leucocyte migration and lymphocyte transformation test. *Br. J. Vener. Dis.* 56:224-229 (1976).
34. P. S. Friedmann and J. L. Turk. A spectrum of lymphocyte responsiveness in human syphilis. *Clin. Exp. Immunol.* 21:59-64 (1975).

35. P. S. Friedmann and J. L. Turk. The role of cell-mediated immune mechanisms on syphilis in Ethiopia. *Clin. Exp. Immunol.* 31:59-63 (1978).
36. D. M. Musher, R. F. Schell, and J. M. Knox. In vitro lymphocyte response to *Treponema refringens* in human syphilis. *Infect. Immun.* 9:654-657 (1974).
37. D. M. Musher, R. F. Schell, R. H. Jones, and A. M. Jones. Lymphocyte transformation in syphilis: An *in vitro* correlate of immune suppression *in vivo*? *Infect. Immun.* 11:1261-1264 (1975).
38. K. W. M. Fulford and J. Brostoff. Leucocyte migration and cell-mediated immunity in syphilis. *Br. J. Vener. Dis.* 48:483-488 (1972).
39. J. Bowszyc and J. Bowszyc. Uber den hemmungstrest der makrophagen im verlauf der unbehandefen lues. *Arch. Dermatol. Forsch.* 251:227-234 (1975)
40. V. Wicher and K. Wicher. Host response to *Treponema pallidum* infection. II. Rabbit leukocyte migration inhibition in the presence of homologous organ extracts. *Int. Arch. Allergy Appl. Immun.* 55:481-486 (1977).
41. M. Metzger, J. Podwinska, and W. Smogor. Cell-mediated immunity in experimental syphilis in rabbits. *Arch. Immun. Ther. Exp.* 25:25-34 (1977).
42. C. S. Pavia, J. D. Folds, and J. B. Baseman. Development of macrophage migration inhibition in rabbits infected with virulent *Treponema pallidum*. *Infect. Immun.* 17:651-654 (1977).
43. H. Noguchi. A cutaneous reaction in syphilis. *J. Exp. Med.* 14:557-568 (1911).
44. L. C. Marshak and S. Rothman. Skin testing with a purified suspension of *Treponema pallidum*. *Am. J. Syph.* 35:35-41 (1951).
45. J. Thivolet, A. Simaray, M. Rolland, and F. Challut. Etude de l'intra dermo-réaction aux suspensions of tréponèmes formolées (souche Nichols pathogène) chez les syphilitiques et les sujets normaux. *Ann. Inst. Pasteur* 85:23-33 (1953).
46. G. Csonka. In *Biology of the Treponematoses* (T. B. Turner and D. H. Hollander, Eds.). World Health Organization, Geneva, 1957, pp. 151-152.
47. S. M. Laird and A. L. Thorburn. Assessment of the "Luotest" in late syphilis. *Br. J. Vener. Dis.* 42:119-121 (1966).
48. A. R. Rich, A. M. Chesney, and T. B. Turner. Experiments demonstrating that acquired immunity in syphilis is not dependent upon allergic inflammation. *Bull. Johns Hopkins Hosp.* 52:179-202 (1933).
48a. S. A. Lukehart. Activation of macrophages by products of lymphocytes from normal and syphilitic rabbits. *Infect. Immun.* 37:64-69 (1982).

49. R. F. Schell and D. M. Musher. Detection of nonspecific resistance to *Listeria monocytogenes* in rabbits infected with *Treponema pallidum*. *Infect. Immun.* 9:658-662 (1974).
50. R. Schell, D. Musher, K. Jacobson, and P. Schwethelm. Induction of acquired cellular resistance following transfer of thymus-dependent lymphocytes from syphilitic rabbits. *J. Immunol.* 114: 550-553 (1975).
51. R. Schell, D. Musher, K. Jacobson, P. Schwethelm, and C. Simmons. Effect of macrophage activation on infection with *Treponema pallidum*. *Infect. Immun.* 12:505-511 (1975).
52. S. R. Graves and R. C. Johnson. Effect of pretreatment with *Mycobacterium bovis* (strain BCG) and immune syphilitic serum on rabbit resistance to *Treponema pallidum*. *Infect. Immun.* 12: 1029-1036 (1975).
53. S. Graves. Susceptibility of rabbits to *Treponema pallidum* after infection with *Mycobacterium bovis*. *Br. J. Vener. Dis.* 55: 394-398 (1979).
54. R. E. Baughn, D. M. Musher, and J. M. Knox. Effect of sensitization with *Propionibacterium acnes* on the growth of *Listeria monocytogenes* and *Treponema pallidum* in rabbits. *J. Immunol.* 118:109-113 (1977).
55. S. Harris, Jr., E. H. Tompkins, H. J. Morgan, and R. S. Cunningham. The effect of lecithin on experimental syphilis in the rabbit. *Am. J. Syph. Neurol.* 18:333-340 (1934).
56. D. L. Harris and C. O. Thoen. Inhibition of skin lesions due to *Treponema pallidum* in BCG-infected rabbits. Abstracts of the Annual Meeting of the American Society for Microbiology, 1977. Abstract E32, page 86 (1977).
57. B. D. Brause and R. B. Roberts. Attachment of virulent *Treponema pallidum* to human mononuclear phagocytes. *Br. J. Vener. Dis.* 54:218-224 (1978).
58. M. Metzger and E. Michalska. *Treponema pallidum* opsonophagocytic test. *Arch. Immun. Ther. Exp.* 22:745-758 (1974).
59. V. Wicher, S. Blakowski, and K. Wicher. Nitroblue tetrazolium test in experimental syphilis. *Br. J. Vener. Dis.* 53:292-294 (1977).

Author Index

Numbers in parentheses are reference numbers and indicate that an author's work is referred to although his name is not cited in the text. Italic numbers give the page on which the complete reference is listed.

A

Aballi, A. J., 350(10), *361*
Abell, E., 105(30), 106(30), *118*
Abood, L. G., 214(43), 221(43), *224*
Abrahams, C., 140(1), 146(1), *153*, 274(20), *293*, 316(6), *327*, 332(16), *344*
Abram, D., 17(55), *27*
Abul-Haj, S. K., 214(43), 221(43), *224*
Ackerman, A. B., 105(29), 106(29), *117*
Adler, J., 17(56), *27*
Akin, D. E., 10(35), *26*
Akutsu, A., 200(21), 217(21), *223*
Alarcon, G., 165(42), *171*
Alden, J., 255(101), 258(101), *269*, 331(6), *344*
Alderete, J. F., 30(9), *35*, 62(60), 63(60), *70*, *98*, 141(17), 143(17), 146(17), 148(17), *154*, 229(3), 231(3,9,10), 232(9), 233(9,10), 235(9), 236(9,10),
[Alderete, J. F.] 237(9,10), *238*, *239*, 244(55), *265*, 279(31), *294*, 325(46), *329*, 343(70), *348*
Allen, R. H., 57(2), *66*, 73(36), *96*
Allen, S. L., 32(25), *36*, 65(56), *70*
Allison, M. J., 113(66), *120*
Anderson, J. R., 107(44), *118*
Anderson, N., 17(57), 18(57), 20(57), *27*
Anderson, N. G., 29(4), 30(4), *34*
Angulo, J. J., 4(7,10), 5(7), 7(10), *24*
Answorth, C. T., 109(45), *118*
Arbeit, R. D., 280(40), *294*
Arko, R. J., 80(44), 87(44), *97*
Armenteros, J. A., 39(10), *52*
Armenteros, T., 39(10), *52*
Armstrong, D., 103(8), *116*
Armuzzi, G., 200(23), *223*
Arnott, H. J., 8(22), *25*
Aronson, I. K., 161(4), 162(4), 163(18), 165(4), 166(4), *168*, *169*

365

Artley, C. W., 73(29), *96*, 308
 (36), *312*
Asboe-Hansen, G., 217(63), *225*
Askonas, B. A., 280(32), 283(32), *294*
Asmar, M., 9(29), *25*
Atkins, E., 166(49), 168(57,58), *171, 172*
Auran, N. E., 33(35,36), *36*
Austin, F. E., 62(59), 65(58), *70*
Avinery, S. H., 163(20), *169*
Awoke, S., *170*, 104(17), *117*
Axelsen, N. H., 21(67), *28*
Azar, H. A., 11(42), *26*, 140(7), 148(7), *153*, 189(15), *192*, 220(86), *227*, 242(10), *262*, 309(39), *313*, 350(16), *361*
Azuma, I., 11(50), *27*, 34(41), *37*

B

Babu, J. P., 129(52), *135*, 246(71), 259(71), 260(71), *267*, 334(49,51), *346, 347*
Backhouse, J. l., 104(10), *116*
Badanoiu, A. L., 352(30), *362*
Bagasra, O., 126(50,51), *135*, 141(87), 152(87), *159*, 297(3), *310*, 334(55), 341(55), 342(55), *347*
Baker-Zander, S. A., 104(19), *117*, 143(48,49), *156*, 190(26), *192*, 206(34), 219(34), *223*, 243(30,38), 244(38,39,40), *263*, 274(23,24), 291(23,24), *293*, 298(7,11,12,13,14), 299(14), 300 (7,11,13,14,19), 301(12,13,14), 302(11,14,20), 303(7,12,14), 304 (11,14), 305(7), 307(20), 308(11 12,13,13,20,33), 309(12,20), *310, 311, 312*, 321(21), 322(21), 323(32), *328*, 349(3,4,5,6), 350(4), 351(4,19a,20), 352(3, 4), *360, 361*

Balows, A., 76(37), *97*
Barber, M. K., 58(11), *67*, 80(40), *97*, 216(49), *224*
Barbieri, J. T., 58(57), 59(22,57), 60(57), 62(22,60), 63(60), 65(22, 50,58), *68, 69, 70*
Barbu, E., 40(18), *53*
Barclay, W. R., 332(24), *345*
Baseman, J. B., 8(18), *25*, 30(5,9), *34, 35*, 58(15), 59(12,15), 60(26), 63-65(43,45,46,49,60), *67, 68, 69, 70*, 72(11,15,19,21), 73(15), 75(15), 79(11,15), 80(42), *95, 96 97, 98*, 141(17), 143(17,37,47), 146(17), 147(66), 148(17), 150 (71), 153(71), *154, 155, 156, 158*, 190(25), *192*, 196(8), 199 (8), 210(8), 214(8), 219(72), 220(81), *222, 226, 227*, 229(1,2, 3), 230(1,6,8), 231(3,8,9,10), 232(8,9), 233(1,8,9), 235(2,8,9), 236(8), 237(9), 238(14,15,16), *238, 239*, 242(16), 243(24,25,28, 29), 244(55), *262, 263, 265*, 274(15,16,17,19), 275(25), 279 (31), *292, 294*, 318(14), 321(14, 16,18), 322(16,18,29,30), 324 (43), 325(14,16,29,46), *327, 328, 329*, 332(31,32,33,37), 343(70,71), *345, 346, 348*, 351(25), 352(26, 28), 353(42), *362, 363*
Baskin, S., 244(66), *266*
Baughn, R. E., 104(14), 105(20, 21), *116, 117*, 140(4), 141(13), 146(4), *153, 154*, 163(17), 165-167(17,41), *169, 170*, 219(73), *226*, 238(13), *239*, 242(18,19,20), *262, 263*, 275-277(28,29), 280-284(28,43), 288(43), 290(28,43), *293, 294*, 304(32), *312*, 323(38), 325(50,51,53), *329, 330*, 332(17, 18), 333(41), 342(17,18), 343 (67), *344, 345, 348*, 356(54), *364*
Becker, F. A., 60(18), 64(18), *67*, 72(16), 73(31), 75(16,31), 79(16), 80(31), 82(31), 83(16), 87(16),

Author Index

[Becker, F. A.]
94(31), *95, 96, 98*, 148(70), *158*, 216(50,51), *224, 225*, 233(12), *239*
Bedi, T. R., 105(27), *117*
Behling, A. H., 220(83), *227*
Bell, P. B., 188(11), *191*
Bell, W. R., 109(46), *118*
Bellanti, J. A., 342(60), *347*
Bendersky, J., 163(20), *169*
Benirschke, K., 113(70), *120*
Bennett, H. D., 107(40), *118*
Bensel, A., 125(41,42), *135*
Bensley, S. H., 217(61), *225*
Berger, B. J., 105(23), *117*
Bergoend, H., 244(64), *266*
Bernheim, H. A., 166(49), *171*
Berry, F. W., 104(16), *116*, 165 (35), *170*
Bertarelli, E., 122(10), *133*
Bessemans, A., 121(2), 131(2), *132*, 334(43), *346*
Beurey, J., 352(32), *362*
Bey, R. F., 31(17), 33(36), *35, 36*, 123(32), *134*, 205(32), 206(32), 215(32), 216(32), 220(32), *223*, 274(14), 275(14), 279(14), *292*, 325(49), *330*, 332(30), *345*
Bharier, M. A., 34(39), *36*
Bhorade, M. S., 109(47), *119*
Bhutani, L. K., 105(27), *117*
Billington, T., 80(47), *97*, 216(55), *225*
Birch-Andersen, A., 4(9), 5(16), 8(9,16), 9(9,29), 11(9,16), 13(9,16), 15(9), 17(9,16), 19 (61), 21(64,65,67,68,), 23(61), *24, 25, 28*, 49(41), 50(41), *54*
Birry, A., 113(68), *120*
Bishop, N. B., 211(40), *224*
Bishop, N. H., 243(31), 244(51), 245(5,67), 247(31), 254(31,96), 255(67), 256(67), 260(67), *264, 265, 266, 268*, 273(4), *292*, 302(21), 303(23,26), 304(30), *311, 312*, 331(1), *343*

Blakowski, S., 141(14), *154*, 357 (59), *364*
Blanden, R. V., 147(69), *158*, 323 (35), *329*
Blasecki, J. W., 336(58), *347*
Bleyman, M. A., 42(30), *54*
Block-Schut, B. J. T., 321(26), *328*
Bloodgood, R. A., 8(23), *25*
Bloom, B. R., 261(102), *269*, 274 (8), 290(8), *292*
Blumershine, R. V., 8(26), *25*
Bocanegra, T., 165(42), *171*
Bodel, P., 168(58), *172*
Boer, A. M., 291(50), *295*
Bokkenheuser, V., 140(1), 146(1), *153*, 274(20), *293*, 316(6), *327*, 332(16), *344*
Bolton, E. T., 42(33), *54*
Bondareff, W., 214(44), 215(44), 217(44), 221(44), *224*
Borel, J. F., 220(84), *227*
Borel, L. J., 144(50,53), *156, 157*
Borstoff, J., 316(7), *327*
Bos, J. D., 141(21), 142(21), *154*, 243(36), *264*
Bowszyc, J., 353(39), *363*
Braunstein, 109(46), *118*
Braunstein, G. D., 166(44), *171*
Brause, B. D., 8(21), *25*, 124(40), *135*, 357(57), *364*
Breznak, J. A., 10(37), *26*, 60 (24), *68*
Brickman, F., 163(18), *169*
Briggs, W., 168(54), *172*
Brimacombe, J. S., 214(42), 216 (42), *224*
Brimble, A. G. S., 274(10), *292*
Britten, R. J., 42(34), *54*
Brodie, A. F., 61(32), *68*
Bromley, D. B., 33(37), *36*
Brooker, B. E., 10(38), *26*
Brostoff, J., 332(34), *345*, 352 (38), *363*
Brown, W. H., 122(15,16,17,18, 19,20,21,22), 124(18,36,37,38), *133, 134*, 298(8,9,10), *311*

Brown, W. J., 242(2), *261*, 297
 (2), *310*
Browning, C. H., 308(34), *312*
Brundell, J., 220(84), *227*
Brunings, E. A., 115(78), *120*
Bruusgaard, E., 248(72), 254
 (72), *267*
Bryceson, A. D. M., 161(7),
 162(13), 163(21), 164(7,13,
 21,26), 165(36), *168, 169, 170*
Bullard, J. C., 76(39), 80(39,
 44), 87(44), *97*, 308(36), *312*
Burkhart, J. E., 113(64), *120*
Butler, T., 164(28), *170*
Butler, T. P., 104(17), *117*
Butterworth, T., 101(1), 104(1),
 114(1), *115*
Butz, W. C., 105(28), *117*
Buzzoni, A., 352(31), *362*
Byrd, L. H., 244(66), *266*

C

Cameron, E., 217(37), *224*
Campbell, R. E., 4(11), *24*
Canale-Parola, E., 11(46), *27*,
 33(38), 34(42), *36, 37*, 41
 (25), 42(32), *53, 54*, 60(24),
 68, 72(12), 79(12), *95*, 216(59),
 225
Cantor, H., 291(49), *295*
Carag, H. B., 109(47), *119*
Carraway, K. L., 188(11), *191*
Casavant, C. H., 143(31), *155*
Castellani, A., 4(12), *24*, 39(9),
 52
Catchpole, H. R., 215(46), 217
 (46), *224*
Catterall, R. D., 113(63), *119*
Chacko, C. W., 144(52), *157*
Challut, F., 244(60), *266*, 316
 (3a), *326*, 354(45), *363*
Chalmers, W. S. R., 60(21), *68*
Chambers, R., 217(65), *226*
Chan, J. K., 126(49,50,51), 129
 (52), *135*, 141(87), 152(86,87),

[Chan, J. K.]
 159, 219(74), *226*, 246(70), 256
 (70), 259(70), 260(70), *266*,
 297(3), *310*, 334(49,50,52,53,54,
 55), 335(52), 336(53), 337(52),
 338(53), 339(54), 341(55), 342
 (55), *346, 347*
Chandler, F. W., Jr., 30(7), *34*,
 152(74), *158*
Chapel. T. A., 102(5), 103(5),
 116
Chapman, G. B., 140(5), *153*
Charon, M. W., 33(37), *36*
Chesney, A. N., 190(28), *193*,
 219(68), *226*, 248(74,75), 252
 (95), *267, 268*, 298(17), 308(17),
 311, 354(48), *363*
Chess, L., 342(61), *347*
Chieregato, G., 352(29), *362*
Christian, C. L., 325(48), *329*
Christiansen, A. H., 165(31), *170*
Christiansen, S., 200(10), 216(10),
 222
Circiumaresco, T., 352(30), *362*
Clark, C. G., 321(27), *328*
Clark, E. G., 110(50), 111(50),
 119, 166(44), *171*
Clark, J. W. Jr., 29(4), 30(4,7),
 34, 73(29), 76(37), *96, 97*, 248
 (78), *267*, 308(36), *312*
Cleveland, P., 8(17), 21(17), *25*,
 30(11), *35*, 147(65), *158*
Cline, G. B., 29(4), 30(4), *34*
Cochems, K. D., 111(52), *119*
Cochran, R. E. J., 105(31), 106
 (31), *118*
Cohen, N. S., 61(32), *68*
Cohen, P. G., 152(75), *158*
Cole, 297(5), *310*, 326(55), *330*,
 334(48), *346*
Collart, P., 144(50,53), 147(56),
 156, 157, 298(18), *311*
Collier, A. M., 8(18), *25*, 72(15),
 73(15), 75(15), 79(15), *95*, 190
 (25), *192*, 196(8), 199(8), 210
 (8), *222*, 229(1), 230(1), 233(1),
 238, 242(16), *262*

Author Index

Cooper, K. E., 163(21), 164(21), 169
Corin, R. E., 62(59), 70
Cormane, R. H., 141(21), 142(21), 154, 243(36), 264
Cortes,, A., 152(77), 158
Costello, M., 351(20), 361
Costerton, J. W., 62(40), 69
Cotram, R. S., 242(17), 245(17), 262
Coutinho, A., 323(33), 328
Cox, C. D., 30(8), 35, 58(11, 57), 59(13, 22, 57), 60(13, 14, 23, 26, 57), 61(13, 14), 62(14, 22, 23, 60), 63(14, 60), 65(13, 22, 50, 58), 67, 68, 69, 70, 72(17), 74(17), 80(40, 41), 82(17), 83(17), 94(17), 95, 96, 216(49), 224
Crilly, K., 98
Csonka, G. W., 332(10), 344, 354(46), 363
Culp, L. H., 188(13), 192
Culter, J. C., 332(11), 344
Cumberland, M. C., 65(51), 70, 190(29), 193, 219(69), 226
Cunningham, R. S., 350(14), 356(55), 361, 364
Cuttler, J. C., 101(4), 102(4), 110(4), 116, 249(89), 254(89), 268
Cwyk, W. M., 42(32), 54

D

Dacres, W. G., 123(31), 134, 249(85, 86), 267, 268
D'Alessandro, G., 142(29), 155
Dalton, H. P., 113(66), 120
Dammin, G. J., 200(24, 25, 26), 215(24), 217(24), 223, 243(34), 264
Danbolt, N., 110(50), 111(50), 119
Dannenberg, A. M., Jr., 105(22), 117, 141(18), 154, 189(20), 190(20), 192, 243(35), 264,

[Dannenberg, A. M., Jr.] 323(41), 329, 349(7), 356(7), 357(7), 361
Daskalopoulos, G., 104(10), 116
Davis, B. D., 65(53), 70
Deeb, S. S., 60(27), 68
de Graciansky, P., 163(23), 169
DeJong, N. H. L., 291(50), 295
Delamater, E. D., 217(36), 224
de Lavergne, E., 352(32), 362
Delbanco, E., 200(19, 20), 222, 223
Delektorskij, V. V., 4(8), 11(40), 17(8, 40, 58), 18(8, 40), 24, 26, 27, 140(10), 153, 189(22), 192, 217(67), 226, 350(19), 361
Deley, J., 61(29, 30), 68
Delgado, D. G., 107(38), 118
de Mello, L., 101(4), 102(3), 104(3), 114(3), 116, 249(89), 254(89), 268, 332(11), 344
DeMoor, A., 121(2), 131(2), 132, 334(43), 346
Denham, S. W., 162(12), 168
Dennie, C. C., 161(3), 168
De Pamphilis, M. L., 17(56), 27
de Sousa, M. A., 321(23), 328
Dessaint, J. P., 244(64), 266
Deubner, B., 200(14), 222
Devemy, P., 244(64), 266
DiChara, G., 142(29), 155
Dickler, H. B., 280(40), 294
Diener, E., 280(33), 294
Diesendruck, J. A., 73(25), 82(25), 96, 243(32), 249(32), 264
Diezel, W., 165(40), 170, 290(48), 295
Dippell, A. L., 113(69), 120
Dismukers, W. E., 107(38), 118
Dixon, F. J., 273(1), 275(1), 291
Doniach, D., 142(27, 30), 155
Doty, P., 41(19), 42(21), 53
Dredergast, R. A., 321(22), 322(22), 328
Drummond, K. N., 109(48), 119
Drusin, 140(5), 153
Drusin, L. M., 103(8), 116

Ducan, W. C., 163(17), 165-167
(17), *169*
Ducan, W. P., 76(39), 80(39),
97
Dunea, B. S., 109(48), *119*
Dunoyer, P., 147(56), *157*
Durel, P., 144(50,53), *156, 157,*
298(18), *311*
Dwyer, J. M., 243(22), *263*, 290
(45), *295*

E

Eagle, H., 40(16), *53,* 57(10),
65(52), 67, 70, 74(33), 75(34),
80(34), *96, 97,* 101(3), 102(3),
104(3), 114(3), *116,* 123(30),
134, 249(80), *267*
East, J., 321(23), *328*
Eggebraten, L., 31(23), 32(23),
35
Ehrlich, I., 107(37), *118*
Eisen, H. N., 280(34), 284(34),
294
Elberg, S. S., 332(14), *344*
Elgin, L. W., 242(1), *261*
Elin, R. J., 104(16), *116,* 165(35),
170
Emanuel, R., 112(58), *119*
Engel, S., 165(40), *170,* 290(48),
295
Ensign, J. C., 11(45), *27*
Erickson, D., 143(42), *156,* 245
(68), 255(68), 258(68), *266,*
303(27), *312,* 331(5), *344*
Escobar, M. R., 113(62,66), *119,*
120
Evans, L. D., 161-163(5), 165
(5,37,38), 166(37,38), 168,
170
Evans, V. J., 75(36), *97*

F

Faine, S., 11(53), *27*
Falcone, V. H., 42(35), *54*

Faldarini, G., 352(29), *362*
Falkow, S., 41(23), *53*
Fallet, G. H., 107(33), *118*
Falls, W. F., Jr., 109(45), *118*
Farmer, T. W., 162(10), *168*
Farr, R. S., 168(54), *172*
Fazzan, F. P., 249(84,90), *267,*
268
Feher, J., 107(42,43), *118*
Feigenbaum, S., 243(31), 247(31),
254(31), *264*
Feldmann, M., 280(33), *294*
Felton, L. D., 220(82), *227*
Ferris, H. W., 151(72,73), *158*
Festenstein, H. C., 140(1), 146
(1), *153,* 274(20), *293,* 316(6),
327, 332(16), *344*
Fichera, G., 142(29), *155*
Fieldsteel, A. H., 32(24,27), *36,*
41(28), 42(29), 47(49), 50(40),
52(50), *54,* 60(18), 64(18), *67,*
72(16,17), 73(13), 74(17), 75(16,
17, 13), 79(16), 80(31), 82(17,31),
83(61,17), 87(16,51), 94(17,31),
95, 96, 98, 148(70), *158,* 216
(50,51), *224, 225,* 233(12), *239*
Finn, M. A., 72(14), 74(14), 76(14),
79(14), *95*
Fitzgerald, J. J., 101(2), 104(2),
114(2), *115*
Fitzgerald, T. J., 8(17,20), 10
(39), 11(39), 21(17), *25, 26,*
30(11,13), *35,* 51(42), *55,* 60(20),
68, 73(23,30), 74(24,30,32), 75
(30,35), 80(23,30,35), 82(30),
87(50), 94(53), *96, 97, 98,* 123
(32,33,34), *134,* 146(58,61), 148
(58,59), *157,* 173(3,4,5,6), 174
(3,4,5,7,8), 187(10), 188(3,4),
189(19), 190(6,23,24), *191, 192,*
196-201(3,4,6,7,17,29,30), 203
(4), 204(29), 205(30,32,33),
206(17,32), 207(3,6,33,38,39),
208(33), 209(39), 210(3,4,6,38),
211(3), 213(33), 214(3,39), 215
(24,32), 216(7,17,32,33,53,58),
219(3,33), 220(17,30,32,33), *221,*
222, 223, 224, 225, 233(11), *238,*

[Fitzgerald, T. J.]
239, 242(14), 244(14,53,53,56),
262, 265, 274(14), 275(14),
279(14,30), 292, 293, 324(45),
325(49), 329, 330, 332(30),
345
Fitzharris, T. P., 8(23), 25
Fiu Mara, N. J., 104(15), 109(49),
111(15), 116, 119
Fleer, A., 321(26), 328
Fleischman, R., 65(52), 70, 74
(33), 96, 101(3), 102(3), 104
(3), 114(3), 116, 123(30), 134,
249(80), 267
Fleming, K. A., 105(31), 106(31),
118
Fleming, W. L., 190(31), 193, 219
(71), 226, 249(81), 267
Fletcher, M., 10(36), 26
Floersheim, G. L., 220(84), 227
Floodgate, G. D., 10(36), 26
Folds, J. D., 143(37,57), 155,
156, 219(72), 220(81), 226,
227, 238(14,15,16), 239, 243
(24,25,28,29), 263, 274(15,16,
17,19), 275(25), 292, 293, 318
(14), 321(14,16,18), 322(16,
18,29,30), 324(43), 325(14,16,
29), 327, 328, 329, 332(31,32,
33,37), 345, 346, 351(25),
352(26,28), 353(42), 362, 363
Folger, C., 72(14), 74(14), 76
(14), 79(14), 95
Fontana, A., 40(13), 53, 71(2),
78(2), 94
Ford, K. L., 109(45), 118
Forsberg, C. W., 62(40), 69
Foster, J. W., 76(37), 97
Franceschini, P., 147(56), 157,
298(18), 311
Francis, L., 166(49), 168(57),
171, 172
Frank, M. M., 104(16), 116,
165(35), 170
Frazier, C. N., 125(41,42), 135
Frederichs, W. R., 21(66), 28
Fredericks, W. R., 34(40), 37

Fribourg-Blanc, A., 152(84), 159,
242(5), 243(5), 262
Friedman, P. S., 105(26), 111(26),
117, 243(27), 263, 317(12,13),
318(13), 327, 352(34,35), 362,
363
From, E., 142(23), 154, 165(39),
166(39), 170, 243(23), 244(23,
63), 263, 266, 274(13), 290(47),
292, 295, 317(11), 325(52), 327,
330, 332(29), 345, 352(33),
353(33), 362
Fujita, T., 62(41), 69
Fulford, K. W. M., 104(18), 117,
166(46), 171, 316(7), 327, 332
(34), 345, 352(38), 363
Fuller, R., 10(38), 26

G

Gager, W. E., 147(55), 157
Galloway, R. E., 170
Galvenek, E.G., 109(46), 118,
166(44), 171
Gamble, C. N., 166(45), 171, 244
(65), 266
Gamboa, D., 244(40), 264, 298(7),
300(7), 303(7), 305(7), 310,
349(6), 360
Garner, M. F., 104(10), 116
Garrard, W. T., 62(42), 69
Gavrilesco, M., 352(30), 362
Gee, B., 290(45), 295
Gelfand, J. A., 104(16), 116,
165(35), 170
Germain, B. F., 165(42), 171
Gel'man, N. S., 60(31), 61(31),
68
Germuth, F. G., 40(17), 53
Gersch, I., 215(46), 217(46), 224
Gershon, R. K., 291(49), 295,
342(62), 347
Gerster, J. C., 107(33), 118
Ginger, C. D., 11(52), 20(52),
27
Giroux, M., 113(68), 120

Gjestland, T., 221(87), 227
Glassman, L. H., 17(59), 18(59), 27, 196(9), 222
Glenn, M. W., 47(37), 54
Glock, R. D., 8(24), 25, 32 (26), 36, 47(36,38), 54, 58 (16), 67
Golden, B., 42(34), 54
Goldman, E. E., 144(54), 157
Goldman, J. N., 189(16), 192, 217(66), 220(66), 226, 242(12), 262, 350(18), 361
Goldsmith, G. H., 170
Goodman, H. M., 230(7), 238
Gordan, J., 8(25), 25
Gospodarowicz, D., 188(12), 191
Gotuzzo, E., 165(42), 170
Grabau, W., 112(58), 119
Graetz, F., 200(19,20), 222, 223
Graham, D. J., 105(22), 117, 141 (18), 154, 189(20), 190(20), 192, 243(35), 264, 323(41), 329, 343(65), 348, 349(7), 356(7), 357(7), 361
Grandidier, M., 352(32), 362
Graves, S. R., 57(5,6), 67, 72(13,20), 73(13,20), 74(20), 75(13), 79(13,20), 80(47), 81(20), 95, 96, 97, 141(12), 154, 216(55), 225, 255(100, 101), 256(100), 258(101), 269, 323(39,40), 329, 331(6), 343(68,69), 344, 348, 356(52, 53), 357(52), 364
Green, R. L., 141(22), 154
Greenwood, R. J., 113(65), 120
Gregoriew, P. S., 189(21), 192, 200(22), 217(22), 223, 243(33), 264
Greisman, S. E., 163(16), 169
Grey, H. M., 168(54), 172
Grigas, D. E., 62(59), 70
Grimble, A. G. S., 146(63), 157, 220(79), 227, 243(21), 244(42),

[Grimble, A. G. S.] 263, 265, 316(4), 325(4), 326, 332(27), 345
Grimble, A. S., 142(27), 155, 166(47), 171
Grin, E. I., 80(43), 97
Grover, A. A., 332(23), 345
Grupper, C., 163(23), 169
Gschwandtner, W. R., 111(51), 119
Gudjonsson, H., 162(5), 166(15), 167(51,52,53), 169, 171
Gueft, B., 121(3), 131(3), 132, 334(45), 346
Guerraz, F. T., 152(83),159, 335 (56), 347
Guest, W. J., 244(48), 265
Guthe, T., 3(4), 5(4), 24, 40(12), 52(43), 53, 55, 57(9), 67, 72(7), 78(7), 95, 114(76), 120
Gyorkey, P., 140(4), 146(4), 153

H

Habte-Michael, A., 104(17), 117
Hackett, C. J., 39(1), 52, 114(75), 120
Hacen, P., 164(28), 170
Haensell, P., 122(9), 133
Hager, L. P., 60(27), 68
Hager, W. D., 113(71), 120
Halbert, S. P., 249(79), 267
Hamerlinck, F., 141(21), 142(21), 154, 243(36), 264
Hamilton, A., 109(46), 118, 166(44), 171
Hampp, E. G., 165(30), 170
Handsfield, H. H., 308(37), 312
Handy, A. H., 47(37), 54
Hanlard, W. A., 8(25), 25
Hannf, P. A., 242-244(3), 250-253 (3), 261
Hardy, P. H., Jr., 10(31), 21(66), 26, 28, 29(2), 30(2,14), 33(30), 34(40), 34, 35, 36, 37, 65(54),

[Hardy, P. H., Jr.]
70, 72(18), 95, 105(22), 117, 141(18), 142(28), 143(39), 154, 155, 156, 165(33), 170, 189(20), 190(20), 192, 200(11,12), 216(11,12), 222, 243(35), 244(44, 45), 255(99), 257(99), 264, 265, 268, 297(5), 303(25), 310, 312, 321(22), 322(22), 323(41), 326(55), 328, 329, 330, 331(4), 334(48), 343(65), 343, 345, 348, 349(7), 352(27), 356(7), 357(7), 361, 362

Harner, R. E., 144(51), 157

Harris, D. L., 8(24), 19(63), 25, 28, 32(26,27), 36, 42(29, 31), 47(29,36,38), 49(39), 57, 58(16,17), 60(25), 67, 68, 343(64), 348, 357(56), 364

Harris, R. A., 60(25), 68

Harris, S., 350(14), 361

Harris, S., Jr., 356(55), 364

Harter, C., 113(70), 120

Hasegawa, T., 140(6), 153

Hattori, S., 34(41), 37

Hattori, Y., 11(50), 27

Hayes, E. C., 150(71), 153(71), 158, 229(2), 230(8), 231(8), 232(8), 233(8), 235(2,8), 236(8), 238, 343(71), 348

Hayes, N. S., 8(18), 25, 30(5), 34, 63-65(43,45), 69, 72(15,19), 73(15), 75(15), 79(15), 80(42), 95, 97, 147(66), 158, 190(25), 192, 196(8), 199(8), 210(8), 214(8), 222, 229(1,2), 230(1, 6), 233(1), 235(2), 238, 242(16), 262

Hazen, C. K., 104(17), 117

Hederstedt, B., 242(6,7,8,9), 243(6,7,8,9), 246(7), 262

Hedge, M., 112(58), 119

Heggtveit, H. A., 112(60), 119

Hellstrom, I., 326(54), 330

Hellstrom, K. E., 326(54), 330

Henkart, P. A., 280(40), 294

Hensen, S. A., 342(60), 347

Herzenberg, L. A., 336(59), 347

Herzig, G. P., 290(46), 295

Heyman, A., 161(5), 162(5,14), 163(5), 165(5,37,38), 166(37,38), 168, 169, 170

Hicklin, M. D., 105(28), 117

Hill, K. R., 125(43), 135

Hill, L. R., 40(22), 53

Hillinger, S. M., 290(46), 295

Hiraoka, K., 112(59), 119

Hoekenga, M. T., 162(10), 168

Hoffman, M. K., 336(57), 347

Hoffmann, E., 3(1,2), 4(1), 23, 39(5,6,7), 52, 122(13), 133

Hollander, D. H., 29(1), 34, 40(11), 53, 72(6), 78(6), 95, 122-126(8,28,29,48), 132, 134, 135, 141(15), 154, 157, 189(1), 191, 195(1), 200(1,27,28), 215-217(1), 219(1,27), 221, 223, 244(43), 248(43), 249(43), 265, 273(6), 274(6), 279(6), 292, 298(6), 308(6), 310, 350(15), 361

Holt, S. C., 11(46,51), 20(51), 27, 34(42), 37

Hooshmand, H., 113(62), 119

Hornick, R. B., 163(16), 169

Horvath, I., 76(39), 80(39,44, 46), 82(46), 87(44), 97, 216(52), 225

Houston, K. J., 336(58), 347

Hovind-Hougen, K., 4(9), 5(16), 8(9,16,19), 9(9,19,28,29), 11(9,16,19,44), 13(9,16,19,44), 15(9,44), 16(44), 17(9,16,19, 44), 18(19), 19(61), 20(19), 21(64,65,67), 23(61), 24, 25, 26, 28, 49(41), 50(41), 54

Howie, J. G. R., 8(25), 25

Hudson, E. R., 39(2), 52(2), 52

Hull, J., 166(50), 171

Hurtado, R. C., 342(60), 347

Hussey, M. S., 214(41), 224

I

Ibrahim, A. N., 30(12), *35*
Idsφe O., 52(43), *55*
Ingall, D., 114(72), *120*
Israel, C. W., 42(35), *54*, 147
  (55), *157*
Isaaca, R., 350(12), *361*
Ishibashi, Y., 18(60), *27*
Ito, K., 205(31), *223*
Iwasaki, Y., 61(35), *68*
Izzat, N. N., 123(31), *134*, 249
  (85,86), *267, 268*

J

Jackson, S. W., 33(34), *36*,
  165(32), *170*
Jacobsen, K., 165(39), 166(39),
  170
Jacobsen, K. U., 142(23), *154*,
  244(63), *266*, 290(47), *295*,
  325(52), *330*
Jacobson, K., 141(11), *153*, 323
  (37), *329*, 332(20), 334(47),
  343(66), *344, 345, 348*, 355
  (50,51), 357(51), *364*
Jaffe, H. W., 113(67), *120*
Jakubowski, A., 121(1), 131(1),
  132, 141(20), *154*, 334(42), *346*
Janot, G., 352(32), *362*
Jarisch, A., 161(1), *168*
Jarisheva, K. G., 200(22), 217
  (22), *223*, 243(33), *264*
Jayawardena, A. N., 290(44),
  295
Jeerapaet, P., 105(29), 106(29),
  117
Jenkin, H. M., 31(15,23), 32(15,
  23), *35*, 57(5,6), 60(19),
  63-65(44,45), *67, 69, 70*, 72
  (13,20), 73(13,20,24), 74(20),
  75(13,24), 79(13,20), 80(24),
  81(21,22), 82(20,22,24), 94(24),
  95, 96, 98, 142(25), (25), *155*,
  216(54), *225*

Jensen, H-J. S., 49(41), 50(41),
  54
Jepsen, O. B., 5(16), 8(16), 11
  (16), 13(16), 17(16), *24*
Jimenez, S., 107(34), *118*
Johnson, N., 104(18), *117*, 166
  (46), *171*
Johnson, R. C., 8(17,20), 10(39),
  11(39,41,49), 13(54), 18(41),
  20(54), 21(17), *25, 26, 27*, 30
  (11,13), 31(16,21,23), 32(16,23,
  25,28), 33(29,31,32,33,35,36),
  34(43), *35, 36, 37*, 51(42), *55*,
  57(5), 65(56), *67, 70*, 72(9,10,
  13), 73(13,30), 74(30,32), 75(13,
  30), 79(9,10), 80(30), 83(30),
  87(50), 94(53), *95, 96, 98*,
  101(2), 104(2), 114(2), *115*,
  122(32,33,34), *134*, 141(12),
  146(61), 147(65), 148(59), *154,
  157, 158*, 196-201(3,4,7,17,29,
  30), 203(4), 205(30,32,33), 206
  (17,32), 207(3,33,38), 208(33,
  39), 209(39), 210(4,38), 211(3),
  213(33), 214(3,39), 215(32),
  216(7,17,32,33,58), 219(3,33),
  220(17,30,32,33), *221, 222, 223,
  224, 225,* 233(11), *238, 239,*
  244(53,54,56), 255(100), 256
  (100), *265, 269*, 274(14), 275(14),
  279(14,30), *292, 293,* 323(39),
  324(45), 325(49), *329, 330,* 332
  (30), 343(68), *345, 348,* 356(52),
  357(52), *364*
Johnson, R. E., 31(17), *35*
Jones, A. M., 10(33), 11(33), *26*,
  30(10), *35*, 94(48), *97*, 141(16),
  154, 200(16), 215(16), 218(16),
  222, 230(4), 233(4), *238*, 244
  (52,62), *265*, 274(12), *292*, 317
  (10), 324(44), *327, 329*, 332(26),
  345, 352(37), *363*
Jones, E. W., 105(30), 106(30),
  118
Jones, R. H., 10(33), 11(33), *26*,
  30(10), *35*, 72(14), 74(14), 76
  (14), 79(14), 94(48), *95, 97*,

Author Index

[Jones, R. H.]
141(16), *154*, 200(16), 215(16), 218(16), *222*, 244(48,52,62), *265*, 274(12), *292*, 317(10), 324 (44), *327, 329*, 332(26), *345*, 352(37), *363*
Joseph, R., 11(46), *27*, 34(42), *37*
Jove, D.F., 113(67), *120*
Jozsa, L., 107(42,43), *118*
Julius, M. H., 336(59), *347*

K

Kadziewicz, E., 104(12), *116*
Kalan, A. J., 4(5), *24*, 140(8), *153*, 189(18), *192*, 242(13,15), *262*, 309(41), *313*, 350(17), *361*
Kalinka, C., 206(35), *223*
Kamanski, D., 146(62), *157*, 275(27), *293*
Kampmeier, R. H., 111(53), *119*, 308(35), *312*
Kantor, F. S., 220(78), *226*, 290(45), *295*, 321(24), *328*, 332(28), *345*
Kaplan, B. I., 101(4), 102(4), 110(4), *116*, 142(26), 145(26), *155*, 249(89), 254(89), *268*, 332(11), *344*
Kaplan, B. S., 109(48), *119*
Kaplan, M. H., 143(33,34), *155*
Kaplan, N. O., 61(33,34), *68*
Karayalain, G., 350(10), *361*
Karimi, Y., 9(29), *25*
Karush, F., 280(34), 284(34), *294*
Kasatiya, S., 113(68), *120*
Kellogg, D. S., Jr., 30(6), *34*, 76(37), *97*
Kemp, J. E., 111(52), *119*, 190 (28), *193*, 219(68), *226*
Keuper, C. S., 125(41,42), *135*
Khan, A. S., 152(78), *158*
Khanijov. A., 350(10), *361*

Kiesel, H. A., 107(40), *118*
Kim, D. U., 244(66), *266*
Kimm, G. E., 57(2), *66*, 73(26), *96*
Kimm, K., 350(10), *361*
Kindmark, C. O., 166(48), *171*
Kinyon, J. M., 8(24), 19(63), *25, 28*, 42(31), 47(38), 49(39), *54*, 58(16,17), 60(25), *67, 68*
Kiraly, K., 31(19), *35*, 216(52), *225*
Kis, Z., 220(84), *227*
Klauder, J. V., 101(1), 104(1), 114(1), *115*
Klaviter, E., 34(43), *37*
Klebanoff, S. J., 143(40), *156*, 255(98), 260(98), *268*, 303(24), *312*, 331(2), *343*
Klein, J. R., 297(5), *310*, 321(22), 322(22), 326(55), *328, 330*, 334 (48), *346*, 352(27), *362*
Klingman, J. D., 142(24), *154*
Klingmüller, G., 18(60), *27*
Kluth, F. C., 242(4), 249(4), *262*
Knerler, C. W., 350(12), *361*
Knight, S. T., 57(6), *67*, 72(20), 73(20), 74(20), 81(22), 82(22), *96*
Knox, J. M., 103(9), 105(20), *116, 117*, 123(31), *134*, 141(13), 143(46), *154, 156*, 242(1), 244(61) (61), 249(85,86), *261, 266, 267, 268*, 274(11), *292*, 317(9), 323 (38), *327, 329*, 332(25), *343*(67), *345, 348*, 352(36), 356(54), *363, 364*
Koch, M., 200(18), *222*
Koehorst, J. A. M., 291(50), *295*
Koffler, H., 17(55), *27*
Kohne, D. E., 42(34), *54*
Kolar, O. J., 113(64), *120*
Kolenbrander, P. E., 11(45), *27*
Kopf, S. W., 113(62), *119*
Kotianinen, S., 280(37,38), *283* (37,38), *294*, 351(23), *362*
Krakenbuhl, J. L., 351(23), *362*
Kraszewski, A., 8(25), *25*
Krauch, J., 104(12), *116*

Kraus, S. J., 141(22), *154*
Krause, R. M., 72(8), 79(8) *95*
Krause Herxheimer, K., 161(2), 165(2), *168*
Krican, M. E., 107(37), *118*
Kubica, K. M., 10(33), 11(33), *26*, 30(10), *35*, 94(48), *97*, 141(16), *154*, 200(16), 215(16), 218(16), *222*, 230(4), 233(4), *238*, 244(52), *265*, 324(44), *329*
Kuhn, U. S. G., III, 42(35), *54*, 152(74,75), *158*, 297(2), *310*
Kumar, V., 142(24), *154*
Kurban, A. K., 11(42), *26*, 140(7), 148(7), *153*, 189(15), *192*, 220(86), *227*, 242(10), *262*, 309(39), *313*, 350(16), *361*

L

Laird, S. M., 354(47), *363*
Lane, F. C., 351(21), *362*
Lapushin, R. W., 140(4), 146(4), *153*
Larsen, S. A., 113(47), *120*
Lascano, E. F., 217(64), *226*
Lascelles, J., 60(28), *68*
Lassus, A., 325(47), *329*
Lauderdale, V., 189(16), *192*, 217(66), *226*, 242(12), *262*, 350(18), *361*
Laurent, T. C., 216(48), *224*
Lawn, A. M., 21(69), *28*
Lazzaro, C., 352(31), *362*
LeClerc, G., 113(68), *120*
Lee, F. D., 8(25), *25*
Lee, H. J., 109(47), *119*
Lee, I., 244(66), *266*
Lee, K. Y., 40(18), *53*
Lee, R., 243(22), *263*
Lees, A. J., 113(65), *120*
Lefford, M. J., 323(35), *329*
LeFrock, J. L., 126(49,50,51), 129(52), *135*, 141(85,87),

[LeFrock, J. L.]
152(85,86,87), *159*, 219(74), *226*, 246(70,71), 256(70), 259(70, 71), 260(70,71), *266*, *267*, 297(3), *310*, 334(49,50,51,52,53, 54,55), 335(52), 336(53), 337(52), 338(53), 339(54), 341(55), 342(55), *346*, *347*
Lejman, K., 105(24), *117*
Lenhoff, H. M., 61(33,34), *68*
León-Blanco, F., 4(7,10), 5(7), 7(10), *24*
Lesinski, J., 104(12), *116*
Lessof, M. G., 142(27), *155*
Levaditi, C., 72(4), 78(4), *95*
Levene, G. M., 140(2), 146(2,63), *153*, *157*, 220(79), *227*, 243(21), *263*, 274(9,10), *292*, 316(4,5), 325(4), *326*, *327*, 332(27), *345*
Levin, J., *170*
Lewis, E. J., 109(46), *118*, 166(44), *171*
Livermore, B. P., 11(41), 18(41), *26*, 31(16,17,21,23), 32(16,23, 28), *35*, *36*
Lloyd, R. M. C., 104(19), *117*, 143(49), *156*, 190(26), *192*, 243(38), 244(38,39), *264*, 298(12,13), 300(13), 301(12,13), 303(12), 308(12,13), 309(12), *311*, 323(32), *328*, 349(4), 350(4), 351(19a), 352(4), *360*, *361*
Lockshin, N. A., 105(23), *117*
Logan, L. C., 143(35), 146(35), 148(35), *155*, 244(48,50), 249(50), *265*
Lopez, B., 113(67), *120*
Loveday, C., 104(18), *117*, 166(46), *171*
Lowenstein, L., 350(11), *361*
Lucas, J. B., 242(2), *261*
Luft, J. H., 10(34), *26*, 214(45,47), 221(45), *224*
Lukehart, S. A., 104(19), *117*, 141(19), 143(48,49), *154*, *156*, 190(26,27), *192*, 206(34), 219(34),

[Lukehart, S. A.]
223, 243(30,37,38), 244(38,40), 245(37), 246(37), 263, 264, 274(23), 291(23), 293, 298(7, 11,12), 300(7,11,19), 301(12), 302(11), 303(7,12,22), 304(1), 305(7), 308(11,12,33,37), 309 (12), 310, 311, 312, 321(21), 322(21), 323(32), 328, 349(2, 3,4,6), 350(4), 351(19a), 352(4), 357(2,3), 359(2), 360, 361
Lukoyanova, M. A., 60(31), 61 (31), 68
Luxon, L., 113(65), 120
Lysko, P. G., 61-63(14,23), 67, 68, 80(41), 97

M

Mackaness, G. B., 147(69), 158, 323(35), 329, 342(63), 348, 351(22), 355(22), 362
Mackenzie, I., 308(34), 312
MacLeod, R. A., 62(40), 69
Magnuson, H. J., 65(52), 70, 74(33), 96, 101(3,4), 102(3,4), 104(3), 110(4), 114(3), 116 123(30), 125(46), 134, 135, 142(26), 143(43), 145(26), 155, 156, 248(76,78), 249(79, 82,88,89), 254(89), 267, 268, 332(11), 344
Magyar, S., 217(62), 225
Mallernee, S. V., 107(38), 118
Mandel, M., 41(23,25), 53
Manejias, R. E., 280(39), 283 (39), 294
Mangi, R. J., 243(22), 263, 290(45), 295
Manikowska-Lesinska, W., 141 (20), 154
Mansfield, J. M., 280(42), 294
Manson-Bahr, P. E. C., 114(77), 120

Maret, S. M., 219(72), 226, 238 (16), 239, 243(29), 263, 274(19), 293,322(30), 328, 352(28), 362
Markes, R., 105(30), 106(30), 118
Marks, M. I., 109(48), 119
Marmur, J., 41(19,23), 42(21), 53
Marshak, L. C., 244(59), 266, 332(9), 344, 354(44), 363
Marshall, R. J., 112(57), 119
Matthews, H. M., 31(15), 32(15), 35, 60(19), 65(55), 67, 70, 73(24), 75(24), 80(24), 82(24), 94(24), 96, 98, 142(25), 155. 216(54), 225
Maurer, K., 107(34), 118
Mayer, M. M., 249(94), 268, 273 (7), 292
McCarthy, B. J., 42(33), 54
McCrory, J. A., 144(51), 157
McDowell, F., 163(19), 169
McIntosh, J. R., 8(23), 25
McLain, J. H., 144(54), 157
McLeod, C. P., 122(26,27), 125 (46,47), 134, 135, 143(43), 152 (79), 156, 158, 242(4), 249(4, 82,83,88), 262, 267, 268
McMichael, A. J., 280(32), 283 (32), 294
McMillian, A., 107(44), 118
McSereney, D., 8(25), 25
Medici, M. A., 143(38), 156, 244 (41), 264, 308(38), 313
Medina, R., 152(75), 158
Mehr, K. A., 105(25), 117
Menke, H. E., 103(6), 115(78), 116, 120
Mercer, S. T., 350(8), 361
Mergenhagen, S. E., 165(30), 168 (56), 170, 172
Mesa, J., 152(77), 158
Metz, G., 11(43), 13(43), 26
Metz, J., 11(43), 13(43), 26
Metzger, M., 10(32), 26, 57(4), 67, 143(44), 156, 200(12), 216 (12), 219(76,77), 221(88), 222,

[Metzger, M.]
  226, 227, 244(45), 249(87,91),
  265, 268, 304(31), 312, 324(42),
  329, 332(38,39,40), 346, 353
  (41), 357(58), 363, 364
Mexxadra, G., 352(31), 362
Meyer, F., 31(22), 32(22), 35
Meyer, H., 31(22), 32(22), 35
Miao, R. M., 32(24,27), 36, 41(28),
  42(29), 47(29), 50(40), 52(40),
  54
Michalska, E., 219(77), 226, 249
  (91), 268, 357(58), 364
Michelson, H. E., 316(3), 326
Mickenberg, I. D., 168(56), 172
Midgley, J. E. M., 64(47), 69
Mifuchi, I., 11(50), 27, 34(41),
  37
Miles, A. A., 121(7), 131(7), 132
Miller C. E., 30(6), 34
Miller, J. D., 147(65), 158
Miller, J. M., 42(35), 54
Miller, J. N., 4(5), 8(17,20),
  21(17), 24, 25, 30(11), 35,
  60(20), 64(48), 65(48), 68,
  69, 73(23,30), 74(23,30), 75
  (30,35), 80(23,30,35), 82(30),
  96, 97, 140(8,9), 141(19), 143
  (45), 146(58), 147(9), 148(58,
  59), 153, 154, 156, 174(7,8),
  189(17,18,19), 190(27), 191,
  192, 193, 196(3,4,6,7), 197(3),
  198(4), 199(3,6), 200(4,13),
  203(4), 207(3,6,38), 210(3,4,
  3,38), 211(3,40), 214(3), 216
  (7,13,53), 219(3), 220(85),
  221(13,89), 221, 222, 224, 225,
  227, 233(11), 239, 242(11,13,
  14), 243(31,37), 244(11,14,
  40,47,49,51,56), 245(37,51,67),
  246(37,51), 247(31), 249(47,
  84,90), 250(51), 251(51),
  254(31,96), 255(67), 256(67),
  260(67), 262, 264, 265, 266,
  267, 268, 273(4), 292, 298(7),
  300(7), 302(21), 303(7,22,23,26),

[Miller, J. N.]
  304(30), 305(7), 309(40,41),
  310, 311, 312, 313, 331(1),
  332(22), 343, 345, 349(2,6),
  350(17), 357(2), 359(2), 360,
  361
Miller, K. R., 8(23), 25
Miller, M. M., 188(11), 191
Milo, S., 103(7), 116
Mitchinson, N. A., 280(38), 283
  (38), 294
Miyao, I., 125(44), 135, 152(80),
  159
Moechli, R. A., 72(17), 74(17),
  75(71), 82(17), 83(17), 94(17),
  95
Mogerley, S., 64(49), 69
Mölbert, E., 4(6), 24
Mollaret, H. H., 152(84), 159
Moller, G., 323(33), 328
Moller, H., 166(48), 171
Monier, J. C., 152(83), 159, 335
  (56), 347
Monjan, A. A., 297(5), 310, 326
  (55), 330, 334(48), 346
Moore, E. B., 174(9), 191
Moore, M. B., Jr., 103(91), 116,
  242(1), 248(73), 254(73), 261,
  267
Morgan, E. L., 280(35), 283(35),
  284(35), 290(35), 294
Morgan, H. J., 73(28), 96, 350
  (13,14), 356(55), 361, 364
Morgan, J. F., 57(2), 66, 73(26),
  96
Morton, H. J., 73(26), 96
Mothershed, S. E., 208(36), 312
Mullin, M. T., 58(16), 67
Mulzer, P., 200(18), 222
Murray, B. A., 188(3), 192
Muschel, L, H., 33(29), 36
Muse, K. E., 8(18), 25, 72(15),
  73(15), 75(15), 79(15), 95,
  190(25), 192, 196(8), 199(8),
  210(8), 214(8), 222, 229(1), 230
  (1), 233(1), 238, 242(16), 262

Author Index

Musher, D. M., 103(7), 104(14), 105(20,21), 106(32), *116, 117, 118*, 140(4), 141(11,13), 143(46), 146(4), 147(68), *153, 154, 156, 158*, 165(41), *170*, 219(73), *226*, 238(13), *239*, 242(18,19,20), 244(61,62), *262, 263, 266*, 273(5), 274(11,12), 275(28), 277(28,29), 278(28,29), 281-284(28,43), 288(43), 290(28,43), *292, 293, 294*, 298(15), 304(32), *311, 312*, 315(1), 317(9,10), 323(34,36,37,38), 325(50,51,53), *326, 327, 328, 329, 330*, 332(17,18,19,20,21,25,26), 333(41), 334(47), 342(17,18,19,21), 343(66,67), *344, 345, 346, 348*, 352(36,37), 355(49,50), 356(54), 357(51), *363, 364*
Mustakallio, K. K., *116*, 161(8), *168*, 325(47), *329*
Myers, T. C., 107(38), *118*

N

Naff, G. B., *170*
Nakayama, T., 61(36), *69*
Nakeeb, S., 206(35), *223*
Nazemi, M. M., 103(7), *116*
Nell, E. E., 10(31), *26*, 21(66), *28*, 29(2), 30(2,14), 33(30), 34(40), *34, 35, 36, 37*, 65(54), *70*, 72(18), *95*, 105(22), *117*, 141(18), 142(28), 143(39), *154, 155, 156*, 189(20), 190(20), *192*, 200(11,12), 216(11,12), *222*, 243(35), 244(44,45), 255(99), 257(99), *264, 265, 268*, 303(25), *312*, 321(22), 322(22), 323(41), *328, 329*, 331(4), 343(65), *343, 348*, 349(7), 352(27), 356(7), 357(7), *361, 362*
Nelson, R. A., Jr., 57(3,8), *67*, 73(25), 82(25), *96*, 152(78),

[Nelson, R. A., Jr.] *158*, 243(32), 248(77), 249(32), 93,94, *264, 267, 268*, 273(7), *292*
Nevin, T. A., 244(48), *265*
Newman, B., 143(39), *156*, 167(52), *171*, 255(99), 257(99), *268*, 303(25), *312*, 331(4), *343*
Nicholas, D. J. D., 61(34), *68*
Nichols, H. J., 122(12), *133*
Nichols, J. C., 30(5), *34*, 58(12,15), 59(15), 63-65(46,49), *67, 69*, 72(21), 80(42), *96, 97*, 146(66), *158*
Nicol, C. S., 104(11), *116*
Nicolau, G., 352(30), *362*
Niel, G., 152(84), *159*
Nielsen, H. A., 21(64), *28*
Nielson, E., 163(24), *169*
Nielson, H. A., 21(65), *28*
Niemel, P. L., 115(78), *120*
Noguchi, H., 3(3), 4(3), *24*, 40(16), *53*, 122(14), *133*, 244(57,58), *266*, 316(2), *326*, 354(43), *363*
Norins, L. C., 112(55,61), 114(72), *119,120*, 297(2), *310*
Norris, S. J., 60(20), 64(48), 65(48), *68, 69*, 75(35), 80(35), *97*, 216(53), *225*
Notowicz, A., 103(6), *116*
Nowinski, W. W., 214(41), *224*
Nowtony, A., 220(83), *227*
Nusseuzweig, U., 280(39), 283(39), *294*

O

Oakes, S. G., 173(3,4,5), 174(3,5), 188(3), *191*
O'Brien, C., 342(61), *347*
O'Farrell, P. H., 230(7), *238*
O'Farrell, P. Z., 230(7), *238*
Ogstand, A. G., 216(48), *224*

Ohta, Y., 121(4), 131(4), *132*, 334(46), *346*
Okawa, S., 112(59), *119*
Olansky, S., 101(4), 102(4), 110(4), 112(54,55,61), *116, 119,* 142(26), 145(26), *155,* 249(89), 254(89), *268,* 332(11), *344*
Olarte, J., 152(76), *158*
Olitzki, L., 163(20), *169*
Olsen, S., 142(23), *154,* 325(52), *330*
O'Neill, P., 104(11), *116*
Oparin, A. I., 60(31), 61(31), *68*
Ørskov, F., 21(68), *28*
Ørskov, I., 21(68), *28*
Osuna, G. G., 152(74), *158*
Ovcinnikov, N. M., 4(8), 11(40), 17(8,40,58), 18(8,40), *24, 26, 27,* 140(10), *153,* 189(22), *192,* 217(67), *226,* 350(19), *361*

P

Pacha, J. M., 219(77), *226*
Pandhi, R. K., 105(27), *117*
Pankratz, H. S., 10(37), *26*
Pariser, R. J., 105(25), *117*
Parker, J., 112(58), *119*
Parodi, U., 122(11), *133*
Parrott, D. M. V., 321(23), *328*
Parry, E. H. O., 162(13), 163(21), 164(13,21,26), *169*
Passaic, N J., 107(41), 111(41), *118*
Paster, B. J., 33(38), *36*
Patterson, R. J., 351(24), *362*
Pavia, C. S., 143(37,47), *155, 156,* 238(14), *239,* 243(24,25), *263,* 274(15,16,17), *292,* 318(14), 321(14,16,18), 322(16,18) 324(43), 325(14,16), *327, 329,* 332(31,32,33,37), *345, 346,* 351(25), 352(26), 353(42), *362, 363*

Payne, A. M., 321(15), *327*
Pdwinska, J., 219(77), *226*
Pearce, L. P., 122(15,16,17,18,19, 20,21,22), 124(18,36, 37,38), *133, 134,* 298(8,9,10), *311,* 349(1), 350(1,9), *360, 361*
Pearsall, N. N., 143(42), *156,* 245(68), 255(68), 258(68), *266,* 303(27), *312,* 331(5), *344*
Pechere, J. C., 147(56), *157*
Pedersen, N. S., 21(67), *28*
Peltier, A., 325(48), *329*
Pepose, J.S., 243(31), 247(31), 254(31,96), *264, 268,* 304(30), *312*
Perine, F. L., 255(98), 260(98), *268*
Perine, P. L., 143(40,42), *156,* 162(13), 163(21), 164(13,21,26), *169,* 245(68), 255(68), 258(68), *266,* 303(24,27), *312,* 313(2,5), *343, 344*
Persson, K., 166(48), *171*
Pesetsky, B. R., 19(62), *28*
Peters, M., 113(67), *120*
Petersen, C. S., 21(67), *28*
Peterson, D., 32(25), *36,* 65(56), *70*
Petrozzi, J. W., 105(23), *117*
Pfau, C. J., 29(3), *34,* 41(24), *53*
Pham, P. H., 220(83,86), *227*
Pham, T. D., 11(42), *26,* 140(7), 148(7), *153,* 189(15), *192,* 242(10), *262,* 309(39), *313,* 350(16), *361*
Piette, F., 244(64), *266*
Pigman, W., 216(56), *225*
Pillot, J., 5(4), 8(14), 11(14,47, 48), *24, 27*
Podivinska, J., 324(42), *329*
Poswinska, J., 249(91), *268,* 324(42), *329,* 332(38), *346,* 353(41), *363*
Pope, H. M., 162(13), 163(25), 164(13,26), *169*
Porter, L., 342(61), *347*
Potter, E. V., 109(47), *119*

Powell, H. C., 302(20), 307(20), 308(20), 309(20), 311, 351(20), 361
Pozos, R. S., 173(3,4), 174(3,4), 188(3,4), 191
Prendergast, R. A., 352(27), 362
Preston, R. H., 107(36), 118
Prewitt, T. A., 112(56), 119
Price, E. V., 242(1), 261
Pupil, P., 352(32), 362
Putkowen, T., 116, 161(8), 166 (50), 168, 171

Q

Qualls, S., 124(40), 135
Quist, E. E., 173(6), 191

R

Rabinovitch, M., 280(39), 283 (39), 294
Radke, K., 18(60), 27
Raiziss, G. W., 123(35), 134
Ramsay, G. C., 115(79), 120
Ratheu, T., 29(3), 34
Rathlev, T., 41(24), 53, 80(45), 97
Reardan, J. B., 244(65), 266
Reardon, J. B., 166(45), 171
Redelman, D., 323(31), 328
Reginato, A. J., 107(34), 118
Rehtijarvik Putkonen, T., 162 (9), 168
Reichman, L. B., 244(66), 266
Remington, J. S., 351(23), 362
Repesh, L. A., 173(3,4,5,6), 174(3,4,5), 188(3,4), 90(6), 191
Restrepo, A., 152(77), 158
Rethy, A., 31(9), 35
Revel, J. P., 188(11), 191
Reynolds, F. W., 190(30), 193, 219(70), 226

Rich, A. R., 354(48), 363
Richter, A., 75(36), 97
Rittenberg, S. C., 34(39), 36, 37
Ritzi, D. M., 10(39), 11(39,41), 18(4), 26, 32(28), 33(31,35), 36, 74(32), 96, 208(39), 209(39), 214(39), 224
Rizvi, S., 216(56), 225
Robbins, S. L., 242(17), 245(17), 262
Roberts, M. S., 60(19), 67, 73 (24), 75(24), 80(24), 82(24), 94(24), 96, 216(54), 225
Roberts, R. B., 8(21), 25, 124 (40), 135, 357(57), 364
Robertson, D. H., 107(44), 118
Rocklin, R., 321(25), 323(25), 328
Rockwell, D. H., 248(73), 254(73), 267
Rola-Pleszczynski, M., 342(60), 347
Rolland, M., 244(60), 266, 316(3a), 326, 354(45), 363
Rollins, B. J., 188(13), 192
Root, R. K., 168(55,56), 172
Rosahn, P. D., 4(11), 24, 121(3), 131(3), 132, 334(45), 346, 349 (1), 350(1,9), 360, 361
Rosales-Quintana, S., 105(28), 117
Rosenau, B. J., 248(76,78), 249 (79), 267
Ross, D., 112(58), 119
Rothblat, G. H., 31(18), 35
Rothman, S., 244(59), 266, 332(9), 344, 354(44), 363
Rouiller, G. C., 140(5), 153
Roux, M. E., 280(32), 283(32), 294
Ruczkowska, J., 10(32), 26, 219 (77), 226
Rudolph. A. H., 104(13), 116
Rumpp. J. W., 30(5), 34, 147(66), 158
Russell, H., 29(4), 30(4), 34

Ryan, J. L., 280(40), *294*
Ryter, A., 5(14), 8(14), 11(14), *24*

S

Saena, B. J. G., 39(10), *52*
Saita, H., *170*
Salo, O. P., *116*, 161(8), *168*
Salussola, D., 143(41), 152(53), *156*, *159*, 255(97), 260(97), *268*, 331(3), 335(56), *343*, *347*
Sandok, P. L., 57(5,6), 60(19), 63-65(44), *67*, *69*, 72(13,20,24), 73(13,20), 74(20), 75(13,24), 79(13,20), 80(24), 81(20,22), 82(20,22,24), 94(24), *95*, *96*, *98*, 216(54), *225*
Sanford, K. K., 75(36), *97*
Sapuppo, A., 352(31), *362*
Sato, R., 62(41), *69*
Saurino, V. R., 217(36), *224*
Savage, D. C., 8(26), *25*
Scales, R. W., 141(22), *154*
Schammel, P., 30(6), *34*
Schaudinn, F., 3(1,2), 4(1), *23*, 39(5,6,7), *52*
Schel. J., 61(30), *68*
Schell, R. F., 103(7), *116*, 126(49, 50,51), 129(52), *135*, 141(11,85, 87), 143(46), 147(68), 152(85, 86,87), *153*, *156*, *159*, 219(74), *226*, 244(61,62), 246(70,71), 256 (70), 259(70,71), 260(70,71), *266*, *267*, 273(5), 274(11,12), *292*, 297(3), 298(15), *310*, *311*, 315(1), 317(9,10), 323(34,36,37), *326*, *327*, *328*, *329*, 332(19,20, 21,25,26), 334(47,49,50,51,52, 53,54,55), 335(52), 336(53), 337(52), 338(53), 339(54), 341 (55), 342(19,21,55), 343(66), *344*, *345*, *346*, *347*, *348*, 352(36, 37), 355(49,50,51), *363*, *364*
Schellekens, P. T. A., 321(26), *328*

Schereschewsky, J., 40(14,15), *53*, 71(1), 78(1), *94*, 121(6), 131(6), *132*
Scherp, H. W., 165(30), *170*
Schiller, N. L., 30(8), *35*, 59(13), 60(13), 61(13), 65(13), *67*
Schlossman, S. F., 342(61), *347*
Schmale, J. D., 30(6), *34*
Schmerold, W., 200(14), *222*
Schobl, O., 125(44), *135*, 152(80), *159*
Schroeter, A. L., 242(2), *261*
Schumacher, H. R., 107(34), *118*
Schwab, J. H., 272(3), *291*
Schwethelm, P., 141(11), *153*, 323 (37), *329*, 332(20), 334(47), 343(66), *344*, *346*, *348*, 355(50, 51), 357(51), *364*
Scott, D. W., 280(36), 283(36), 290(36), *294*
Scott, V., 166(43), *171*, 200(24, 25,26), 215(24), 217(24), *223*, 243(34), *264*
Seldeen, M. J., 9(30), *26*
Sell, K. W., 342(60), *347*
Sell, S., 104(19), *117*, 143(48,49), *156*, 190(26), *192*, 206(34), 219 (34), *223*, 243(30,38), 244(38, 39,40), *263*, *264*, 274(23,24), 291(23,24), *293*, 298(7,11,13,14), 299(14), 300(7,11,13,14,19), 301(13,14), 302(11,14,20), 303 (7,14,29), 304(11,14), 305(7), 307(20), 308(11,13,14,20,33,37), 309(20), *310*, *311*, *312*, 321(20, 21), 322(21), 323(31,32), *327*, *328*, 349(3,4,5,6), 350(4), 351 (5,19a,20), 352(3,4), *360*, *361*
Senear, F. E., 107(35), *118*
Sepetjian, M., 143(41), 152(83), *156*, *159*, 255(97), 260(97), *268*, 331(3), 335(56), *343*, *347*
Severac, M., 123(35), *134*
Shaffer, B., 162(11), *168*
Sheldon, W. H., 161-163(5,14), 165 (5,37,38), 166(37,38), *168*, *169*, *170*
Shekin, H. A., 162(11), *168*

Sheppard, H. W., 323(31), 328
Shore, R. N., 107(40), 118
Sidman, C. L., 280(41), 294
Simeray, A., 244(60), 266, 316(3a), 326, 354(45), 363
Simmons, C. B., 105(21), 117, 304(32), 312, 333(41), 343(66), 346, 348
Simpson, E., 336(59), 347
Singer, C., 103(8), 116
Singer, I. I., 189(14), 192
Skanse, B., 216(57), 225
Skog, E., 162(15), 166(15), 167(51), 169, 171
Skovgaard, H. J., 19(61), 23(61), 28
Skovgaard, J. J., 4(9), 8(9), 9(9), 11(9), 13(9), 15(9), 17(9), 24
Smibert, R. M., 5(15), 9(15), 24, 31(20), 35, 41(26,27), 42(35), 53, 54
Smith, D. W., 332(23), 345
Smith, E. B., 249(86), 268
Smith, H. E., 8(22), 25
Smith, J. L., 19(62), 28, 144(51, 54), 147(55), 157
Smith L., 61(37), 62(39), 69
Smith, M., 51(42), 55, 101(2), 104(2), 114(2), 115
Smith, P. F., 31(18), 35
Smogar, W., 57(4), 67, 143(44), 156, 219(77), 221(88), 226, 227, 249(87,91), 268, 304(31), 312, 324(42), 329, 332(38), 333(40), 346, 353(41), 363
Snyderman, R., 168(56), 172
Sobel, H. J., 107(41), 111(41), 118
Soborg, M., 316(8), 327
Sølling, J., 142(23), 154, 165(39), 166(39), 170, 244(63), 266, 290(47), 295, 325(52), 330
Sølling, K., 142(23), 154, 165(39), 166(39), 170, 244(63), 266, 290(47), 295, 325(52), 330

Soltani, K., 161(4), 162(4), 163(18), 165(4), 166(4), 168, 169
Somogyi, T., 107(42,43), 118
Sondel, P. M., 342(61), 347
Spitznagel, J. K., 229(2), 235(2), 238
Starzycki, Z., 105(24), 117
Steinhardt, E., 71(3), 78(3), 94
Steinman, H. G. 57(8,10), 67
Stobel, P. L., 196(9), 222
Storey, J., 166(46), 171
Storre, J., 104(18), 117
Stout, J. G., 60(18), 64(18), 67, 72(16), 73(31), 75(16,31), 79(16), 80(31), 82(31), 83(16), 87(16,51), 94(31), 95, 95, 98, 148(70), 158, 216(50,51), 224, 225, 233(12), 239
Streitfeld, M. M., 30(12), 35
Strempel, R., 200(23), 223
Strobel, P. L., 17(59), 18(59), 27
Strong, A. M. M., 105(31), 106(31), 118
Sueoka, N., 41(20), 53
Suguira, M., 112(59), 119
Sundblad, L., 216(57), 225
Swain, R. H. A., 5(13), 9(13), 17(57), 18(57), 20(57), 24, 27, 200(15), 222
Sykes, J. A., 4(5), 8(17,20), 21(17), 24, 30(11), 35, 60(20), 64(48), 65(48), 68, 69, 73(23, 30), 74(23,30), 75(30,35), 80(23,30,35), 82(30), 96, 97, 140(8,9), 146(58), 147(9,65), 148(58,59), 153, 157, 158, 174(7, 8,9), 189(17,18,19), 191, 192, 196(3,4,6,7), 197(3), 198(4), 199(3,6), 200(4), 203(4), 207(3,6,38), 210(3,4,6,38), 211(3), 214(3), 216(7,53), 219(3), 220(85), 221, 222, 224, 225, 227, 233(11), 239, 242(11,13,14,15), 244(11,14,56), 262, 265, 309(40,41), 313, 350(17), 361
Szabo, G., 217(62), 225

T

Takeuchi, A., 8(27), 25
Taniyama, T., 11(50), 27, 34(41), 37
Taylor-Robinson, D., 60(21), 68
Tedder, R. S., 104(18), 117, 166(46), 171
Tempelis, C. H., 280(35), 283(35), 284(35), 290(35), 294
Thayer, J. O., 30(6), 34
Theofilopoulos, A. N., 272(1), 275(1), 291
Thestrup-Pedersen, K., 243(23), 244(23), 263, 274(13), 292, 317(11), 327, 332(29), 345, 352(33), 353(33), 362
Thivolet, J., 143(41), 156, 244(60), 255(97), 260(97), 266, 268, 316(3a), 326, 331(3), 343, 354(45), 363
Thoen, C. O., 343(64), 348, 357(56), 364
Thomas, E. V., 142(26), 145(26), 155
Thomas, E. W., 101(4), 102(4), 110(4), 116, 249(89), 254(89), 268, 332(11), 344
Thomas, J. J., 72(14), 74(14), 76(14), 79(14), 95
Thomas, M. L., 29(4), 30(4), 34
Thomas, T. L., 352(32), 362
Thompson, F. A., 249(88), 268
Thompson, J., 243(22), 263
Thompson, R. G., 107(36), 118
Thomson, J., 105(31), 106(31), 118
Thorburn, A. L., 354(47), 363
Thulin, H., 243(23), 244(23), 263, 274(13), 292, 317(11), 327, 332(29), 345, 352(33) 353(33), 362
Tight, R. R., 107(39), 118
Timmer, M., 107(42,43), 118
Tinelli, R., 11(48), 27

Titus, R. G., 245(69), 255(69), 266, 303(28), 312, 331(7) 344
Tolliver, E. A., 297(2), 310
Tompkins, E. H., 350(14), 356(55), 361, 364
Tourville, D. R., 244(66), 266
Tung, K. S. K., 165(41), 170, 238(13), 239, 242(20), 263, 281-284(43), 288(43), 290(43), 294, 325(53), 330
Turk, J. L., 140(2), 142(27), 146(2,63), 153, 155, 157, 220(79), 227, 243(21,27), 263, 274(10), 292, 316(4,5), 317(12, 13), 318(13), 325(4), 326, 327, 332(27), 345, 352(34,35), 362, 363
Turner, D. R., 140(3), 146(3), 153, 274(21), 293, 332(15), 344
Turner, R. H., 242(2,4), 249(4), 261, 262
Turner, T. B., 29(1), 34, 40(12), 53, 65(51), 70, 76(6), 78(6), 95, 122-126(8,23,24,25,26,27,28, 29,45,47,48), 132, 133, 134, 135, 141(15), 143(39), 151(72,73), 152(78,79,81,82), 154, 156, 157, 159, 167(52), 171, 189(1,2), 190(29), 191, 193, 195(1,2), 200(1,27,28), 215-219(1,2,28,69), 221, 223, 226, 244(43), 248(43, 77), 249(43,92), 255(99), 257(99), 265, 267, 268, 273(6), 274(6), 279(6), 292, 298(6), 303(25), 308(6), 310, 312, 331(4,8), 332(12), 343, 344, 350(15), 354(47), 361, 363
Turner, T. R., 76(38), 97

U

Udris, Z., 41(25), 53
Uhlenhuth, P., 200(18), 222

Unanue, E. R., 280(41), *294*, 351(21), *362*
Updyke, E. L., 122(27), 126(48), *134, 135*, 152(79), *158*
Urbach, F., 217(36), *224*

V

Vaczi, L., 31(19), *35*
Vaisman, A., 121(5), 131(5), *132*, 334(44), *346*
Valenti, A. J., 103(8), *116*
VanderHart, M., 321(26), *328*
Vander Sluis, J. J., 291(50), *295*
Varela, G., 4(7,10), 5(7), 7(10), *24*, 152(72,76), *158*
Vasey, F. B., 165(42), *171*
Vatter, A. E., 17(55), *27*
Vegas, M., 152(75), *158*
Vincent, M. M., 342(60), *347*
Vischer, T. L., 107(33), *118*
Volpino, G., 40(13), *53*, 71(2), 78(2), *94*
Vryonis, G. P., 73(28), *96*

W

Wachter, M. S., 11(49), *27*, 33(31,32), *36*
Wager, O., 321(47), *329*
Wahl, R., 40(18), *53*
Waksman, B. D., 280(36), 283(36), 290(36), *294*
Waksman, B. K., 290(44), *295*
Wallace C. K., 164(28), *170*
Wallace J. A., 280(42), *294*
Wallace, S., 104(17), *117*
Walsh, J. L., 104(10), *116*
Wang, M. C. C., 297(4), *310*
Ware, J. L., 220(81), *227*, 238(15), *239*, 243(28), *263*, 275(25), *293*, 322(29), 325(29), *328*

Waring, G. W., 190(31), *193*, 219(71), *226*, 249(81), *267*
Warner, J. F., 107(39), *118*
Warner, R. W., 104(11), *116*
Warrell, D. A., 162(13), 163(21), 164(13,21,26), *169*
Wattre, W., 244(64), *266*
Watson, J. H. L., 4(7,10), 5(7), 7(10), *24*
Watts, J. C., 105(28), *117*
Weber, J. M., 214(42), 216(42), *224*
Weber, M. D., 73(27), *96*
Wedderburn, C. C., 4(7,10), 5(7), 7(10), *24*
Weigeshaus, E., 332(23), *345*
Weingarten, N., 163(17), 165-167(17), *169*
Weintraub, A., 107(33), *118*
Weiser, R. J. Jr., 112(57), *119*
Weiser, R. S., 143(40,42), *156*, 245(68,69), 255(68,69,98), 258(68), 260(98), *266, 268*, 303(24,27,28), *312*, 331(2,5,7), *343, 344*
Wende, R., 249(85), *267*
Werth, J. A., 123(31), *134*
Whang, S. J., 249(84,90), *267, 268*
Wharton, C. M., 162(12), *168*
Whitaker, M. G., 321(27), *328*
White, D. C., 61(38), 62(39), *69*
Whittle, H. C., 163(25), *169*
Wicher, K., 121(1), 131(1), *132*, 141(14), 142(24), 143(31,32,36), 146(36,62), 147(64), *154, 155, 157, 158*, 206(35), 219(75), 220(80), *223, 226, 227*, 243(26), *263*, 274(18,22), 275(26,27), *293*, 297(4), *310*, 321(17,19), 322(17,28), 324(19), 325(28), *327, 328*, 332(35,36), 334(42), *346*, 353(40), 357(59), *363, 364*
Wicher, V., 141(14), 143(31,32,36), 146(36,62), 147(64), *154*,

[Wicher, V.]
  155, 157, 158, 206(35), 219(75), 220(80), 223, 226, 227, 243(26), 263, 274(18,22), 275(26,27), 293, 297(4), 310, 321(17,19), 322(17,28), 324(19), 325(28), 327, 328, 332(35,36), 346, 353(40), 357(59), 363, 364
Wiegand, S. E., 17(59), 18(59), 27, 196(9), 222
Wiesinger, D., 220(84), 227
Wiglesworth, F. W., 109(48), 119
Wile, U. J., 107(35), 118, 350(12) 361
Willcox, R. R., 3(4), 5(4), 24, 39(4), 40(3,12), 52(43), 52, 53, 55, 57(9), 67, , 72(7), 78(7), 95
Williams, H. U., 114(73), 115(73), 120, 124(39), 135
Williams, R. G., 217(60), 225
Wilson, G. S., 121(7), 131(7), 132
Wilson, J., 114(74), 120
Windsor, C. P., 242(4), 249(4), 262
Witherbee, W. D., 124(36,37,38), 134
Woese, C. R., 42(30), 54
Wolf, E. H., 107(41), 111(41), 118
Wolf, E. T., 94(53), 98, 200(29), 204(29), 215(29), 216(58), 223, 225, 244(53), 265, 279(30), 293
Wolff, S. M., 163(22), 164(22), 168(55,56), 169, 172
Woody, J. N., 342(60), 347
Worton, H. J., 57(2), 66
Wright, D. J. M., 105(26), 111(26), 117, 140(2,3), 142(27), 146(57,63), 153, 155, 157, 166(47), 171, 243(21), 244(42), 263, 265, 274(9,10,21), 292, 293, 316(4,5), 325(4), 326, 327,

[Wright, D. J. M.]
  332(15,27), 344, 345
Wright, D. L., 220(79), 227
Wright, M. I., 72(5), 78(5), 95

Y

Yamamura, Y., 11(50), 27, 34(41), 37
Yanagawa, R., 11(53), 27
Yanagihara, Y., 11(50), 27, 34(41), 37
Yang, T. K., 31(15), 32(15), 35, 65(55), 70, 142(25), 155
Yasuda, S., 11(50), 27, 34(41), 37
Yeagle, N., 206(35), 223
Yobs, A. R., 248(73), 254(73), 267, 308(36), 312
Yogeswari, L., 144(52), 157
Youmans, G. P., 332(13), 344, 351(24), 362
Young, E. J., 163(17), 165-167(17), 169

Z

Zachar, Z., 238
Zachariae, H., 163(24), 169
Zaffiro, P., 142(29), 155
Zajd, D., 244(66), 266
Zeigler, J. A., 10(33), 11(33), 26, 30(10), 35, 141(16), 154, 200(16), 215(16), 218(16), 222, 324(44), 329
Zeltzer, P. M., 243(31), 247(31), 254(31,96), 264, 268, 304(30), 312
Zeleznikar, R., 173(6), 190(6), 191

Zelger, J., 111(51), *119*
Zeller, J. A., 8(27), *25*
Zey, P. N., 33(34), *36*, 165(32), *170*

Zhukova, I. G., 60(31), 61(31), *68*
Ziegler, J. A., 94(48), *97*, 230(4), 233(4), *238*, 244(52), *265*
Zweifach, B. W., 217(65), *226*

Subject Index

A

Animal models of experimental treponemal infection, 121
 hamster, 126, 152, 260, 297
 mouse, 121, 297, 336
 rabbit, 72, 122, 248, 272, 297, 321, 333, 350
 relevance to human disease, 131
Antibodies (See Humoral mechanisms)
 cardiolipin, 103, 141
 FTA-ABS, 103, 124, 141, 273
 treponemal, 104, 141, 244, 273
 VDRL (Venereal Disease Research Laboratories), 103, 124, 273
Attachment of treponemes, 195
 cell surfaces, 8, 21, 187, 195, 299
 healing response, 218
 immunosuppression, 201, 205, 206, 219
 in vitro, 196

[Attachment of treponemes]
 ligand-receptor interaction, 229
 mucopolysaccharide capsule, 10, 30, 87, 147, 199
 mucopolysaccharide enzyme, 207
 role of capsule and mucopolysaccharidase, 214
 surface receptors, 207
 treponemal receptors, 210

B

Binding proteins of treponemes, 235

C

Cell-mediated immunity, 315, 331
 animals, 321
 direct evidence for, 333
 human, 312
 indirect evidence for, 332

[Cell-mediated immunity]
  passive transfer of resistance, 333
  resistance, 331
  T-cell mediated, 298, 336
Cellular reactions in syphilitic lesions, 139, 297
Composition of treponemes, 29
  cell wall, 34
  deoxyribonucleic acid, 32, 40
  envelope, 32
  filaments, 33
  flagella, 33
  lipids, 31
  mucopolysaccharides, 30, 190
  protein content, 30
Cross-immunity among treponemes, 129
Cultivation, 71
  cell-free systems of incubation, 85
  cell types, 76, 80, 81, 82, 83, 233
  estimation of treponemal numbers, 73
  mammalian cell-treponeme coincubation, 80
  motility, 74, 75, 86, 92, 93
  oxygen requirements, 80, 83, 85, 90, 92, 93
  passage and harvest in rabbits, 72
  preparation and constitutents of media, 75
  virulence, 74, 83

E

Endemic syphilis, 126, 150, 334

F

Frambesial disease (*See* Yaws)
  animal models, 129

G

Genetic relationship among treponemes, 40
  deoxyribonucleic acid base composition, 40
  T. pallidum and cultivable treponemes, 42
  T. pallidum and *T. hyodysenteriae*, 47
  T. pallidum and *T. pertenue*, 49

H

Histopathology, 139, 297 (*See* Immunopathology)
  effects of cortisone on experimental lesions, 308
  latency and tertiary lesions, 297
  local manifestations, 300
  phases of experimental syphilis, 298
  systemic manifestations, 298
Humoral immune mechanism, 143, 241
  immunity by infection and vaccination, 248
  mechanisms of resistance, 249
  neutralizing activity of serum, 250
  passive immunity, 254
  role in acquired resistance, 248
  role in pathogenesis, 242
  suppression, 271, 300
  treponemicidal factors, 250

I

Immune complexes, 165, 284, 325
Immune responses (*See* Humoral immune mechanisms)

Subject Index

[Immune responses]
  antibodies, 103, 124, 141, 241, 271, 331
  autoimmune, 142
  cell-mediated resistance, 315, 331
  complement, 250
  cross-resistant studies, 129
  immunoregulation, 271
  immunosuppression, 146, 201, 206, 219, 244, 271
  macrophages, 349
  T-cell-mediated resistance, 331
Immunopathology, 139, 297 (See Histopathology)
  cellular location, 140
  histopathology, 140
  immune response, 141
  immunopathologic mechanisms, 145
  Jarisch-Herxheimer reaction, 142, 161
  other pathogenic treponemes, 148
  persistence of, 144
  reactivation, 145
Immunoregulation of immune response, 271
  host-parasite relationship (See Animal models)
  immune complexes, 284
  immunosuppression, 146, 201, 206, 219, 244, 271
  impaired lymphocyte function (See Lymphocytes)
  unresponsiveness, 271

J

Jarisch-Herxheimer reaction, 142, 161
  clinical characteristics, 161
  experimental models of, 166

[Jarisch-Herxheimer reaction]
  Herxheimer-like reaction in other diseases, 163
  theories of etiology, 164

L

Lymphocytes, 140, 242, 274, 298, 316, 333, 350
  blast transformation, 205, 220, 300, 317, 318, 321
  T-cells, 274, 300, 336, 350

M

Macrophage involvement, 297, 342, 349
  activated, 349, 351, 355, 360
  destruction of treponemes, 358
  histologic evidence for macrophage function, 350
  macrophage-activating factor, 355
  migration inhibition factor, 352
  nonspecific resistance, 141, 322, 342, 355
  phagocytosis, 357
  sensitized lymphocytes, 351
Metabolic activity, 57
  anabolic, 63
  anaerobic nature, 58, 66
  catabolism, 58
Morphology, 3, 32
  basal body, 15
  cell envelope, 9, 32
  cytoplasm, 17
  cytoplasmic membrane, 11
  cytoplasmic tubules, 17
  division, 19
  filament, 13
  fimbriae, 9
  flagella, 13
  hook, 15
  outer membrane, 10

[Morphology]
  peptidoglycan layer, 11
  size and shape, 5
  zone differentiation, 8
Mucopolysaccharide (*See* Attachment of treponemes)

P

Parasitic strategies, 229
  attachment, 229, 233
  evidence for ligand-receptor interaction, 229
  immunogenicity, 230
Phagocytosis, 141, 350, 357
  (*See* Macrophage involvement)
Pinta, 5, 151

S

Serological tests (*See* Antibodies), 103, 109, 111, 124, 141, 151, 241, 271, 331
Syphilitic disease
  animal models (*See* Animal models)
  antibody response, 103, 104, 141
  chancre, 102
  congenital, 113
  endemic syphilis, 126, 150, 334
  human, 102
  latent, 109
  neurosyphilis, 113

[Syphilitic disease]
  primary, 102
  reactivation, 145
  secondary (disseminated), 104
  tertiary, 111

T

Treponemes (related)
  T. carateum, 4, 5, 39
  T. hyodysenteriae, 47
  T. pallidum Bosnia A, 126, 148, 334
  T. pallidum endemicum, 126, 148, 334
  T. pertenue, 4, 5, 7, 9, 10, 11, 19, 39, 83, 148
  T. refringens, 41
  T. strain *reiter*, 11, 21
Toxic effects of, 173
  application to clinical manifestations, 187
  attachment, 187
  in vitro toxic effects, 174
  tissue pathology of, 173

V

Virulence, 74, 83, 229

Y

Yaws, 4, 101, 114
  animal models, 129